P9-AFZ-613

dvances in Neurochemistry

VISORY EDITORS

Axelrod	H. R. Mahler	P. Morell	M. Rapport
M. Gál	P. Mandel	J. S. O'Brien	E. Roberts

A Continuation Order Plan is available for this series. A continuation order will bring
delivery of each new volume immediately upon publication. Volumes are billed only upon
actual shipment. For further information please contact the publisher.

Advances in

Neurochemistry

Volume

Advances in
Neurochemistry

Volume 3

Edited by

B. W. Agranoff
*Mental Health Research Institute and
Department of Biological Chemistry
University of Michigan
Ann Arbor, Michigan*

and

M. H. Aprison
*Institute of Psychiatric Research and
Department of Psychiatry and Biochemistry
Indiana University School of Medicine
Indianapolis, Indiana*

PLENUM PRESS • NEW YORK AND LONDON

The Library of Congress cataloged the first volume of this series as follows:

Advances in neurochemistry/edited by B.W. Agranoff and M.H. Aprison.
 —New York: Plenum Press, [1975-
 v.   : ill.; 24 cm.
 Includes bibliographies and index.
 ISBN 0-306-39221-6 (v. 1)

 1. Neurochemistry. I. Agranoff, Bernard W., 1926-   II. Aprison, M. H.,
 1923-
 [DNLM: 1. Neurochemistry – Period. W1 AD684E]
 QP356.3.A37   612'.822   75-8710

Library of Congress Card Catalog Number 75-8710
ISBN 0-306-39223-2

© 1978 Plenum Press, New York
A Division of Plenum Publishing Corporation
227 West 17th Street, New York, N.Y. 10011

CONTRIBUTORS

M. H. APRISON • *Section of Applied and Theoretical Neurobiology, The Institute of Psychiatric Research and Departments of Biochemistry and Psychiatry, Indiana University Medical Center, Indianapolis, Indiana*

JOHN W. BIGBEE • *Department of Pathology, Stanford University School of Medicine, Stanford, California, and Veterans Administration Hospital, Palo Alto, California*

PATRICK ROBERT CARNEGIE • *The Russell Grimwade School of Biochemistry, University of Melbourne, Parkville, Victoria, Australia*

E. C. DALY • *Section of Applied and Theoretical Neurobiology, The Institute of Psychiatric Research and Departments of Biochemistry and Psychiatry, Indiana University Medical Center, Indianapolis, Indiana*

LAWRENCE F. ENG • *Department of Pathology, Stanford University School of Medicine, Stanford, California, and Veterans Administration Hospital, Palo Alto, California*

LEWIS T. GRAHAM, JR. • *Department of Biochemistry and Molecular Biology, Louisiana State University Medical Center, Shreveport, Louisiana*

SAHEBARAO P. MAHADIK • *Division of Neuroscience, New York State Psychiatric Institute, and Department of Biochemistry, Columbia University College of Physicians and Surgeons, New York, New York*

MAURICE M. RAPPORT • *Division of Neuroscience, New York State Psychiatric Institute, and Department of Biochemistry, Columbia University College of Physicians and Surgeons, New York, New York*

RICHARD P. SHANK • *Department of Physiology, Temple University School of Medicine, Philadelphia, Pennsylvania*

NEIL RAYMOND SIMS • *The Russell Grimwade School of Biochemistry, University of Melbourne, Parkville, Victoria, Australia*

HADASSAH TAMIR • *Division of Neuroscience, New York State Psychiatric Institute, and Department of Biochemistry, Columbia University College of Physicians and Surgeons, New York, New York*

PREFACE

The original premise of the Editors in initiating this series was that there existed a readership of neurochemists with considerable biochemical background who would make use of a series dedicated to both new developments and specialized reviews in neurochemistry. Having selected our authors, we have offered them virtually complete freedom to reflect and speculate in a field in which they have achieved prominence. The response to the first two volumes has been rewarding. The present one continues in this tradition. While we have not attempted to publish specialized volumes, the present volume contains two somewhat related chapters (Chapters 4 and 5, on the role of amino acid neurotransmitters). The first three chapters examine three diverse approaches, each of current interest, in neurochemical approaches to the molecular bases of neuronal and glial structure.

B. W. Agranoff
M. H. Aprison

CONTENTS

CHAPTER 2

IMMUNOHISTOCHEMISTRY OF NERVOUS SYSTEM-SPECIFIC ANTIGENS

LAWRENCE F. ENG AND JOHN W. BIGBEE

CHAPTER 3

MOLECULAR COMPOSITION AND FUNCTIONAL ORGANIZATION OF SYNAPTIC STRUCTURES

SAHEBARAO P. MAHADIK, HADASSAH TAMIR, and MAURICE RAPPORT

CHAPTER 4

THE MULTIPLE ROLES OF GLUTAMATE AND ASPARTATE IN NEURAL TISSUES

RICHARD P. SHANK and LEWIS T. GRAHAM, JR.

CHAPTER 5

BIOCHEMICAL ASPECTS OF TRANSMISSION AT INHIBITORY
SYNAPSES: THE ROLE OF GLYCINE

M. H. APRISON and E. C. DALY

Erratum: In Volume 2 of this series, Chapter 2, Table 5 (page 147), the units of V_{max} for brain slices taken from the work of Kiely and Sourkes (1972) and Denizeau and Sourkes (1977) should all be mmol liter^{-1} min^{-1}.

2',3'-CYCLIC NUCLEOTIDE 3'-PHOSPHODIESTERASE

NEIL RAYMOND SIMS AND PATRICK ROBERT CARNEGIE

The Russell Grimwade School of Biochemistry
University of Melbourne
Parkville, Victoria, Australia

1. INTRODUCTION

2',3'-Cyclic nucleotide 3'-phosphodiesterase (CNPase, EC 3.1.4.37*) has been widely used for several years as a marker for the presence of myelin in the central nervous system, but no review is available on its application and limitation as a marker enzyme and there is no information on its role in myelin. This was the first enzyme to be unequivocally characterized as a myelin component; previously it had been thought that myelin was enzymatically inert (Adams *et al.*, 1963). Several other enzymes have now been

---

*2',3'-Cyclic nucleotide 3'-phosphodiesterase was recently assigned the enzyme commission number 3.1.4.37. (IUPAC-IUB Enzyme Commission, 1976). Several workers had erroneously assigned the number 3.1.4.16 (2',3'-cyclic nucleotide 2'-phosphodiesterase) because of an error in the previous reference list for this entry. We have chosen the abbreviation CNPase for this enzyme following the style used for a number of enzymes (e.g., ATPase, RNase). Several other abbreviations have been used including CNP and CNPH.

proposed as being myelin-associated (for references see Carnegie and Sims, 1977; Norton, 1977), but evidence of myelin association is incomplete for some of these, such as protein kinase (Carnegie *et al.*, 1974; Miyamoto and Kakiuchi, 1974; Steck and Appel, 1974; Miyamoto, 1976) and phosphoprotein phosphatase (Miyamoto and Kakiuchi, 1975). In the case of nonspecific esterase (Keoppen *et al.*, 1969; Frey *et al.*, 1971; Rumsby *et al.*, 1973; Mitzen *et al.*, 1974) and arylamidase (Banik and Davison, 1969; Riekkinen and Clausen, 1970; Riekkinen and Rumsby, 1972; Mezei and Palmer, 1974) there is some controversy as to whether the enzymes are truly myelin-associated or are bound as an artifact of the preparation of myelin. There is strong evidence that cholesterol ester hydrolase is a myelin enzyme (Eto and Suzuki, 1973). The evidence that CNPase is a true myelin component is presented herein.

The physiological function of the enzyme is unknown but activity is measured by determining conversion of $2',3'$-cyclic nucleotides to $2'$-nucleotides. CNPase-like activity has been found in other tissues and other nervous system subfractions but specific activities are generally much lower. This widespread distribution of activity could be an indication of a role of some general importance for the enzyme. The relationship of the enzyme to myelin and the properties of isolated and membrane-bound forms of CNPase are examined.

Since much of this chapter is concerned with CNPase in central nervous system (CNS) myelin a brief comment on the structure of this type of myelin is included. CNS myelin coats nerve axons and provides an insulating material which allows for more rapid transmission of electrical signals within the axon than would otherwise be possible. The myelin sheath is composed of a number of layers of membranous material which produces a characteristic multilamellar pattern in electron micrographs. Myelin has a high lipid-to-protein ratio (4:1 wt/wt) and the protein content would appear from gel electrophoresis to be simplified when compared to other membranes. Two major proteins, basic protein (18,000 daltons) and proteolipid protein (25,000 daltons), account for approximately 80% of the total myelin protein, the remainder being high-molecular-weight components. Among the lipid fraction, the cerebrosides are the most characteristic constituent, being present in much higher levels in myelin than in any other nervous system fraction or subfraction. The oligodendroglial cell is responsible for production of myelin. Since the composition of myelin from developing animals is different from that of the adult, it is possible that some of the components may be incorporated into myelin after it has been formed and deposited by the oligodendroglia. (For a more detailed review on myelin structure see Norton, 1972.)

2. ASSAY OF CNPase

2.1. Need for Activation

Early work on CNPase demonstrated that pretreatment of material using sonication or detergents resulted in an increase in the measured specific activity of the enzyme and allowed more reproducible results to be obtained. The significance of this activation is discussed fully in Section 5.1. It must be stressed that the assay values obtained are dependent on the method used for activating the enzyme. Treatment with the detergents Triton X-100 and sodium deoxycholate has been the most widely used activation procedures. However, sodium deoxycholate is not readily soluble at pH values below neutrality and activation at pH 7.5 followed by dilution and assay at pH 6.2 is necessary, whereas activation with Triton X-100 is unaffected by a change from pH 7.5 to 6.2 and both activation and assay can be performed at the lower pH.

2.2. Comparison of Assays

CNPase activity is assayed by measuring the conversion of 2',3'-cyclic nucleotides to 2'-nucleotides by estimation of either the product formed or the substrate remaining. Both fixed-time assays and continuous monitoring systems have been used. Although continuous monitoring assays are essential for accurate kinetic studies these have not been favored where the enzyme is used as a marker because they usually require more sophisticated equipment and in some cases are not as sensitive as fixed-time assays.

The major features of the assay methods available for CNPase are summarized in Table 1. None of these methods is applicable to all situations and the choice of a suitable assay is dependent on the nature of the samples being examined, the equipment and materials available, the number of assays required, and the sensitivity desired. Early methods (for references see Table 1) can be separated into two groups. The first involved determination of either substrate or product following separation by techniques including paper electrophoresis, paper chromatography, and thin-layer chromatography. These suffer from the disadvantage that spotting and elution are fairly tedious and time-consuming and limit the reproducibility. Furthermore the number of assays that can be handled at one time is limited by facilities for chromatography. The second group of assays involved determination of product formed by selectively removing the phosphate from the 2'-nucleotides with alkaline phosphatase followed by

TABLE 1. Comparison of CNPase Assays

Assay method	Substrate ([mM] in assay)	Total hours[a] (20 samples)	Actual man-hours[a] (20 samples)	Sensitivity (cf. I_{a1})	Separation of 2'- and 3'-nucleotides	Reference[c]
I. Fixed-time assays						
a. Spectrophotometric determination after:						
Paper chromatography	2',3'-Cyclic AMP (7.5)	≈20	2.5–3.5		Yes	Kurihara and Tsukada, 1967
Thin-layer chromatography	2',3'-Cyclic AMP (7.5)	4–6	2–3	Equal	Yes	Zanetta et al., 1972; Glastris and Pfeiffer, 1974
Column chromatography	2',3'-Cyclic CMP (na)	na	na		No	Lundblad and Moore, 1969
Alkaline phosphatase treatment for selective release of phosphate from product	2',3'-Cyclic AMP (7.5)	1.25–2.5[b]	1–2[b]	Equal	No	Olafson et al., 1969; Prohaska et al., 1973; Kurihara and Takahashi, 1973
b. Fluorometric determination after:						
Precipitation	2',3'-Cyclic AMP (7.5)	1.25–1.5	1–1.25	Equal	No	Sims and Carnegie, 1976
Precipitation	$1,N^6$-Ethenoadenosine-2',3'-cyclic monophosphate (5)	1–1.25	0.75–1	Greater	No	Trams, 1973
Alkaline phosphatase treatment and separation of substrate and dephosphorylated product on column chromatography	$1,N^6$-Etheno-2-aza-adenosine-2',3'-cyclic monophosphate (4.95)	2–2.5	1.5–2	Greater	No	Lo et al. 1975
II. Continuous monitoring assays						
a. ΔOD_{286}	2',3'-Cyclic CMP (1)	2–3	≈2	Less	No	Hugli et al., 1973
b. pH stat titration of release of second phosphoryl group	2',3'-Cyclic AMP (7.5)	≥2	≈2	Less	No	Kurihara and Takahashi, 1973
c. ΔOD_{340} after coupled reaction with glucose-6-phosphate dehydrogenase	2',3'-Cyclic NADP (1)	1–1.5	≈1.25	Equal	Yes	Sogin, 1976

[a] Approximate values determined from information in literature or from authors' own experience (na, not available).
[b] Time required dependent on variation of method used.
Source: Modified from Sims and Carnegie (1976).

determination of the phosphate by colorimetric analysis. This was originally proposed as a one-step reaction (CNPase and alkaline phosphatase acting simultaneously), but was later modified to two separate steps
because the enzymes have different pH optima and K_m values. Although
these assays do not suffer the drawbacks of chromatographic separation,
their applicability is limited because a number of additives in the assay
(e.g., some detergents) interfere with the action of alkaline phosphatase or
the phosphate analysis.

CNPase acts on all naturally occurring 2',3'-cyclic nucleotides with
optimal activity toward 2',3'-cyclic adenosine monophosphate (2',3'-cyclic
AMP—Section 6.1). Generally this is the substrate of choice and was the
substrate used in the assays just described. Several fixed-time assays have
been proposed which utilize other substrates. One such method, based on a
ribonuclease assay, used 2',3'-cyclic cytidine monophosphate and separation of the reaction mixture on an ion exchange column (Lundblad and
Moore, 1969). Two fluorometric methods have also been proposed using
derivatives of 2',3'-cyclic AMP, $1,N_6$-ethenoadenosine-2',3'-cyclic monophosphate (Trams, 1973) and $1,N_6$-etheno-2-azaadenosine-2',3'-cyclic
monophosphate (Lo et al., 1975). Separation of the substrate and product
was achieved by selective precipitation in the first case and by an involved
procedure requiring alkaline phosphatase treatment and chromatographic
separation in the other. Although these substrates improved sensitivity
they have not been widely used, probably because of the need to prepare
these unusual derivatives. Furthermore, the K_m values for these substrates
are very high (about 10 mM) compared to that of 2',3'-cyclic AMP (0.2–1.2
mM). Since the substrate is used at around 5 mM for reasons of cost and
solubility this will affect the linearity of response. The greater sensitivity of
these assays is of little consequence when dealing with myelin or whole
brain homogenates but may be useful in examining the much smaller levels
of activity in nonmyelin subfractions and tissues from outside the nervous
system.

Continuous monitoring assays have been difficult to devise because of
the similarities between the substrate and product in properties which can
be readily measured. The use of pH stat titration to determine hydrolysis of
the phosphoryl ester bond has been described but is insensitive and uses
comparatively large amounts of substrate (Kurihara and Takahashi, 1973).
A second method used 2',3'-cyclic cytidine monophosphate as substrate
and involved measurement of small changes in the absorption spectrum at
286 nm as the product was formed (Hugli et al., 1973).

Two other assays have recently been published and would seem to
offer advantages for the assay of CNPase under most conditions. An assay
that has been successfully used under widely ranging conditions in this

laboratory (Sims and Carnegie, 1976) for several years is based on the early fixed-time methods of Drummond *et al.* (1962) and Kurihara and Tsukada (1967). However, chromatographic separation of the reaction mixture was replaced by selective coprecipitation of 2'-AMP with cadmium carbonate (Figure 1). Because the absorbance of substrate remaining is measured directly, substances which absorb at 260 nm may interfere with the assay. However, the large dilutions involved in the procedure mean that only substances with high absorption maximum in this region show any effect. In most cases, these effects are small enough to be easily controlled, e.g.,

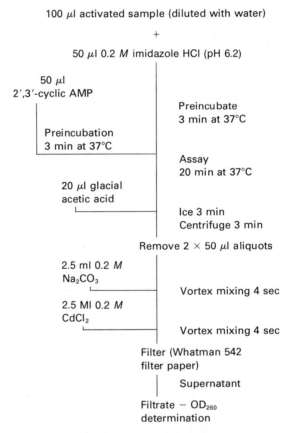

FIGURE 1. Precipitation assay for CNPase (Sims and Carnegie, 1976). Assay at 37°C has been used as a routine in this laboratory but assay at 30°C may be substituted to obtain slightly higher results.

by measurement of blanks with no enzyme or inactivated enzyme. Even with Triton X-100, correction is needed only when the concentration is greater than 0.2% in the final assay mixture. In our experience interference is a greater problem in the alternative assay involving alkaline phosphatase, and in addition two incubations are required in the latter. Since spotting, development, and elution of chromatograms are also eliminated the assay is faster and less open to introduction of error than the chromatographic methods. Furthermore, the number of assays performed is not limited by facilities for chromatography, and the method is relatively inexpensive.

The second new method (Sogin, 1976) involves the use of 2',3'-cyclic NADP as substrate and is suitable for continuous monitoring. The modification to the substrate does not result in a change of measured K_m. Activity was determined by using 2'-NADP formed from CNPase action as a substrate for glucose-6-phosphate dehydrogenase in a combined reaction mixture. NADPH formed in this reaction was measured by a change in absorbance at 340 nm.

In Table 1 the ability of the methods to distinguish between 2'- and 3'-AMP is listed. This is important since certain ribonuclease enzymes (pancreatic RNase A type) hydrolyze 2',3'-cyclic nucleotides to form 3' derivatives and if the assay method does not allow separate recognition of the 2' and 3' derivatives, such hydrolysis can lead to spurious results. This does not represent a problem when CNPase is used as a myelin marker, for Drummond *et al.* (1962) have shown the absence of such RNase activity in central nervous system. If CNPase activities are examined in other tissues, a check for RNase activity using a suitable chromatographic method (e.g., Kurihara and Tsukada, 1967; Glastris and Pfeiffer, 1974) must be performed before more rapid assays can be used routinely. Interference of this nature is not a problem with the continuous monitoring method of Sogin (1976) just outlined since the 3'-NADPH produced is not a suitable substrate for glucose-6-phosphate dehydrogenase.

3. ASSOCIATION OF CNPase WITH MYELIN

3.1. Historical

CNPase activity was first demonstrated in bovine spleen (Whitfeld *et al.,* 1955) and pancreas (Davis and Allen, 1956) but Drummond and co-workers in 1962 examined tissue distribution of the enzyme in the dog and showed that central nervous system material contained at least ten times the levels of other tissues. Regional distribution of the enzyme within the

CNS of several vertebrates seemed to correlate fairly closely with the distribution of myelinated fibers (Kurihara and Tsukada, 1967). Unmyelinated invertebrate nerves contained no activity (Drummond *et al.*, 1971). These results suggested an association of CNPase with myelin. Evidence to corroborate this was obtained from three major approaches: subcellular fractionation and production of pure myelin; developmental studies; and examination of myelin-deficient neurological mutant mice.

3.2. Subcellular Fractionation

Subcellular fraction of both rabbit brain (Kurihara and Tsukada, 1967) and bovine brain (Olafson *et al.*, 1969) demonstrated localization in myelin subfractions. Although some activity was found in other fractions this could be largely attributed to myelin contamination. Discontinuous gradient centrifugation of purified myelin (0.62 *M* sucrose layered over 0.70 *M*) indicated that the enzyme was not uniformly distributed in myelin but occurred with higher specific activity in heavier material. A similar distribution was seen for the myelin-associated glycoprotein and other high-molecular-weight components while myelin basic protein increased in lighter fractions (Matthieu *et al.*, 1973; Zimmerman *et al.*, 1975). This uneven distribution may be of functional significance and perhaps may reflect a tendency of higher molecular weight proteins to be associated with oligodendroglial fractions and newly formed loose myelin.

3.3. Development

A rapid increase in the level of CNPase during the main period of myelination was first demonstrated in the chicken (Kurihara and Tsukada, 1968) and later in the rat (Olafson *et al.*, 1969) and mouse (Kurihara *et al.*, 1970) (Figure 2). CNPase appeared to develop more rapidly than myelin basic protein in whole rat brain for it reached a level 65% of the adult value by day 20 (Olafson *et al.*, 1969) whereas basic protein attained 30% in most brain regions (Cohen and Guarnieri, 1976). Detering and Wells (1976) have stressed the nonsynchronous appearance of myelin components and, at least for the optic nerve, showed that CNPase activity appeared early during myelination. In the rabbit CNPase specific activity in isolated myelin did not change during rapid myelination whereas other myelin proteins generally exhibited changes (Matthieu *et al.*, 1975*b*).

These studies indicate that not only is CNPase a true myelin component but it appears early in myelination and is maintained at a high level as myelin is produced, suggesting a possible role of the enzyme in the myelination process.

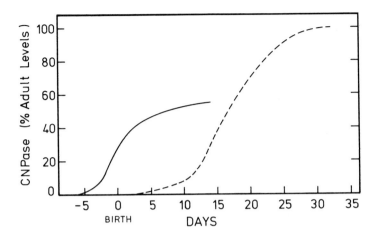

FIGURE 2. Development of CNPase activity in the chicken (solid line) and mouse (dashed line) in relation to adult levels. (From Kurihara and Tuskada, 1968, and Kurihara *et al.*, 1970.) In the rat a pattern similar to that of the mouse was observed, reaching greater than 80% adult levels by day 30 (Olafson *et al.*, 1969).

3.4. Mutant Mice

Sidman *et al.* (1964) described two neurological mutant mice, Quaking and Jimpy, which suffer from a deficiency of myelination as determined from chemical and histological analysis. CNPase levels in whole brain homogenates were reduced to 25–50% in Quaking (Olafson *et al.*, 1969; Kurihara *et al.*, 1970) and 10–15% in Jimpy (Kurihara *et al.*, 1969; Drummond *et al.*, 1971; Matthieu *et al.*, 1974*b*). This is consistent with the latter showing more severe defects leading to death at about 30 days, and is strong evidence for CNPase being a myelin component.

In normal mice CNPase levels rise rapidly between days 10 and 30. By contrast in Quaking mice the increase occurred at a slower rate and did not change beyond 21 days. In Jimpy, levels rose very little and no change at all occurred beyond day 15. Myelin isolated from the Quaking mutant has been reported to show a decrease in several major myelin proteins, in particular proteolipid protein, and also had an altered lipid content. This myelin had the same specific activity of CNPase as normal myelin (Gregson and Oxberry, 1972). Since several major proteins are reduced in Quaking myelin it seems likely that CNPase levels must also be reduced in order that the myelin specific activity appear unchanged.

Two groups (Kurihara *et al.*, 1971; Matthieu *et al.*, 1974*b*) have attempted purification of Jimpy myelin, and on the basis of CNPase specific activities the same degree of purification was achieved as with normals. Since Jimpy has a much lower myelin content an increased enrichment of CNPase would be expected, and both groups of authors suggested that the lack of this was the result of greater contamination in the Jimpy myelin. This has been confirmed by microscopy, and Matthieu *et al.* (1974*b*) further demonstrated the lack of a number of other characteristic myelin proteins from this material. The observed deficiencies in a number of myelin components seen in both these mutants suggest that the site of the defect may be in oligodendroglial cells.

3.5. Use as a Myelin Marker

As has been indicated there is unequivocable evidence that CNPase is a component of myelin. As such it is now widely used as a "marker" or indicator of myelin in a number of situations: determining purity of isolated myelin, following myelin development, determining myelin contamination in other fractions during subcellular fractionation, and detecting myelin deficiencies in disease (induced or natural). There would be little achieved by cataloging the increasing number of papers in which CNPase has been found useful as a marker but examples are presented in later sections of this chapter, in particular in relation to the study of pathological conditions affecting myelin. Use of CNPase as a marker enzyme is not completely without its drawbacks. CNPase activity is not exclusive to myelin, existing as it does both in other nervous system fractions and in other tissues (Section 4). However, with the exception of oligodendroglial cells and some myelinlike or myelin-related fractions (Section 3.6), the levels in other material represent only a few percent or less than those in myelin. As such, although it is advisable to remain aware of this nonmyelin activity, it does not usually represent a problem in practice.

Determination of CNPase–cerebroside ratios from homogenates of several CNS regions in the dog has produced a wide range of values (Drummond *et al.*, 1971). Since cerebroside in the nervous system exists mainly in myelin this led to the suggestion that CNPase did not necessarily represent a quantitative marker for myelin. Support for the notion that differences in these ratios were due, at least in part, to variations in CNPase levels in different regions comes from two sources. First, myelin isolated from the bovine CNS showed specific activity differences, in particular between brain and spinal cord (Lees and Paxman, 1974). Second, as already discussed, CNPase levels varied in myelin subfractions obtained on discontinuous gradients (Section 3.2), suggesting nonuniform distribution of the enzyme. Until a function for this enzyme is determined it is not possible to propose a reason for these variations in distribution. Although these results eliminate the use of CNPase for the direct quantitation and comparison of myelin yields from different regions, it does not affect the uses outlined previously which are dependent on the existence of high and consistent levels of CNPase within a given region.

Drummond *et al.* (1971) also determined CNPase–cerebroside ratios in a number of vertebrates which represent varying stages on the evolutionary scale. CNPase content was very low in dogfish and increased several hundredfold in the dog. CNPase cannot therefore be used to compare myelin content from animals at different evolutionary stages. This indicates that CNPase and cerebrosides have undergone different evolutionary development (with CNPase appearing later) and probably reflects an increasing sophistication of myelin in higher animals. More recently it has been shown that myelin isolated from dogfish contained no CNPase (N. L. Banik, personal communication). A closer examination of CNPase in elasmobranchs and teleosts showed an enzyme with properties similar to those of the mammalian enzyme; interestingly, however, the levels in the interrenal body of the brown shark and sting ray as well as in the liver and kidney of the ray were the same (on a wet weight basis) as those in brain (Trams and Brown, 1974). This would suggest that the association of high activities of CNPase in brain (and myelin) compared to those in other fractions is a relatively recent evolutionary development.

3.6.   Myelin-Related Fractions and Peripheral Nerve Myelin

Using different isolation procedures two subfractions that contain high specific activities of CNPase have been prepared from developing animals; it was thought that these preparations represented precursor material for myelin. These subfractions, termed "myelinlike" fraction (Banik and Davison, 1969; Agrawal *et al.*, 1970) and "membrane" fraction (Agrawal *et al.*, 1974) consisted primarily of single-walled vesicles and differed markedly from myelin in lipid and protein composition. These fractions showed differences in their lipid composition and it has been suggested, on the basis of gel electrophoresis, that both contained myelin basic protein (Agrawal *et al.*, 1973, 1974). Tryptophan was rapidly incorporated into the myelinlike and the membrane fractions and more slowly into myelin, thus supporting the idea of a precursor–product relationship for these fractions (Agrawal *et al.*, 1974).

In attempting to extend the observations a stage further, Sabri *et al.* (1975) examined subcellular localization of CNPase activity from birth to the end of the rapid myelination phase in rats. The low levels of CNPase which were present up to 10 days were predominantly associated with microsomal and myelinlike fractions. It was proposed that the microsomal fraction may be responsible for the synthesis of a precursor membrane which is incorporated into myelinlike fragments and finally into myelin.

Waehneldt and Mandel (1972) isolated a microsome-free fraction (called SN4) following osmotic shock of purified myelin from mature rat brains. This fraction was largely single membranes and contained low levels of the major myelin proteins by electrophoresis. Subsequent work (Waenheldt, 1975) showed that it can also be isolated from young animals. The specific activity of CNPase in the fraction increased with age and was higher than in the pure myelin from which it was derived. These authors have suggested that this material, which was obtained in very low yields when compared to myelin, may represent an intermediate stage in myelin formation and could be related to the myelinlike fraction.

In summary then it would seem that a number of subfractions can be isolated which are morphologically different from myelin but which resemble myelin by the presence of small amounts of myelin-specific proteins and high levels of CNPase. It has been proposed that these represent intermediate stages in myelin formation.

The oligodendroglial cell is the site of myelin production and it might be expected that high levels of CNPase would exist in these cells. Until recently difficulty has been encountered in studying oligodendroglia because of a lack of suitable techniques for separation of these from other types of brain cells. Poduslo and Norton (1972) recently described a method for bulk isolation of oligodendroglial cells of high purity and reported a CNPase specific activity in the whole cell approximately half that of myelin. CNPase levels in isolated oligodendroglial, astroglial, and neuronal cells during development (16–29 days) in rat brain have been examined (Deshmukh *et al.*, 1974). Greater than twofold increases in specific activity were found for oligodendroglia whereas neuronal cells exhibited only 10% of the level, percentage that was not altered during development. Astroglial cells showed an activity change between days 19 and 26. However, this fraction was shown by light microscopy to be heavily contaminated with cell debris and broken cell products, and hence the observed change may have arisen from oligodendroglial contamination.

Oligodendroglial cells were fractionated to yield plasma membrane and material resembling myelin but attached to plasma membrane. The specific activity of CNPase was approximately twice as high in the myelin-type fraction as in the plasma membrane fraction and both exhibited levels lower than those for true myelin (Poduslo, 1975). Enzyme markers typical of plasma membranes were also present in both fractions, although these were lower in the myelin type, while enzyme markers usually associated with other subcellular fractions were present only at low levels.

A procedure has been described for the isolation of an axolemma-enriched fraction from bovine brain; this was found to have a CNPase specific activity equal to approximately 45% of that of myelin (De Vries, 1976). The most obvious explanation is that this fraction was contaminated with myelin or myelin-related membranes. However, if there is a genuinely elevated level of CNPase in axolemma it may have some importance in the interaction, which appears to occur early in myelination, between the processes of oligodendroglial cells and the axon.

Discussion so far has largely been concerned with CNPase in CNS myelin. This enzyme also exists in peripheral nervous system myelin but at only about 10% of the level at which it is found in the CNS (Uyemura *et al.*, 1972). In the sciatic nerve of the chicken CNPase increased rapidly from day 14 *in ovo* to day 1 after hatching (i.e., day 22) thus marginally preceding the period of rapid myelination in the CNS (Dreiling and Newburgh, 1972; Mezei and Palmer, 1974). Braun and Barchi (1972) reported no change of CNPase in sciatic nerve of rats between birth and adult and suggested CNPase may not be associated with myelin in this species.

4. CNPase IN NONMYELIN FRACTIONS

The existence of the major amount of CNPase activity in myelin and related fractions has been adequately established, and not surprisingly most studies of the enzyme have used this material. However, low levels of CNPase-type activity have also been demonstrated in other tissues (Whitfeld *et al.*, 1955; Davis and Allen, 1956; Drummond *et al.*, 1962) and in other cell fractions from the brain (e.g., astroglia and neurons; Deshmukh *et al.*, 1974), and this activity has been examined in some detail in human erythrocytes (Sudo *et al.*, 1972) and spleen (Konings and Pierce, 1974). In both cases CNPase was shown to be totally associated with particulate fractions and also demonstrated the same pH optima as the brain enzyme. Furthermore, in the erythrocyte membrane the enzyme showed similar substrate specificity and response to metal ions. It would seem, therefore, that CNPase-type activity in other cells is primarily membrane-bound and is produced by an enzyme similar to that in brain. This may mean that the function of the enzyme is related to a general membrane phenomenon. (For studies on CNPase in tumor cells see Section 7.6.)

5. ACTIVATION AND ISOLATION

5.1. Introduction

Despite the widespread use of CNPase as a biological marker little work has been reported on characterization of the enzyme in myelin or its isolation and purification from myelin. These studies are useful in providing further information in relation to the marker role of the enzyme and may also be useful in providing clues to the function of the enzyme. Because of the high lipid–protein ratio of myelin it might be expected that the problems associated with isolation of proteins from other membranes would be accentuated in dealing with myelin proteins. Techniques suitable for isolation of CNPase may be applicable for other minor myelin proteins and may provide a useful insight into procedures suitable for use with enzymes present in other membranes.

5.2. Activation

Kurihara and Tsukada (1967) reported that higher and more reproducible levels of CNPase in brain homogenates and subcellular fractions could be obtained if material was disrupted by sonication prior to assay, presumably as a result of increasing access of the substrate to the active sites. It was later demonstrated that activation was also achieved with several detergents including sodium deoxycholate (Kurihara *et al.*, 1969), Triton X-100 (Agrawal *et al.*, 1970), and lysolecithin (Gregson and Oxberry, 1972). Once activation of the enzyme was achieved subsequent dilution of the detergent–enzyme mixture did not affect the activation.

Lees *et al.* (1974) examined the effects of the detergents Triton X-100, sodium deoxycholate, cetyltrimethylammonium bromide (cetavlon), and sodium dodecyl sulfate (SDS) on CNPase in lyophilized myelin, fresh myelin suspensions, and erythrocyte ghosts. Activation of myelin CNPase was achieved with all detergents except SDS, which inactivated the enzyme. By contrast CNPase from erythrocyte ghosts was not affected by Triton X-100 and sodium deoxycholate and was inactivated partially by cetavlon and totally by SDS. These results suggest that the brain and red blood cell CNPase are localized differently in the membranes, the latter being more exposed to substrate in the absence of prior disruptive treatment, and perhaps may not be as deeply buried in the membrane lipid. Work in this laboratory (N. R. Sims and P. R. Carnegie, unpublished observations) has also examined the activating effects of several detergents on myelin suspensions; the results obtained (Figure 3) are in general agreement with those of Lees and co-workers when the same concentrations were examined. Since SDS is a strong protein denaturant it is not surprising that enzyme activity was lost in its presence. However, at concentrations lower than those used by Lees' group, this compound also produced activation, again probably by solubilizing the lipid and disrupting the membrane, and thereby increasing the exposure of enzyme to the substrate. The neutral detergents sulfobetaine DLH (lauryl ammonium sulfonic acid betaine) and Empigen BB (R $-$ N$^+$(CH$_3$)$_2$CH$_2$CO$_2^-$, where R is mainly C$_{12}$ and C$_{14}$) produced the greatest activation among the detergents examined.

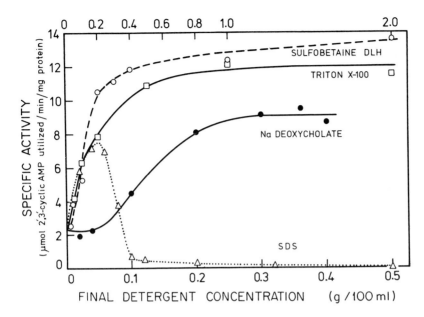

FIGURE 3. Activation of CNPase in myelin suspensions by detergents. Myelin in water (100 μl; 0.5 mg protein/ml) was mixed with 100 μl of detergent and 50 μl 0.05 M Tris-HCl, pH 7.5, at 4°C and CNPase assayed at pH 6.2 after appropriate dilution with water. The actual activation achieved was dependent on the method of myelin preparation and its history with respect to freeze–thawing, but the order of effectiveness of the detergents remained the same. The results presented were obtained with myelin prepared by the method of Mokrasch (1971) and stored at −20°C. A second neutral detergent (Empigen BB) produced an activation similar to that of sulfobetaine DLH (lauryl ammonium sulfonic acid betaine). The upper horizontal axis corresponds to the curves for sulfobetaine DLH and Triton X-100, the lower, to those for sodium deoxycholate and SDS.

5.3. Solubilization and Fractionation

Drummond *et al.* (1962) demonstrated that CNPase activity was detectable in a powder from bovine brain, prepared by successive extraction with acetone, *n*-butanol, and petroleum ether. Extraction of this powder with 0.02 M phosphate buffer released less than 5% of the activity and 50% of the protein. The enzyme was extracted from the powder with 3 M sodium chloride containing the nonionic detergent Tween 20 (6%) and was lyophilized and reextracted with acetone to remove detergent. It was claimed that the final powder contained 90% of the activity of the brain and a relative specific activity of 50; however, since no activation of the enzyme was used for the assays, and extraction would increase the exposure of the enzyme, these figures probably represent a considerable overestimation.

Hugli *et al.* (1973) found that 2 *M* guanidinium chloride containing 6% Tween 20 was three times more effective in extracting CNPase from acetone-dried powder into low-speed supernatants (35,000 × *g* for 30 min). Partial fractionation of the enzyme was achieved by gel filtration of the resultant supernatant on Sepharose 4B although most of the activity was eluted coincidently with the front of the major protein peak, which appeared to be extremely heterogeneous.

Systematic examination of the solubilization of CNPase from myelin suspensions with respect to the effects of ionic strength and concentration of the detergent Triton X-100 has been performed (Sims and Carnegie, 1975) (Figure 4). Solubilization in these studies was measured as the ability to remain in 100,000 × *g* (1 hr) supernatants, conditions which represent minimal criteria for solubilization.* The plateau level of solubilization achieved was independent of the severity of the extraction method (mild mixing being as effective as extensive homogenization) but was dependent on the salt used for adjustment of ionic strength. The negative chaotropic ion, thiocynanate, produced slightly lower release (45%), whereas 2 *M* guanidinium chloride (a positive chaotrope) released 75%, although the enzyme was denatured fairly rapidly in the presence of this salt. This dependence of extraction on the salt used is a common phenomenon in membrane destabilization processes (Hatefi and Hanstein, 1974). Gel filtration of solubilized supernatants produced results similar to those of Hugli *et al.* (1973) and attempts to reduce ionic strength or remove Triton X-100 resulted in a loss of soluble activity.

It is interesting that maximum activation of CNPase is achieved at high Triton X-100 concentrations without the need for high ionic strength, conditions which result in almost no solubilization. This further supports the contention that activation occurs by exposure of the active sites as a result of disruption of the membrane but does not necessarily involve release of CNPase into solution.

Several studies have now been reported in which CNPase has been solubilized in the absence of detergent. In early work fairly vigorous treatments were employed but solubilization of native enzyme from acetone-dried powders was achieved when dilute basic buffers or "sulfito-

---

*Supernatants obtained by centrifugation at 100,000 × *g* for 1 hr are considered, by convention, to contain only "soluble" material. Quite large protein aggregates are not pelleted under these conditions and they should therefore be regarded as minimal criteria for defining the constituents in soluble fractions. Milder centrifugation conditions have been used in some studies and these may lead to a failure to sediment membrane subunits adequately; e.g., Miyamoto and Kakiuchi (1975) used 22,000 × *g* for 15 min in the preparation of soluble phosphoprotein phosphatase from myelin. Clearly, use of a more rigorous centrifugation procedure in this case would have helped confirm that the enzyme was truly released from the membrane.

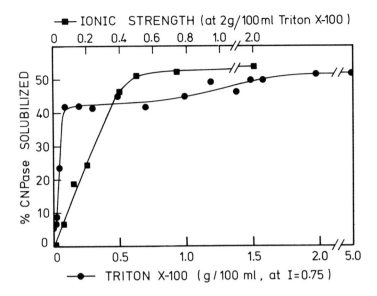

FIGURE 4. Solubilization of CNPase by Triton X-100: dependence on detergent concentration and ionic strength. Myelin was adjusted to 0.5 mg protein/ml with solutions containing imidazole HCl (pH 6.2, $I = 0.0125$) and appropriate concentrations of Triton X-100 and sodium chloride (for ionic strength adjustment) and mixed by hand. Mixtures were left for 10 min at 4°C and centrifuged at 105,000 × g for 1 hr. CNPase activity was determined in the supernatant by the method of Sims and Carnegie (1976).

lysis'' (involving treatment with sodium sulfite, guanidinium chloride, and EDTA) was used with long incubations at 37°C (Lundblad and Moore, 1969). Since no activation process was used in the assay procedure it is not possible to determine the extent of solubilization.

Guha and Moore (1975) reported high levels of solubilization of CNPase, again from acetone-dried powder by treatment with dithiothreitol, EDTA, and guanidinium chloride in 2-(*N*-morpholino)ethanesulfonic acid (MES) buffer (outlined in Figure 5). Activity was retained in solution only if the guanidinium chloride concentration was reduced stepwise, presumably by eliminating material that combined with CNPase and precipitated it. Following purification the final material had a specific activity 500 times that of the starting powder. This method of solubilization was also used on fresh myelin (Sogin, 1976) but the product required detergent activation to express full activity, suggesting that it was released in combination with other membrane components.

Myelin has been solubilized in an active form which was suitable for gel electrophoresis and detectable by histological enzyme staining (Braun and Barchi, 1972). Rat myelin was treated with Triton X-100, urea, and

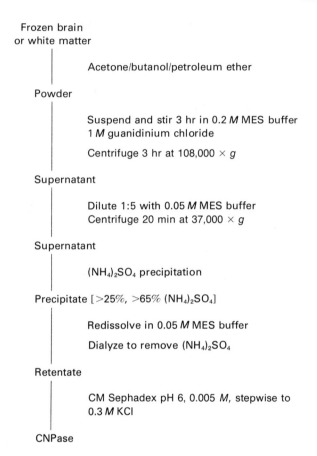

Frozen brain
or white matter

| Acetone/butanol/petroleum ether

Powder

| Suspend and stir 3 hr in 0.2 *M* MES buffer
| 1 *M* guanidinium chloride
|
| Centrifuge 3 hr at 108,000 × *g*

Supernatant

| Dilute 1:5 with 0.05 *M* MES buffer
| Centrifuge 20 min at 37,000 × *g*

Supernatant

| $(NH_4)_2SO_4$ precipitation

Precipitate [>25%, >65% $(NH_4)_2SO_4$]

| Redissolve in 0.05 *M* MES buffer
|
| Dialyze to remove $(NH_4)_2SO_4$

Retentate

| CM Sephadex pH 6, 0.005 *M,* stepwise to
| 0.3 *M* KCl

CNPase

FIGURE 5. Purification of CNPase without detergent (Guha and Moore, 1975).

mercaptoethanol; the activity migrated with the high-molecular-weight region of the gel although exact localization to a single band could not be achieved. (Attempts to repeat this procedure in our laboratory using bovine and rat myelin resulted in rapid inactivation of the CNPase activity on exposure to the solvent.) Recently Kurihara *et al.* (1977) found that non-aqueous chloroform–methanol could be used to delipidate freeze-dried brain with minimal loss of enzyme activities. CNPase activity was retained provided all the chloroform–methanol was completely removed prior to assay.

In conclusion, solubilization of the enzyme is possible but only under conditions which remove lipids and disrupt the protein structure of the membrane. This would suggest that CNPase is embedded in myelin and represents a true intrinsic membrane enzyme. Purification of the enzyme can be achieved by standard techniques if solubilization is performed without the use of detergent.

6. PROPERTIES

6.1. Substrate Specificity

CNPase was shown to hydrolyze 2',3'-cyclic nucleotide derivatives of each of the four common bases examined, with the greatest rate for adenine and decreasing through guanine and cytidine to uridine (17.5% of adenosine derivatives); 2'-nucleotides are the exclusive product. The general reaction is

(Drummond and Perrott-Yee, 1961: Drummond *et al.*, 1962). K_m values for the enzyme have been determined by a number of workers and values from 0.22 to greater than 6 mM have been obtained depending on the assay conditions and possibly also the nature and source of the enzyme (Olafson *et al.*, 1969; Zanetta *et al.*, 1972, Kurihara and Takahashi, 1973; Hugli *et al.*, 1973; Prohaska *et al.*, 1973; Sogin, 1976). Two values recently reported for the soluble forms of the enzyme were 0.22 mM with 2',3'-cyclic AMP as substrate at pH 6, 25°C (Sogin, 1976), and 0.8 mM for 2',3'-cyclic CMP, pH 6, 25°C (Hugli *et al.*, 1973).

Simple nucleoside phosphate esters and 3',5'-cyclic derivatives were not hydrolyzed nor were internucleotide bonds of RNA; however, oligonucleotides with 2',3'-cyclic phosphate terminals were converted to 2'-ended oligonucleotides although the rate of hydrolysis was less than for free 2',3'-cyclic AMP. 2',3'-Cyclic phosphorothioate derivatives of free nucleotides were also hydrolyzed at a rate less than that for 2',3'-cyclic AMP (Drummond *et al.*, 1962; Olafson *et al.*, 1969). As a result of work performed in designing assays for CNPase it has been shown that 2',3'-cyclic NADP (Sogin, 1976) and the fluorometric derivatives 1,N^6-ethenoadenosine-2',3'-cyclic monophosphate (Trams, 1973) and 1,N^6-etheno-2-azaadenosine-2',3'-cyclic monophosphate (Lo *et al.*, 1975) are also hydrolyzed, the first of these with a K_m similar to that of 2',3'-cyclic AMP (0.23 mM, pH 6, 25°C) and the fluorometric compounds at a higher K_m (6–10 mM, pH 6.5, 30°C).

6.2. Inhibition

A wide variety of substances have been tested as possible inhibitors of CNPase, many of which produced no effect (Drummond *et al.*, 1962; Olafson *et al.*, 1969; Hugli *et al.*, 1973). Those substances which were inhibitory to the enzyme and some of the more interesting noninhibitory compounds are summarized in Table 2. Difficulties arise when the effects of these inhibitors are compared because the studies were performed with different enzyme preparations, using various assays and substrates. Continuous monitoring assays are more suitable for detecting inhibition than fixed-time methods. Early studies reported no inhibition of 2',3'- or 5'-AMP on the enzyme at levels as high as 1.5 times those of the substrate (2',3'-cyclic AMP) whereas Hugli *et al.* (1973), using 2',3'-cyclic CMP as substrate, obtained 50% inhibition with all three compounds at approximately half the substrate concentration. In part this probably reflects the higher affinity of the enzyme for purine compared to pyrimidine bases (2',3'-cyclic AMP being hydrolyzed at approximately three times the rate of 2',3'-cyclic CMP). A further factor which probably contributed to the difference was the pH of assay which was 7.5 in the early studies and 6.0 when inhibition was detected. The pK_{a_2} of phosphate in 2'- and 3'-AMP is 5.9 and 6.2, respectively, and since the monodissociated form more closely resembles 2',3'-cyclic AMP on charge considerations, it is not surprising that inhibition was more readily detectable at the lower pH. Despite these problems the observation that 2',3'- and 5'-AMP produce very similar inhibitions is interesting since it may have been expected, if 2',3'-cyclic AMP was the true substrate, that the product, 2'-AMP, would inhibit more strongly (Hugli *et al.*, 1973). The ability of all three compounds to block activity almost equally suggests that the binding site region may not be completely filled.

As substrate is utilized and 2'-nucleotide accumulates it may be expected that the reaction would be increasingly inhibited and linearity of assay lost, but there is contention as to what amount of product formation

TABLE 2.   Inhibition of CNPase

Compound	Compound concentration (mM)	Substrate	Substrate concentration (mM)	Percent inhibition	Reference[a]
Cupric sulfate	2	2',3'-Cyclic AMP	7.5	26	1
Zinc acetate	2	2',3'-Cyclic AMP	7.5	75	1
Mercuric chloride	1	2',3'-Cyclic AMP	7.5	100	1
Guanidinium chloride	0.22	2',3'-Cyclic CMP	1	50	3
Sodium acetate	0.16	2',3'-Cyclic CMP	1	50	3
Diisopropyl fluoroacetate	1	2',3'-Cyclic AMP	7.5	0	1
Physostygmine	1	2',3'-Cyclic AMP	7.5	0	1
Iodoacetamide	1	2',3'-Cyclic AMP	7.5	0	1
Arsenite, arsenate	1	2',3'-Cyclic AMP	7.5	0	1
Theophyllin	2	2',3'-Cyclic AMP	4	0	2
Tubercidin	2	2',3'-Cyclic AMP	4	0	2
2'-AMP	0.5	2',3'-Cyclic CMP	1	50	3
3'-AMP	0.5	2',3'-Cyclic CMP	1	50	3
5'-AMP	0.52	2',3'-Cyclic CMP	1	50	3
5'-ATP	0.96	2',3'-Cyclic CMP	1	50	3
3',5'-Cyclic AMP	4.4	2',3'-Cyclic CMP	1	50	3
Orthophosphate	8.5	2',3'-Cyclic CMP	1	50	3
Adenosine	16.0	2',3'-Cyclic CMP	1	50	3

[a] Drummond et al. (1962) (1) and Olafson et al. (1969) (2) assayed CNPase at pH 7.5 using paper electrophoresis and paper chromatography, respectively, to separate substrate and product. Hugli et al. (1972) (3) used a continuous monitoring assay at pH 6.0 involving changes in absorbance at 286 nm.

is required before the assay is affected. A continuous monitoring assay using 2',3'-cyclic CMP (Hugli *et al.*, 1973) and a fixed-time assay with 2',3'-cyclic NADP as substrate (Sogin, 1976) found inhibition at 15 and 18% substrate utilization, respectively. By contrast fixed-time assays performed at pH 7.5 (Drummond *et al.*, 1962; Olafson *et al.*, 1969) and 6.2 (Kurihara and Tsukada, 1967; Glastris and Pfeiffer, 1974; Sims and Carnegie, 1976) found linearity to at least 50% utilization. Although not specifically investigated this may be a genuine effect resulting from the nature of the enzyme preparation used, since the studies in which marked inhibition was observed were performed on solubilized enzyme from acetone-dried powders while all other investigations, performed at comparable pH (6.2), utilized CNS homogenates or myelin suspensions.

6.3. Optima

The optimal pH of CNPase from mammalian brain is 6.2 (Kurihara and Takahashi, 1973; Prohaska *et al.*, 1973) but activity measured is dependent on the buffer used, activity being higher in imidazole and glutarate than in citrate, phosphate, or dimethyl glutarate (Kurihara and Takahashi, 1973). Optimal temperature is 30°C; at 37°C the measured activity is reduced by 10% (Prohaska *et al.*, 1973).

CNPase in spleen and erythrocyte ghosts exhibited the same pH optima as the brain enzyme. CNPase activity detected in the brown shark had both the same pH and temperature optimum (Trams and Brown, 1974).

6.4. Comparison with Other Myelin Proteins

CNPase activity would appear not to be associated with the two major myelin proteins, basic protein and proteolipid protein, from several lines of evidence. Gel electrophoresis (Braun and Barchi, 1972) showed CNPase activity exclusively associated with the high-molecular-weight region of the gel, with a mobility less than either of the major proteins. In the purification procedure of Guha and Moore (1975) the enzyme appeared to have a molecular weight of approximately 65,000 (by SDS electrophoresis) which is far greater than basic protein monomer or proteolipid protein monomer. Discontinuous gradient centrifugation of myelin resulted in several subfractions with different protein composition, and CNPase varied between these fractions similarly to myelin glycoprotein but differently to the two major proteins (Matthieu *et al.*, 1973; Zimmerman *et al.*, 1975).

The molecular weight of 65,000 suggested for CNPase indicates that the activity is not associated with the major myelin glycoprotein since the latter imigrated in SDS electrophoresis with an apparent molecular weight of 110,000 (Quarles *et al.*, 1973). Furthermore, solubilized CNPase was not bound to concanavalin A–Sepharose, suggesting that carbohydrate residues with affinity for this lectin are absent or inaccessible on the enzyme (N. R. Sims and P. R. Carnegie, unpublished observations).

When synthetic phosphorylated peptides (homologous to amino acid residues 106–113 of human basic protein) were incubated with myelin, phosphate was released as a result of the action of phosphoprotein phosphatase. Partially purified CNPase (Guha and Moore, 1975) showed no such effect, indicating that phosphatase activity was not associated with CNPase and that phosphoprotein phosphatase has been removed by the purification procedure (N. R. Sims and P. R. Carnegie, unpublished observations).

6.5. Comparison with Other Nucleases

Several endoribonucleases produce 2',3'-cyclic nucleotides as intermediates in the hydrolysis of ribonucleic acid. Extensive studies have been performed on ribonuclease I (pancreatic ribonuclease, EC 3.1.4.22) because of the relative ease of obtaining preparations of high purity, and a number of reviews have been devoted to this protein (e.g., Richards and Wyckoff, 1971). The enzyme was specific for pyrimidine nucleotides and ultimately hydrolyzed the cyclic intermediates to 3' derivatives. Extensive characterization of the substrate requirements has been performed largely by the use of nucleotide analogues. Guanoribonuclease (EC 3.1.4.8) and ribonuclease II (EC 3.1.4.23) both performed the same reaction but the former was specific for guanylate residues whereas the latter attacked both purines and pyrimidines.

Besides CNPase, several other enzymes exist which hydrolyze 2',3'-cyclic nucleotides but do not degrade ribonucleic acid. A wide range of microorganisms contained an enzyme which produced 3' derivatives from 2',3'-cyclic nucleotides with the base type having little effect on the rate. The same enzyme also appeared to contain 3'-nucleotidase activity, although probably at a second active site, and the ultimate products were thus free orthophosphate and nucleoside. Several properties of the enzyme (e.g., pH optimum and metal ion effects) were dependent on the organism from which it was derived, but in all cases both activities were exhibited (for a review see Drummond and Yamamoto, 1971). A cyclic nucleotide phosphodiesterase from silkworm likewise catalyzed hydrolysis of 2',3'-cyclic nucleotides to 3' derivatives but this enzyme also converted 3',5'-cyclic nucleotides to the 5'-nucleotides (Morishima, 1974).

Hence, hydrolysis of 2',3'-cyclic nucleotides is not peculiar to CNPase. However, within our knowledge CNPase as found in the mammalian tissues is the only enzyme which converts this substrate exclusively to the 2'-mononucleotide.

6.6. Antibody

Antibody to CNPase was produced in rabbits using solubilized CNPase. The antibody inhibited the enzyme activity but the extent of inhibition varied with different enzyme preparations. Proteins of high molecular weight present in normal serum increased the activity of CNPase (Sims and Carnegie, 1977).

7. CNPase IN PATHOLOGICAL CONDITIONS

7.1. Introduction

Use of CNPase as a myelin marker has been widely applied to the examination of diseases and treatments affecting myelination, thus providing in many cases a sensitive indication of myelin deficiency. Detection of myelin deficiency is usually achieved by comparing CNPase levels in homogenates of unfractionated material obtained from test and control groups, a simple approach which has proven satisfactory in the majority of cases. Small lesions of demyelination or those localized to a narrow region of the brain may sometimes pass undetected although this can often be overcome by determining levels for different regions of the CNS rather than the brain as a whole, and by selecting likely areas from the clinical and histological presentation. A further difficulty in using CNPase as a marker of myelin deficiency could arise if the defect were selective, resulting in loss or malfunction of one or more myelin components without an effect on CNPase, analogous to the occurrence in some leukodystrophies of regions of defective myelination which appear normal by histologic methods. In most cases in which CNPase levels have been examined in regions of known defective myelination such a problem has not arisen, a situation which is probably a reflection of the simplicity of the myelin structure resulting in a close dependency among the constituents. Some exceptions, in which demyelination has been demonstrated without affecting the level of CNPase, are now discussed.

In a number of studies in which a myelin deficiency has been demonstrated, purified myelin has been prepared to determine whether it is normal with respect to characteristic properties including CNPase activity. Although useful information can be obtained from such an approach it suffers from the inherent disadvantage that the nature of the myelin prepared is determined by the isolation procedure which is, by necessity, designed on the basis of the properties of normal myelin. Hence defective myelin may be discarded during the processing. A finding of no abnormalities in the myelin composition (as has often been the case) can only be taken as an indication that some of the myelin produced is normal and leaves open the question as to whether an abnormal type of myelin is also produced.

Apart from examining these pathological states as an important example of the use of CNPase as a marker, further interest in these situations arises from the possibility that inhibition or malfunction of CNPase itself may be the primary defect in some of the cases. Detection and analysis of such abnormalities could provide valuable information on the role of the enzyme in myelin.

The results for a number of conditions studied are summarized in Table 3. To avoid confusion due to the use of different assay procedures, species, and brain regions in the various studies, the results are expressed in terms of the qualitative changes observed rather than the absolute values determined by the original authors. A number of studies which provide good examples of the uses (and pitfalls) of CNPase as a marker, or which bear directly on the role of CNPase in myelin are considered in detail.

7.2. Genetic Abnormalities

The changes in myelin levels and CNPase in the mutant mice Quaking and Jimpy which exhibit dysmyelination as a primary disorder have already been discussed (Section 3.4).

Another mutant mouse which has been studied for deficient myelination is Snell's dwarf mouse which suffers from hereditary pituitary dwarfism (Reier et al., 1975). Although the primary site of action of the defect is at the level of the pituitary, it is recognized that one secondary effect is hypothyroidism. Total brain homogenates from these mice showed a decrease to 76% of the control level but isolated myelin showed a normal composition of all components examined, including CNPase. This condition serves to illustrate the care required when CNPase levels are examined in isolated myelin. The yield of myelin was only 44% of the control which leaves a discrepancy of 30% between CNPase detected in whole homogenates and in isolated myelin. This may result from the existence of an "abnormal-type" myelin which was not isolated under the conditions used.

Autopsy material from patients with Down's syndrome (mongolism), caused by a congenital chromosome abnormality, also showed a decreased yield of myelin. The myelin had a normal composition (by gel electrophoresis) for the major myelin proteins and for characteristic lipids. However, specific activities of CNPase were decreased by 20–35% in isolated myelin and the authors suggested that this was indicative of a fault in the structure of myelin (Banik et al., 1975). It was not possible to determine whether the

TABLE 3. Effect of Pathological Conditions on CNPase Levels in Whole Brain Homogenates and Isolated Myelin

Condition	Comment	Material studied[a]		Reference
		Unfractionated homogenate	Isolated myelin	
Genetic abnormalities				
Jimpy mice	Defective myelination	∨	0	Kurihara et al., 1969, 1971; Drummond et al., 1971; Matthieu et al., 1974b
Quaking mice	Defective myelination	∨	0	Olafson et al., 1969; Kurihara et al., 1970; Gregson and Oxberry, 1972
Snell's mice	Pituitary dwarfism (secondary hypothyroidism)	∨	0	Reier et al., 1975
Down's syndrome	Chromosome defect causing mental retardation		∨	Banik et al., 1975
Chemical treatments				
Hexachlorophene ingestion	Vacuolation of myelin			
Adult rat		0	0	Cammer et al., 1975
Newborn rat			< Floating fraction 0	Matthieu et al., 1974a
Acute triethyllead intoxication		< Sciatic nerve 0 CNS	0 Floating fraction	Konat et al., 1976
1,1,3-Tricyano-2-amino-1-propene				Dreiling and Newburgh, 1972
Conditions affecting development				
Protein deficiency				
a. Postnatal		∨	∨	Nakhasi et al., 1975
b. Prenatal and postnatal		∨		Simons and Johnston, 1976

Condition	Notes	Effect		Reference
Neonatal hypothyroidism	Cretinism	<		Tsukada and Nomura, 1971; Wysocki and Segal, 1972; Valcana et al., 1975; Matthieu et al., 1975a
			0	Matthieu et al., 1975a
			0	Wysocki and Segal, 1972
Neonatal hyperthyroidism	Earlier development	>		Bondy and Madsen, 1972
Excision of innervating eye	Examined for effect on myelination in optic nerve	< Contralateral, 0 Ipsilateral		Grundt and Hole, 1974
p-Chlorophenylalanine injection	Experimental phenylketonuria	0		
p-Chlorophenylalanine + phenylalanine injection		<		Prohaska and Wells, 1974a
Copper deficiency	Model for human Menkes' disease and swayback in sheep	<	0	Zimmerman et al., 1976; Prohaska and Wells, 1974b
Zinc deficiency		< Gestational–lactational deficiency, 0 Lactational deficiency only		Prohaska et al., 1974
Hypoxia	Born and raised at high altitude (3800 m)	< Day 22		Dalal et al., 1973
Diseases				
Experimental autoimmune encephalomyelitis	Model for multiple sclerosis (?)	0 Whole white matter		Drummond et al., 1971
		> Whole white matter		Pechan and Simekova, 1972
		< Plaques of demyelination		Govindarajan et al., 1974

(Continued)

TABLE 3.   (Continued)

Condition	Comment	Material studied[a] Unfractionated homogenate	Material studied[a] Isolated myelin	Reference
Diseases (cont.)				
Multiple sclerosis		0 Apparently normal white matter < Plaques of demyelination		Braun and Barchi, 1972; Riekinnen et al., 1972
Schilder's disease	Gangliosidosis	0 Apparently normal white matter < Demyelinating regions	<	Komiya and Kasahara, 1971; Kurihara and Takahashi, 1972
Subacute sclerosing panencephalitis	Measles-virus-induced	< Whole white matter < Plaques of demyelination	< Floating fraction	Riekinnen et al., 1972; Ramsey et al., 1974
Wallerian degeneration	Degeneration of myelin and axon distal to sectioned nerve fiber	<Distal } Sciatic 0 Proximal } nerve		Mezei et al., 1974

[a] CNPase levels determined in comparison to controls. Changes shown as > greater, < less, 0 no change. Blanks indicate situations not examined.

CNPase deficiency and the lack of development of the full myelin complement were related but it would seem that more detailed work on this disease might be helpful to understanding the function of CNPase.

7.3. Chemical Treatments

In hexachlorophene intoxication an abnormal "floating" fraction was isolated which appeared related to myelin. In the adult rat, CNPase levels in this fraction when compared to myelin were lowered and the lipid content increased (Cammer *et al.*, 1975) while in the young animal the only significant difference observed was a decrease in a major myelin-associated glycoprotein (Matthieu *et al.*, 1974*a*). A similar fraction was isolated from triethyltin-treated rats which also show edema of myelin. Triethyltin had no effect on CNPase *in vitro* (Wassenaar and Kroon, 1973), but levels of enzyme from treated animals have not been reported. Floating fractions have also been obtained in cases of subacute sclerosing panencephalitis (Norton *et al.*, 1966), Schilder's disease (Suzuki *et al.*, 1970), Wallerian degeneration (Bignami and Eng, 1973), Tay–Sachs disease, and G_{M1} gangliosidosis (Suzuki *et al.*, 1969). In these cases the floating fraction contained cholesterol esters which were absent in the fractions induced by hexachlorophene and triethyltin. This would suggest that where floating fractions are isolated from diseased brains the composition may be a guide to the mechanism involved in the production of defective myelin.

Injection of 1,1,3-tricyano-2-amino-1-propene increases neuronal metabolism (Hyden and Hartelius, 1948) and affects RNA composition in oligodendroglia (Egyhazi and Hyden, 1961). Treatment of 13-day-old chick embryos with this compound produced a fourfold increase in CNPase activity in sciatic nerve within 24 hr of injection, although no change was seen in a number of other enzymes including CNPase in the CNS (Dreiling and Newburgh, 1972). This was not the result of direct activation of the enzyme; radiotracer studies and gel electrophoresis of isolated nerve suggested that increased CNPase levels resulted from specific increases in the synthesis of CNPase although the results were far from conclusive. Further work is necessary on the effects of this compound in both the peripheral nervous system and CNS.

7.4. Conditions Affecting Development

Undernutrition during brain development produces wide-ranging effects including deficient myelin production (see Dobbing, 1972; Krigman and Hogan, 1976; Wiggins *et al.*, 1976). Nakhasi *et al.* (1975) reported on the composition of myelin isolated from rats fed protein-deficient diets from birth. Myelin yield (as measured from levels of total protein and several lipids) was decreased and CNPase levels were lowered by 44% compared to controls. Furthermore, specific activity of CNPase in the myelin was 25% less, suggesting that this enzyme was more severely affected than other myelin proteins in undernutrition.

Effects of undernutrition on brain development are seen as a secondary phenomenon in a number of pathological conditions affecting young animals and difficulty is often experienced in separating primary effects from those resulting from the undernutrition. In cases in which the sites and mechanisms of action of administered substances or agents are under examination this represents a real problem. Care is therefore required in interpreting results when defective myelination is detected in animals which have been subjected to treatment in the critical period just prior to myelination. In cases in which animal models are required for evaluating treatment of a human condition the existence of effects from undernutrition would be desirable where these were also a feature of the human clinical presentation, and effects on the myelination pattern could be used as one method of monitoring the effectiveness of treatments. Neonatal hypothyroidism is one disease for which animal models are readily produced and in which the clinical presentation is partially dependent on undernutrition. CNPase levels in neonatal hypothyroidism in rats have been well studied (Tsukada and Nomura, 1971; Wysocki and Segal, 1972; Valcana *et al.*, 1975; Matthieu *et al.*, 1975*a*) and there is a decreased level in whole homogenates. However, when isolated myelin was assayed one group found no change in specific activity (Matthieu *et al.*, 1975*a*) while another reported a 20% decrease (Valcana *et al.*, 1975), which is similar to that reported in postnatal protein deficiency.

A particularly interesting example of the use of CNPase as a myelin marker is seen in a study of the effects in newborn chickens of excision of an innervating eye on myelination in the contralateral optic lobe (Bondy and Madsen, 1972). CNPase specific activities decreased between days 10 and 20 whereas in control material from the ipsilateral optic lobe and from untreated animals an increase was observed in this period. The level in the contralateral optic lobe at day 20 was approximately 30% of that of controls and cerebrosides were also decreased but not as dramatically as CNPase. The authors suggested that these data are consistent with axonal migration of neurohumors which act as effectors in differentiation of adjacent cells, in this case the oligodendroglia.

7.5. Demyelinating Diseases

Experimental autoimmune encephalomyelitis (EAE) is an autoimmune disease induced in animals by injection of myelin basic protein or whole myelin. This disease is widely used for examining autoimmunity and on the basis of similarities in gross pathological presentation has been proposed as a model for the human demyelinating condition multiple sclerosis, although there are a number of dissimilarities between the two (Mackay *et al.*, 1973). EAE produces histologically observable lesions of demyelination in some species. Drummond *et al.* (1971) observed no change in CNPase levels in whole homogenates of spinal cord from guinea pigs but obtained a slight increase in levels of cerebrosides when compared to controls. CNPase levels in guinea pigs with EAE, induced by injection of freeze-dried whole brain and spinal cord, have also been examined by Pechan and Simekova (1972) in two regions of the spinal cord as well as in the cerebral cortex. Small increases over controls were found as rapidly as 6 hr after injection and these were maintained for at least 13 days. These unexpected observations have not been investigated further and no explanation has been offered beyond a suggestion that they may arise as an early reaction to the encephalitogenic mixture. In multiple sclerosis and in EAE in monkeys demyelinating lesions or plaques are easily discernible and CNPase levels can be determined and compared with surrounding normal-appearing white matter and corresponding material from control animals. Lesions in both EAE in the monkey (Govindarajan *et al.*, 1974) and multiple sclerosis (Braun and Barchi, 1972; Riekkinen *et al.*, 1972) showed markedly diminished CNPase activity at the center of the plaques with smaller decreases at the edges where demyelination was still progressing.

It has been shown (Bornstein and Raine, 1970) that myelination in explant cultures is inhibited by addition of sera from multiple sclerosis patients or animals with EAE. CNPase appearance was inhibited by this procedure and both myelin and CNPase increased in parallel on removal of the sera (Fry *et al.*, 1973). Tsukada *et al.* (1972, 1973) found that myelination in cultures increased up to 20 days before plateauing; addition of EAE or multiple sclerotic sera at 20 days resulted in demyelination and CNPase activity fell by 80% within a few hours. No CNPase activity was detected in the culture medium, suggesting that the enzyme was being rapidly blocked or destroyed. This group could find no direct effect of the sera on CNPase in mouse brain homogenates, with or without Triton X-100 activation, or in myelin. We also obtained no inhibitory effect of such sera with bovine myelin and with CNPase isolated from bovine brain by the method of Guha and Moore (1975) and with the Triton X-100 method as described in Section 5.3 (N. R. Sims and P. R. Carnegie, unpublished observations). Thus the effect in cultures would not seem to result from direct interaction of the sera with CNPase. The observed loss of CNPase activity may have resulted from an effect on oligodendroglial cells which in turn might produce rapid changes in myelin, but it is difficult to envisage a mechanism for this.

In addition to multiple sclerosis and EAE, plaques with reduced CNPase levels have also been observed in Schilder's disease (Komiya and

Kasahara, 1971; Kurihara and Takahashi, 1972) and subacute sclerosing panencephalitis (SSPE) (Riekkinnen *et al.*, 1972). Homogenates of brains from patients with SSPE produced an abnormal floating myelin fraction and both this floating fraction and the apparently normal myelin had a decreased CNPase level (Ramsey *et al.*, 1974). The possible association of CNPase with the primary defect in SSPE requires further investigation.

When nerves are sectioned Wallerian degeneration results, in which the axon and associated myelin sheath distal to the section rapidly degenerate while the proximal portion undergoes only temporary demyelination (Adams and Liebowitz, 1969). CNPase changes mirror the observed demyelination pattern, showing dramatic decreases in the distal portion with little change in the proximal stump (Mezei *et al.*, 1974).

7.6. Tumors and Cultured Cells

In addition to the conditions outlined in Table 3, a number of other pathological situations have also been studied. In a limited series of tumors from brain it was shown that CNPase activity was highest for an oligodendroglioma although levels in this material were much lower than in white matter from normal brain (Kurihara *et al.*, 1974). By contrast a lymphosarcoma obtained from spleen had twice the levels of the normal spleen tissue. A second spleen enzyme, 3',5'-cyclic nucleotide phosphodiesterase, showed decreased levels in the tumor (Konings and Pierce, 1974). Further work is required to determine the generality of this observation in spleen and to see whether this is also true for other nonneural tumors.

Zanetta *et al.* (1972) reported that the C_6 cell line, derived from a chemically induced tumor of rat brain, contained CNPase activity at about 10% of the level of normal myelin. Further work on this clone has shown that it produces several myelin proteins and as such resembles oligodendroglial cells. Interestingly fractionation of these cells indicated that 12% of the CNPase activity was contained in the soluble fraction (100,000 × g supernatant) in contrast to all normal tissues studied where the enzyme has been found only in the membrane fraction (Volpe *et al.*, 1975). Physiological concentrations of norepinephrine induced an increase of CNPase in C_6 cells and this response was mediated by a β-adrenergic receptor and cAMP (McMorris, 1977).

CNPase has also been demonstrated in a clone derived from a rat schwannoma at levels above other lines derived from peripheral nervous system (Pfeiffer and Wechsler, 1972) and at widely ranging levels in a variety of cell lines established from a number of animal tumors (Pfeiffer, 1973) and from human brain material obtained at biopsy and autopsy, including several samples from multiple sclerosis patients (Duch *et al.*, 1975). A number of the human lines were transformed with PML-SV40 virus, a manipulation which resulted in a three- to twelvefold increase in the measured CNPase levels. Sundarraj *et al.* (1975) examined six clonal lines from a transplantable mouse glioma (G-26) which contained detectable CNPase activity. The enzyme could not be detected in clones grown *in vitro* but when these were regrown as subcutaneous tumors the ability to express CNPase was regained. Cultures of fetal brain tissue prepared from explants (Fry *et al.*, 1973) or by cell aggregation (Schmidt, 1975) produced myelin, and CNPase activity increased in parallel providing a ready marker for the formation. The use of these and other cell lines and tissue cultures derived from human and animal material should prove invaluable for examining the processes of myelination and may provide an insight into the function of CNPase.

8. CONCLUSIONS AND SPECULATIONS

Use of CNPase as a marker for myelin has increased rapidly in recent years but information on the enzyme and its role in myelin is still lacking. Further development of techniques for purification of the enzyme should provide for more rapid progress in this direction.

From early work (Drummond *et al.*, 1962; Olafson *et al.*, 1969) the substrate specificity with respect to nucleotides is fairly well established. However, it has not yet been demonstrated that 2',3'-cyclic nucleotides are the true substrate for the enzyme. As far as we can ascertain there are no reports of 2',3'-cyclic nucleotides in mammalian tissues despite numerous chromatographic identifications of 3',5'-cyclic AMP.

A nuclease has been reported in brain nuclei which hydrolyzed RNA to produce 2',3'-cyclic nucleotides but did not hydrolyze these further (Niedergang *et al.*, 1974), and it has been suggested (Sogin, 1976) that CNPase may utilize this source of substrate material. However, it is more likely that this nuclease activity is related to salvage pathways for the nucleotides to enable their reuse within the nuclei. Even if the hydrolysis products from the nuclease were released from the nuclei it is difficult to envisage why an enzyme would evolve in myelin to deal with them, especially as the nuclease produces only free 2',3'-cyclic pyrimidines whereas CNPase shows a preference for purine substrates. It might be worthwhile to look for a similar nuclease in other subcellular fractions and in oligodendrocytes.

As described in Section 6.2, 2'-, 3'-, and 5'-nucleotides produce similar inhibition, a result that would seem unlikely to arise if 2'-AMP were the *in vivo* product of CNPase action. In contrast, pancreatic RNAase I, which converts 2',3'-cyclic nucleotides to 3' derivatives, is inhibited by the product ten times more effectively than the 2' derivative (Hugli *et al.*, 1973).

Myelin basic protein can be phosphorylated by a myelin kinase and by a cytoplasmic kinase at only a few serine and threonine residues (Carnegie *et al.*, 1974). It is conceivable that these phosphoesters constrained by the protein structure could provide a substrate for CNPase, possibly as a phosphotransferase. Such a mechanism could allow fine control over basic protein conformation in myelin. Initial experiments with basic protein phosphorylated by cytoplasmic kinase *in vitro* have provided no support for this speculation but the possibility remains that there could be a role for CNPase in association with the myelin kinase.

Several potential cyclic phosphate substrates such as cyclic inositol phosphates (T. Kurihara, personal communication; B. W. Agranoff, personal communication) have also been tested but these are not hydrolyzed by CNPase. The possibility remains that the observed hydrolysis is artifactually produced by an enzyme or protein in myelin with a function unrelated to hydrolysis or synthesis of cyclic phosphoesters. Even if the activity were shown to be without physiological significance, this would not detract from the value of the enzyme as a myelin marker. Furthermore, the fact that CNPase activity is widespread would suggest that it is indicative of a protein of general importance in membrane function or structure.

An interesting picture is emerging when CNPase is examined in relation to the process of myelination. It appears not to be present in significant quantities in myelin of lower animals, including the dogfish (Drummond *et al.*, 1971; N. L. Banik, personal communication). This suggests that its development is related to recent refinements of myelin which either enable it to cope better in its accepted role as an insulator, or reflect the appearance of the development within myelin of functions unrelated to its role in assisting nervous transmissions. Information has been presented (Section 3.6) showing that CNPase is found at high levels in the oligodendroglia and is present through the proposed intermediate forms of myelin (oligodendroglial myelin, myelin-like and membrane fractions, etc.) into mature myelin. In development CNPase attains adult levels more rapidly than myelin basic protein when whole homogenates are examined and there is a relatively high content of CNPase in myelin isolated from young animals. Taken overall these data would seem to suggest that CNPase has a role in the process of myelination, possibly in relation to the alteration of oligodendroglial membrane into the stable closely packed layers seen in mature myelin. It is difficult to see why an enzyme apparently related to the myelination process would also be found in other membranes. It is interesting, however, that CNPase activity is increased in at least one nonneural tumor and in viral transformation of normal tissue, and is lost when a rat tumor is transferred from the animal to cell culture but is regained on reimplantation, all of which are situations in which the membrane structure is known to be altered (for references see Section 7).

In conclusion, CNPase is associated with a wide range of tissues but is primarily contained in CNS myelin and as such is a good enzymatic marker for this material. Its function remains an enigma, however. Further studies on the purified forms of the enzyme and its role in myelination will likely lead to a breakthrough in this area.

9. REFERENCES

Adams, C. W. M., and Liebowitz, S., 1969, The general pathology of demyelinating disease, in: *The Structure and Function of Nervous Tissue* (G. H. Bourne, ed.), pp. 309–382, Academic Press, New York.

Adams, C. W. M., Davison, A. N., and Gregson, N. A., 1963, Enzyme inactivity of myelin: Histochemical and biochemical evidence, *J. Neurochem.* **10**:383–395.

Agrawal, H. C., Banik, N. L., Bone, A. H., Davison, A. N., Mitchell, R. F., and Spohn, M., 1970, The identity of a myelin-like fraction isolated from developing brain, *Biochem. J.* **120**:635–642.

Agrawal, H. C., Trotter, J. L., Mitchell, R. F., and Burton, R. M., 1973, Criteria for identifying a myelin-like fraction from developing brain, *Biochem. J.* **136**:1117–1119.

Agrawal, H. C., Trotter, J. L., Burton, R. M., and Mitchell, R. F., 1974, Metabolic studies on myelin. Evidence for a precursor role of a myelin subfraction, *Biochem. J.* **140**:99–109.

Banik, N. L., and Davison, A. N., 1969, Enzyme activity and composition of myelin and subcellular fractions in the developing rat brain, *Biochem. J.* **115**:1051–1062.

Banik, N. L., Davison, A. N., Palo, J., and Savolainen, H., 1975, Biochemical studies on myelin isolated from the brains of patients with Down's syndrome, *Brain* **98**:213–218.

Bignami, A., and Eng, L. F., 1973, Biochemical studies of myelin in Wallerian degeneration of rat optic nerve, *J. Neurochem.* **20**:165–173.

Bondy, S. C., and Madsen, C. J., 1972, Arrested development of myelin in chick optic tectum following deafferentation, *Brain Res.* **47**:177–184.

Bornstein, M. B., and Raine, C. S., 1970, Experimental allergic encephalomyelitis. Antiserum inhibition of myelination *in vitro, Lab. Invest.* **23**:536–542.

Braun, P. E., and Barchi, R. L., 1972, 2',3'-Cyclic nucleotide 3'-phosphodiesterase in the nervous system. Electrophoretic properties and development studies, *Brain Res.* **40**:437–444.

Cammer, W., Rose, A. L., and Norton, W. T., 1975, Biochemical and pathological studies of myelin in hexachlorophene intoxication, *Brain Res.* **98**:547–559.

Carnegie, P. R., and Sims, N. R., 1977, Proteins and enzymes of myelin, in: *Multiple Sclerosis, A Critical Conspectus* (E. J. Field, ed.), pp. 165–206, Medical and Technical Publ., London.

Carnegie, P. R., Dunkley, P. R., Kemp, B. E., and Murray, A. W., 1974, Phosphorylation of selected serine and threonine residues in myelin basic protein by endogenous and exogenous protein kinases, *Nature* **249**:147–150.

Cohen, S. R., and Guarnieri, M., 1976, Immunochemical measurement of myelin basic protein in developing rat brain: An index of myelin synthesis, *Dev. Biol.* **49**:294–299.

Dalal, K. B., Petropoulos, E. A., and Timiras, P. S., 1973, Effects of hypoxia on 2',3'-cyclic nucleotide 3'-phosphohydrolase activity in brain myelin of the developing rat, *Environ. Physiol. Biochem.* **3**:117–119.

Davis, F. F., and Allen, F. W., 1956, A specific phosphodiesterase from beef pancreas, *Biochim. Biophys. Acta* **21**:14–17.

Deshmukh, D. S., Flynn, T. J., and Pieringer, R. A., 1974, The biosynthesis and concentration of galactosyl diglyceride in glial and neuronal enriched fractions of actively myelinating rat brain, *J. Neurochem.* **22**:479–485.

Detering, N. K., and Wells, M. A., 1976, The nonsynchronous synthesis of myelin components during early stages of myelination in the rat optic nerve, *J. Neurochem.* **26**:253–257.

De Vries, G. H., 1976, Isolation of axolemma-enriched fractions from bovine central nervous system, *Neurosci. Lett.* **3**:117–122.

Dobbing, J., 1972, Vulnerable periods of brain development, in: *Lipids, Malnutrition and the Developing Brain,* Ciba Foundation Symposium, pp. 9–29, Elsevier, Amsterdam.

Dreiling, C. E., and Newburgh, R. W., 1972, Effect of 1,1,3-tricyano-2-amino-1-propene on 2′,3′-cyclic AMP 3′-phosphohydrolase in the sciatic nerve of the chick embryo, *Biochim. Biophys. Acta* **264**:300–310.

Drummond, G. I., and Perrott-Yee, S., 1961, Enzymatic hydrolysis of adenosine 3′,5′-phosphoric acid, *J. Biol. Chem.* **236**:1126–1129.

Drummond, G. I., and Yamamoto, M., 1971, Nucleoside cyclic phosphate diesterases, in: *The Enzymes* (P. D. Boyer, ed.), Vol. IV, pp. 355–371, Academic Press, New York.

Drummond, G. I., Iyer, N. T., and Keith, J., 1962, Hydrolysis of ribonucleoside 2′,3′-cyclic phosphates by a diesterase from brain, *J. Biol. Chem.* **237**:3535–3539.

Drummond, G. I., Eng, D. Y., and McIntosh, C. A., 1971, Ribonucleoside 2′,3′-cyclic phosphate diesterase activity and cerebroside levels in vertebrate and invertebrate nerve, *Brain Res.* **28**:153–163.

Duch, D., Mandel, P., and Koprowski, H., 1975, Demonstration of enzymes related to myelinogenesis in established human brain cell cultures, *J. Neurol. Sci.* **26**:99–105.

Egyhazi, E., and Hyden, H., 1961, Experimentally induced changes in the base composition of the ribonucleic acids of isolated nerve cells and their oligodendroglial cells, *J. Biophys. Biochem. Cytol.* **10**:403–410.

Eto, Y., and Suzuki, K., 1973, Cholesterol ester metabolism in rat brain. A cholesterol ester hydrolase specifically localized in the myelin sheath, *J. Biol. Chem.* **248**:1986–1991.

Frey, H. J., Arstila, A. U., Rinne, U. K., and Riekkinen, P. J., 1971, Esterases in developing CNS myelin, *Brain Res.* **30**:159–167.

Fry, J. M., Lehrer, G. M., and Bornstein, M. B., 1973, Experimental inhibition of myelination in spinal cord tissue cultures: Enzyme assays, *J. Neurobiol.* **4**:453–459.

Glastris, B., and Pfeiffer, S. E., 1974, Mammalian membrane marker enzymes: Sensitive assay for 5′-nucleotidase and assay for mammalian 2′,3′-cyclic-nucleotide-3′-phosphohydrolase, in: *Methods in Enzymology* (S. Fleischer and L. Packer, eds.), Vol. 32, pp. 124–131, Academic Press, New York.

Govindarajan, K. R., Rauch, H. C., Clausen, J., and Einstein, E. R., 1974, Changes in cathepsins B-1 and D, neutral proteinase and 2′,3′-cyclic nucleotide-3′-phosphohydrolase activities in monkey brain with experimental allergic encephalomyelitis, *J. Neurol. Sci.* **23**:295–306.

Gregson, N. A., and Oxberry, J. M., 1972, The composition of myelin from the mutant mouse "Quaking," *J. Neurochem.* **19**:1065–1071.

Grundt, I. K., and Hole, K., 1974, *p*-Chlorophenylalanine treatment in developing rats: Protein and lipids in whole brain and myelin, *Brain Res.* **74**:269–277.

Guha, A., and Moore, S., 1975, Solubilization of 2′,3′-cyclic nucleotide 3′-phosphohydrolase from bovine brain without detergents, *Brain Res.* **89**:279–286.

Hatefi, Y., and Hanstein, W. G., 1974, Destabilization of membranes with chaotropic ions, in: *Methods in Enzymology* (S. Fleischer and L. Packer, eds.), Vol. 31, pp. 770–790, Academic Press, New York.

Hugli, T. E., Bustin, M., and Moore, S., 1973, Spectrophotometric assay of 2′,3′-cyclic nucleotide 3′-phosphohydrolyase: Application to the enzyme in bovine brain, *Brain Res.* **58**:191–203.

Hyden, H., and Hartelius, H., 1948, Stimulation of nucleoprotein production in nerve cells by malonitrile and its effect on psychic functions in mental disorders, *Acta Psychiatr. Neurol. (Suppl.)* **48**:1–117.

IUPAC–IUB Enzyme Commission, 1976, Enzyme nomenclature, Supplement 1: Corrections and additions (1975), *Biochim. Biophys. Acta* **429**:1–45.

Koeppen, A. H., Barron, K. D., and Bernsohn, J., 1969, Redistribution of rat brain esterases during subcellular fractionation, *Biochim. Biophys. Acta* **183**:253–264.

Komiya, Y., and Kasahara, M., 1971, 2'3'-Cyclic nucleotide 3'-phosphohydrolase activity in myelin fractions from one patient with Schilder's disease, *J. Biochem.* **70**:371–374.

Konat, G., Offner, H., and Clausen, J., 1976, Triethyllead-restrained myelin deposition and protein synthesis in the developing rat forebrain, *Exp. Neurol.* **52**:58–65.

Konings, A. W. T., and Pierce, D. A., 1974, Hydrolysis of 2',3'-cyclic adenosine monophosphate and 3',5'-cyclic adenosine monophosphate in subcellular fractions of normal and neoplastic mouse spleen, *Life Sci.* **15**:491–499.

Krigman, M. R., and Hogan, E. L., 1976, Undernutrition in the developing rat: Effect upon myelination, *Brain Res.* **107**:239–255.

Kurihara, T., and Takahashi, Y., 1972, 2',3'-Cyclic nucleotide 3'-phosphohydrolase activity in cerebral white matter of demyelinating disease, *Annu. Rep. Niigata Univ. Brain Res. Inst.* **5**:57–58.

Kurihara, T., and Takahashi, Y., 1973, Potentiometric and colorimetric methods for the assay of 2',3'-cyclic nucleotide 3'-phosphohydrolase, *J. Neurochem.* **20**:719–727.

Kurihara, T., and Tsukada, Y., 1967, The regional and subcellular distribution of 2',3'-cyclic nucleotide 3'-phosphohydrolase in the central nervous system, *J. Neurochem.* **14**:1167–1174.

Kurihara, T., and Tsukada, Y., 1968, 2',3'-Cyclic nucleotide 3'-phosphohydrolase in the developing chick brain and spinal cord, *J. Neurochem.* **15**:827–832.

Kurihara, T., Nussbaum, J. L., and Mandel, P., 1969, 2',3'-Cyclic nucleotide 3'-phosphohydrolase in the brain of the "Jimpy" mouse, a mutant with deficient myelination, *Brain Res.* **13**:401–403.

Kurihara, T., Nussbaum, J. L., and Mandel, P., 1970, 2',3'-Cyclic nucleotide 3'-phosphohydrolase in brains of mutant mice with deficient myelination, *J. Neurochem.* **17**:993–997.

Kurihara, T., Nussbaum, J. L., and Mandel, P., 1971, 2',3'-Cyclic nucleotide 3'-phosphohydrolase in purified myelin from brain of Jimpy and normal young mice, *Life Sci.* **10**:421–429.

Kurihara, T., Kawakami, S., Ueki, K., and Takahashi, Y., 1974, 2',3'-Cyclic nucleotide 3'-phosphohydrolase activity in human brain tumours, *J. Neurochem.* **22**:1143–1144.

Kurihara, T., Nishizawa, Y. and Takahashi, Y., 1977, The use of nonaqueous chloroform/methanol extraction for the delipidation of brain with minimal loss of enzyme activities, *Biochem. J.* **165**:135–140.

Lees, M. B., and Paxman, S. A., 1974, Myelin proteins from different regions of the central nervous system, *J. Neurochem.* **23**:825–831.

Lees, M. B., Sandler, S. W., and Eichberg, J., 1974, Effect of detergents on 2',3'-cyclic nucleotide 3'-phosphohydrolase activity in myelin and erythrocyte ghosts, *Neurobiology* **4**:407–413.

Lo, K. W., Yip, K. F., and Tsou, K. C., 1975, Fluorometric assay of 2',3'-cyclic adenosine monophosphate 3'-phosphohydrolase with $1,N^6$-etheno-2-aza-adenosine 2',3'-monophosphate, *J. Neurochem.* **25**:181–183.

Lundblad, R. L., and Moore, S., 1969, Studies on the solubilization of 2',3'-cyclic nucleotide 3'-phosphohydrolase from bovine brain, *Brain Res.* **12**:227–229.

Mackay, I. R., Carnegie, P. R., and Coates, A. S., 1973, Immunopathological comparisons between experimental autoimmune encephalomyelitis and multiple sclerosis, *Clin. Exp. Immunol.* **15**:471–482.

Matthieu, J.-M., Quarles, R. H., Brady, R. O., and Webster, H. de F., 1973, Variation of proteins, enzyme markers and gangliosides in myelin subfractions, *Biochim. Biophys. Acta* **329**:305–317.

Matthieu, J.-M., Zimmerman, A. W., Webster, H. de F., Ulsamer, A. G., Brady, R. O., and Quarles, R. H., 1974*a*, Hexachlorophene intoxication: Characterization of myelin and myelin-related fractions in the rat during early postnatal development, *Exp. Neurol.* **45**:558–575.

Matthieu, J.-M., Quarles, R. H., Webster, H. de F., Hogan, E. L., and Brady, R. O., 1974*b*, Characterization of the fraction obtained from the CNS of Jimpy mice by a procedure for myelin isolation, *J. Neurochem.* **23**:517–523.

Matthieu, J.-M., Reier, P. J., and Sawchak, J. A., 1975*a*, Proteins of rat brain myelin in neonatal hypothyroidism, *Brain Res.* **84**:443–451.

Matthieu, J.-M., Moyat, G., Koellreutter, B., and Gautier, E., 1975*b*, Changes in the protein and glycoprotein composition of rabbit brain myelin during early postnatal development, *Exp. Brain Res. (Suppl.)* **23**:138.

McMorris, F. A., 1977, Norepinephrine induces glial-specific enzyme activity in cultured glioma cells, *Proc. Natl. Acad. Sci. USA* **74**:4501–4504.

Mezei, C., and Palmer, F. B. St. C., 1974, Hydrolytic enzyme activities in the developing chick central and peripheral nervous system, *J. Neurochem.* **23**:1087–1089.

Mezei, C., Mezei, M., and Hawkins, A., 1974, 2′,3′-Cyclic AMP 3′-phosphohydrolase activity during Wallerian degeneration, *J. Neurochem.* **22**:457–458.

Mitzen, E. J., Barron, K. D., Koeppen, A. H., and Harris, H. W., 1974, Enzyme activity of human central nervous system myelin, *Brain Res.* **68**:123–131.

Miyamoto, E., 1976, Phosphorylation of endogenous proteins in myelin of rat brain, *J. Neurochem.* **26**:573–577.

Miyamoto, E., and Kakiuchi, S., 1974, *In vitro* and *in vivo* phosphorylation of myelin basic protein by exogenous and endogenous adenosine 3′,5′-monophosphate-dependent protein kinases in brain, *J. Biol. Chem.* **249**:2769–2777.

Miyamoto, E., and Kakiuchi, S., 1975, Phosphoprotein phosphatases for myelin basic protein in myelin and cytosol fractions of brain, *Biochim. Biophys. Acta* **384**:458–465.

Mokrasch, L. C., 1971, Purification and properties of isolated myelin, in: *Methods of Neurochemistry* (R. Fried, ed.), Vol. 1, pp. 1–29, Dekker, New York.

Morishima, I., 1974, Cyclic nucleotide phosphodiesterase in silkworm: Purification and properties, *Biochim. Biophys. Acta* **370**:227–241.

Nakhasi, H. L., Toews, A. D., and Horrocks, L. A., 1975, Effects of a postnatal protein deficiency on the content and composition of myelin from brains of weanling rats, *Brain Res.* **83**:176–179.

Niedergang, C., Okazaki, H., Ittel, M. E., Munoz, D., Petek, F., and Mandel, P., 1974, Ribonucleases of beef brain nuclei. Purification and characterization of an alkaline RNAase, *Biochim. Biophys. Acta* **358**:91–104.

Norton, W. T., 1972, Myelin, in: *Basic Neurochemistry* (R. W. Albers, G. J. Siegel, R. Katzman, and B. W. Agranoff, eds.), pp. 365–386, Little, Brown, Boston, Mass.

Norton, W. T., 1977, Isolation and Characterization of myelin, in: *Myelin* (P. Morell, ed.), pp. 161–199, Plenum Press, New York.

Norton, W. T., Poduslo, S. E., and Suzuki, K., 1966, Subacute sclerosing leukoencephalitis, II. Chemical studies including abnormal myelin and an abnormal ganglioside pattern, *J. Neuropathol. Exp. Neurol.* **25**:582–597.

Olafson, R. W., Drummond, G. I., and Lee, J. F., 1969, Studies on 2′,3′-cyclic nucleotide-3′-phosphohydrolase from brain, *Can. J. Biochem.* **47**:961–966.

Pechan, I., and Simekova, J., 1972, 2′,3′-Cyclic nucleotide 3′-phosphohydrolase activity of the central nervous tissue in experimental allergic encephalomyelitis, *J. Neurochem.* **19**:557–558.

Pfeiffer, S. E., 1973, Clonal lines of glial cells, in: *Tissue Culture of the Nervous System* (G. Sato, ed.), pp. 203–230, Plenum Press, New York.

Pfeiffer, S. E., and Wechsler, W., 1972, Biochemically differentiated neoplastic clone of Schwann cells, *Proc. Natl. Acad. Sci. U.S.A.* **69**:2885–2889.

Poduslo, S. E., 1975, The isolation and characterization of a plasma membrane and a myelin fraction derived from oligodendroglia of calf brain, *J. Neurochem.* **24**:647–654.

Poduslo, S. E., and Norton, W. T., 1972, Isolation and some chemical properties of oligodendroglia from calf brain, *J. Neurochem.* **19**:727–736.

Prohaska, J. R., and Wells, W. W., 1974a, Effect of phenylalanine and p-chlorophenylalanine administration on the development of rat brain 2',3'-cyclic nucleotide 3'-phosphohydrolase, *Proc. Soc. Exp. Biol. Med.* **147**:566–571.

Prohaska, J. R., and Wells, W. W., 1974b, Copper deficiency in the developing rat brain: A possible model for Menkes' steely-hair disease, *J. Neurochem.* **23**:91–98.

Prohaska, J. R., Clark, D. A., and Wells, W. W., 1973, Improved rapidity and precision in the determination of brain 2',3'-cyclic nucleotide 3'-phosphohydrolase, *Anal. Biochem.* **56**:275–282.

Prohaska, J. R., Luecke, R. W., and Jasinski, R., 1974, Effect of zinc deficiency from day 18 of gestational and/or during lactation on the development of some rat brain enzymes, *J. Nutr.* **104**:1525–1531.

Quarles, R. H., Everly, J. L., and Brady, R. O., 1973, Evidence for the close association of a glycoprotein with myelin in rat brain, *J. Neurochem.* **21**:1177–1191.

Ramsey, R. B., Banik, N. L., Bowen, D. M., Scott, T., and Davison, A. N., 1974, Biochemical and ultrastructural studies on subacute sclerosing panencephalitis and demyelination, *J. Neurol. Sci.* **21**:213–225.

Reier, P. J., Matthieu, J.-M., and Zimmerman, A. W., 1975, Myelin deficiency in hereditary pituitary dwarfism: A biochemical and morphological study, *J. Neuropathol. Exp. Neurol.* **34**:465–477.

Richards, F. M., and Wyckoff, H. W., 1971, Bovine pancreatic ribonuclease, in: *The Enzymes* (P. D. Boyer, ed.), Vol. IV, pp. 647–806, Academic Press, New York.

Riekkinen, P. J., and Clausen, J., 1970, Peptidase activity of purified myelin, *Acta Neurol. Scand.* **46**:93–101.

Riekkinen, P. J., and Rumsby, M. G., 1972, Aminopeptidase and neutral proteinase activity associated with central nerve myelin preparations during purification, *Brain Res.* **41**:512–517.

Riekkinen, P. J., Rinne, U. K., Arstila, A. U., Kurihara, T., and Pelliniemi, T. T., 1972, Studies on the pathogenesis of multiple sclerosis. 2',3'-Cyclic nucleotide 3'-phosphohydrolase as marker of demyelination and correlation of findings with lysosomal changes, *J. Neurol. Sci.* **15**:113–120.

Rumsby, M. G., Getliffe, H. M., and Riekkinen, P. J., 1973, On the association of nonspecific esterase activity with central nerve myelin preparations, *J. Neurochem.* **21**:959–967.

Sabri, M. I., Tremblay, C., Banik, N. L., Scott, T., Gohil, K., and Davison, A. N., 1975, Biochemical and morphological changes in the subcellular fractions during myelination of rat brain, *Biochem. Soc. Trans.* **3**:275–276.

Schmidt, G. L., 1975, Development of biochemical activities associated with myelination in chick brain aggregate cultures, *Brain Res.* **87**:110–113.

Sidman, R. L., Dickie, M. M., and Appel, S. H., 1964, Mutant mice (Quaking and Jimpy) with deficient myelination in the central nervous system, *Science* **144**:309–311.

Simons, S. D., and Johnston, P. V., 1976, Prenatal and postnatal protein restriction in the rat: Effect of some parameters related to brain development, and prospects for rehabilitation, *J. Neurochem.* **27**:63–69.

Sims, N. R., and Carnegie, P. R., 1975, Release of 2',3'-cyclic nucleotide 3'-phosphohydrolase from myelin: A useful model of membrane protein solubilisation, *Proc. Aust. Biochem. Soc.* **8**:75.

Sims, N. R., and Carnegie, P. R., 1976, A rapid assay for 2',3'-cyclic nucleotide 3'-phosphohydrolase, *J. Neurochem.* **27**:769–772.

Sims, N. R., and Carnegie, P. R., 1977, Antibody to 2',3'-cyclic nucleotide 3'-phosphohydrolase from myelin, *Proceedings of the International Society of Neurochemistry* **6**:550.

Sogin, D. C., 1976, 2',3'-cyclic NADP as a substrate for 2',3'-cyclic nucleotide 3'-phosphohydrolase, *J. Neurochem.* **27**:1333–1337.

Steck, A. J., and Appel, S. H., 1974, Phosphorylation of myelin basic protein, *J. Biol. Chem.* **249**:5416–5420.

Sudo, T., Kikuno, M., and Kurihara, T., 1972, 2',3'-Cyclic nucleotide 3'-phosphohydrolase in human erythrocyte membranes, *Biochim. Biophys. Acta* **355**:640–646.

Sundarraj, N., Schachner, M., and Pfeiffer, S. E., 1975, Biochemically differentiated mouse glial lines carrying a nervous system specific cell surface antigen (NS-1), *Proc. Natl. Acad. Sci. U.S.A.* **72**:1927–1931.

Suzuki, K., Suzuki, K., and Kamoshita, S., 1969, Chemical pathology of G_{M1}-gangliosidosis (generalized gangliosidosis), *J. Neuropathol. Exp. Neurol.* **28**:25–73.

Suzuki, Y., Tucker, S. H., Rorke, L. B., and Suzuki, K., 1970, Ultrastructural and biochemical studies of Schilder's disease, *J. Neuropathol. Exp. Neurol.* **29**:405–419.

Trams, E. G., 1973, A rapid fluorometric assay for 2',3'-cyclic adenosine monophosphate 3'-phosphoesterhydrolase, *J. Neurochem.* **21**:995–997.

Trams, E. G., and Brown, E. A. B., 1974, The activity of 2',3'-cyclic adenosine monophosphate 3'-phosphoesterhydrolase in elasmobranch and teleost brain, *Comp. Biochem. Physiol. (B)* **48**:185–189.

Tsukada, Y., and Nomura, M., 1971, Neurochemical studies on the developing rat brain after neonatal thyroidectomy, in: Abstracts 3rd International Meeting of the International Society for Neurochemistry, Budapest, p. 194.

Tsukada, Y., Shibuya, M., and Ogawa, Y., 1972, Studies on 2',3'-cyclic nucleotide 3'-phosphohydrolase on myelinating cerebellar tissue grown in cultures, *Shinkei Kagaku* **11**:60–63.

Tsukada, Y., Shibuya, M., and Ogawa, Y., 1973, Changes in 2',3'-cyclic nucleotide 3'-phosphohydrolase on myelinating neural tissue grown in culture, in: Abstracts 4th International Meeting of the International Society for Neurochemistry, Tokyo, Japan, p. 299.

Uyemura, K., Tobari, C., Hirano, S., and Tsukada, Y., 1972, Comparative studies on the myelin proteins of bovine peripheral nerve and spinal cord, *J. Neurochem.* **19**:2607–2614.

Valcana, T., Eistein, E. R., Csejtey, J., Dalal, K. B., and Timiras, P. S., 1975, Influence of thyroid hormones on myelin proteins in the developing rat brain, *J. Neurol. Sci.* **25**:19–27.

Volpe, J. J., Fujimoto, K., Marasa, J. C., and Agrawal, H. C., 1975, Relation of C-6 glial cells in culture to myelin, *Biochem. J.* **152**:701–703.

Waehneldt, T. V., 1975, Ontogenetic study of a myelin-derived fraction with 2',3'-cyclic nucleotide 3'-phosphohydrolase activity higher than that of myelin, *Biochem. J.* **151**:435–437.

Waehneldt, T. V., and Mandel, P., 1972, Isolation of rat brain myelin, monitored by polyacrylamide gel electrophoresis of dodecyl sulfate-extracted proteins, *Brain Res.* **40**:419–436.

Wassenaar, J. S., and Kroon, A. M., 1973, Effects of triethyltin on different ATPases, 5'-nucleotidase and phosphodiesterases in grey and white matter of rabbit brain and their relation with brain edema, *Eur. Neurol.* **10**:349–370.

Whitfeld, P. R., Heppel, L. A., and Markham, R., 1955, The enzymic hydrolysis of ribonucleoside-2' : 3'-phosphates, *Biochem. J.* **60**:15–19.

Wiggins, R. C., Miller, S. L., Benjamins, J. A., Krigman, M. R., and Morell, P., 1976, Myelin synthesis during postnatal nutritional deprivation and subsequent rehabilitation, *Brain Res.* **107**:257–273.

Wysocki, S. J., and Segal, W., 1972, Influence of thyroid hormones on enzyme activities of myelinating rat central nervous tissues, *Eur. J. Biochem.* **28**:183–189.

Zanetta, J. P., Benda, P., Gombos, G., and Morgan, I. G., 1972, The presence of 2',3'-cyclic AMP 3'-phosphohydrolase in glial cells in tissue culture, *J. Neurochem.* **19**:881–883.

Zimmerman, A. W., Quarles, R. H., Webster, H. de F., Matthieu, J.-M., and Brady, R. O., 1975, Characterization and protein analysis of myelin subfractions in rat brain: Developmental and regional comparisons, *J. Neurochem.* **25**:749–757.

Zimmerman, A. W., Matthieu, J.-M., Quarles, R. H., Brady, R. O., and Hsu, J. M., 1976, Hypomyelination in copper-deficient rats: Prenatal and postnatal copper replacement, *Arch. Neurol.* **33**:111–119.

IMMUNOHISTOCHEMISTRY OF NERVOUS SYSTEM-SPECIFIC ANTIGENS

LAWRENCE F. ENG AND JOHN W. BIGBEE

Department of Pathology
Stanford University School of Medicine
Stanford, California
and
Veterans Administration Hospital
Palo Alto, California

1. INTRODUCTION

In recent years, immunohistochemical detection and localization of specific antigens in tissue sections have had important clinical and experimental applications. Morphological information derived from these studies combined with biochemical data is proving to be an extremely valuable means for studying structural and functional components of tissue. Biochemical data describing brain antigens have prompted many immunohistochemical studies attempting to localize these factors. Whereas most studies have employed the immunofluorescence technique, the increasing requirement for high-resolution localization offered by electron microscopy (EM) necessitates the use of immunoperoxidase methods. Immunocytochemical localization of brain antigens is lending a great deal to our understanding of brain morphology, organization, and function. Many but not all of the nervous system antigens being studied by immunohistochemical techniques have been cited in this chapter. The authors have attempted to concentrate on areas of most recent advances and of broad general interest.

2. IMMUNOFLUORESCENT MARKERS

The immunofluorescence method was first introduced by Coons *et al.* (1941) and later simplified by Riggs *et al.* (1960). Fluorescein isocyanate, the fluorochrome used to label the antibody, was soon replaced by fluorescein isothiocyanate (FITC) (Riggs *et al.,* 1960), which proved to be much more stable and is still the predominant marker used in immunofluorescence. New methods of conjugation (Chantler, 1975; McKinney *et al.,* 1976; Vinogradov, 1974; Bergquist, 1971; Green *et al.,* 1976; Thomason and Herbert, 1974), introduction of new fluorochromes (Clayton, 1954; Brandtzaeg, 1975; Rothbarth *et al.,* 1975), improvements in fluorescent microscopy, and attempts at standardization (McKinney and Spillane, 1975; Taylor, 1975; Haaijman and Van Dalen, 1974; Taylor and Heimer, 1974; Fagraeus and Bergquist, 1975) all combine to make immunofluorescence a significant tool with both research and clinical applications. Immunofluorescence has been incorporated into many standard clinical laboratory procedures for diagnostic use and research in diseases of the skin (Bauer, 1976; Dobzhanski and Tabakova, 1974; Luders and Adam, 1972; Beutner, 1975; Holubar *et al.,* 1976), excretory system (Humair, 1969; McCluskey, 1971; Wilson, 1975), and endocrine system (Kawaoi, 1975), parasitic diseases (Kalis *et al.,* 1975; Dayan and Stokes, 1971, 1973; Koshi and Chacko, 1971; Joncas *et al.,* 1974; Wajgt, 1971; Liu, 1975; Knight *et al.,* 1975; Aycock, 1973; Goldman, 1971; Rombert, 1974; Stauffer *et al.,* 1975; Hunter, 1975; Wilkinson, 1973; Iakovleva, 1975; Shinski and Rusina, 1975), and cancer (Nairn *et al.,* 1975). The reader is directed for more complete coverage of techniques and procedures to reviews on immunofluorescence (Faulk and Hijmans, 1972; Borek, 1961; Coons, 1956, 1958; Pearse, 1968; Nairn and Marrack, 1969; Hijams and Schaeffer, 1975; Blundell, 1970; Beutner, 1961).

3. HEAVY METAL MARKERS

Inherent problems and limitations in the immunofluorescence technique such as impermanency of the preparation, difficulty in counterstaining, endogenous or fixation-induced autofluorescence, complex microscopic requirements, and limitation to light microscopic (LM) study prompted development of alternative immunohistochemical methods.

Ferritin (Striker *et al.*, 1966; Wagner and Wagner, 1972; Bretton *et al.*, 1972; Marucci *et al.*, 1974; Yokota and Nagata, 1974; Linthicum and Sell, 1975; Singer, 1975), uranium and other heavy metals (Sternberger *et al.*, 1966; Wilson *et al.*, 1966; Sternberger 1969), and viruses (Morgan *et al.*, 1961) conjugated to antibodies were developed mainly to permit visualization of antigens at the electron microscopic level. Immunofluorescence can be used to detect surface antigens by scanning electron microscopy (Springer *et al.*, 1974), but cannot be used to detect intracellular antigens. Thus these electron-dense conjugates, when allowed to diffuse into cells, could display antigens with a very high degree of resolution. Limitations with these conjugates include the large size of the conjugate, which reduces penetration (ferritin and viruses), high levels of nonspecific staining (ferritin), and low-contrast electron microscopic images (metals). These methods are still being employed, especially ferritin, and are valuable for use in double staining or localization of two antigens at the electron microscopic level.

4. ENZYME MARKERS

4.1. General

Attempts to improve immunohistological localization further have relied on enzyme-conjugated antibodies (immunoglobulins, IgG) that could produce reaction products at the site of the antigen which are visible at both LM and EM levels. Enzymes used include acid and alkaline phosphatase (Gordienko and Kosmach, 1973; Storch, 1972), cytochrome *c* (Kraehenbuhl *et al.*, 1971), and by far the most popular, horseradish peroxidase (HRPO) (Nakane and Pierce, 1966, 1967).

4.2. Horseradish Peroxidase–Antibody Markers

Initial attempts to produce an HRPO conjugate met with varying degrees of success (Boorsma and Kalsbeek, 1975; Modesto and Pesce, 1973; Mannik and Downey, 1973; Avrameas and Guilbert, 1971; Clyne *et al.*, 1973; Avrameas and Ternynck, 1971; Avrameas 1969*a,b*, 1972). Conjugation procedures often destroyed HRPO activity and produced conjugates of varying specificity and inactive polymeric species. Reproducibility of the conjugation procedure came when Nakane and Kawaoi (1974) used the nonenzymatic carbohydrate portion of the HRPO molecule to link to the

Fab portion of the immunoglobulin. Also, blocking the amino groups of the HRPO molecule prior to conjugation assured that only HRPO–IgG or HRPO–Fab conjugates would be formed. The HRPO itself lends no color to the antigen site; it is only after the HRPO is incubated with an appropriate substrate that the HRPO, and hence the antigen, can be visualized. The most common substrate for HRPO is 3′,3′-diaminobenzidine (DAB) which, in the presence of HRPO and hydrogen peroxide, yields a permanent brown deposit which can be made electron-dense by reaction with osmium. Other substrates for HRPO, α-naphthol and chloronaphthol (Nakane, 1968), 3-amino-9-ethylcarbazole (Rojas-Espinosa *et al.*, 1974), and benzidine (Straus, 1972), produce pink, blue, or red deposits but are not entirely permanent nor visible at the EM level.

The immunoperoxidase method, or any of the other immunohistochemical methods, can be used either by a direct or indirect procedure. The direct or one-step technique utilizes a primary antibody–HRPO conjugate, whereas the indirect or two-step technique utilizes an immunoglobulin or Fab fragment–HRPO conjugate directed against the primary antiserum.

4.3. Peroxidase–Antiperoxidase Marker

The most recent development in enzyme immunohistochemistry is the peroxidase–antiperoxidase (PAP) technique of Sternberger *et al.* (1970). It is a three-step, indirect method utilizing a bridge antibody between the primary antiserum and the PAP complex. The PAP technique offers two immediate advantages. First, the addition of the third layer greatly increases sensitivity, thus allowing antigen localization in tissue fixed in formalin and paraffin embedded, fixed and embedded in EM resins, or tissue inherently containing small amounts of antigen. Second, the nature of the PAP complex increases staining specificity. Unlike the chemically linked HRPO conjugates, the PAP complex utilizes an anti-HRPO antibody to bind the HRPO. This assures maximum activity of the HRPO and reduces nonspecific staining since the immunoglobulin binding is highly specific for the HRPO and does not cross-react with the tissue (Sternberger, 1974). Details of the PAP technique are more extensively discussed elsewhere (Petrali *et al.,* 1974; Bocker, 1974; Petrusz *et al.,* 1975; Moriarty *et al.,* 1973) including its use on formalin-fixed, paraffin-embedded tissue (Taylor and Mason, 1974; Burns, 1975*a,b*; Taylor and Burns, 1974).

A point unique to the PAP procedure is the possibility of obtaining false negative results. Positive staining can be safely accepted, assuming pure and specific reagents are used, but negative results must be interpreted with caution. In addition to problems of fixation (see later), false negatives can also be a function of improper primary antiserum dilution. This is due to the complete binding of the bivalent bridge antibody by the primary antiserum. As the bridge antibody is used to bind the PAP complex, excessively bound primary antibody will bind both Fab ends of the bridge antibody leaving no binding site free to attach the PAP complex. This will result in negative or nonspecific background staining.

Primary antiserum dilution is therefore much more critical with the PAP technique than with either the one- or two-step immunoperoxidase technique, both of which lack the bridge antibody. This factor becomes most important when dealing with lightly fixed material or frozen sections which may contain large amounts of antigen and thus are capable of binding excessive amounts of the primary antibody (Bigbee *et al.*, 1977). Attempts at using a four-layer technique with the intent to employ rabbit PAP with primary human antiserum (Marucci and Dougherty, 1975) produced sections with excessively high background.

5. MULTIPLE ANTIGEN LOCALIZATION

Multiple staining of tissue antigen in the same section can be performed either with immunofluorescence (Brandtzaeg, 1973; Klein *et al.*, 1971; Pernis *et al.*, 1970; Bubenik *et al.*, 1976a) or immunoperoxidase (Nakane, 1968). Immunofluorescence uses fluorochrome conjugates with different emission spectra and immunoperoxidase uses different substrates which react with the HRPO (see earlier). Multiple staining with immunofluorescence is less cumbersome for it involves different staining reagents and conjugates whereas immunoperoxidase uses the same enzyme to develop the color of all four substrates. To perform multiple staining with the immunoperoxidase or PAP method, the first antigen is labeled and visualized with DAB. Acid or concentrated salt solution is used to remove the immunoglobulins and HRPO while leaving the DAB deposit in place. A second antigen can then be localized using another antibody and visualized with any of the other three substrates. For multiple staining, it is best to use DAB first followed by one or more of the other colors since DAB introduces more general darkening or staining of the tissue and tends to discolor or obscure the first color. Multiple staining combining HRPO/DAB with autoradiography has been successfully accomplished (Gonatas *et al.*, 1974), as has immunoperoxidase combined with immunofluorescence (Dal Canto *et al.*, 1975).

Multiple staining can be used at the EM level by using combinations of ferritin, cytochrome *c*, acid phosphatase, heavy metals, and HRPO conjugates directed against different antigens. In this case, differential staining is judged by the physical appearance of the deposit.

6. TISSUE PREPARATION

Immunofluorescence, immunoperoxidase, and PAP can all be used at the LM level on fixed or fresh frozen sections, aldehyde-fixed and paraffin-embedded tissue, Vibratome sections, and tissue culture. At the EM level, immunoperoxidase, PAP, ferritin, and heavy metals procedures are used. Antigens are most often localized in vibratome sections or ultrathin sections mounted on grids. Frozen sections introduce too severe freeze–thaw artifacts unless cryotomy is performed below −30°C. The most difficult problem in immunoelectron microscopy is achieving optimum balance between retention of antigen specificity and tissue fixation. These problems among others have been thoroughly treated (McLean and Nakane, 1974; Miller, 1972; Smit *et al.,* 1974; Kraehenbuhl and Jamieson, 1974; Kuhlmann and Miller, 1971; Kraehenbuhl *et al.,* 1971; Kuhlmann *et al.,* 1974; Avrameas and Bouteille, 1968; Avrameas, 1969*a,b*); fixation is always a compromise between preserving ultrastructure and antigenicity. Aldehyde fixation is generally best. Penetration of reagents can be increased by using Fab antibody conjugates, extending exposure times in the antisera, or avoiding the problem altogether by staining directly on ultrathin sections (postembedding staining) (Sternberger, 1974; Kawarai and Nakane, 1970; Hardy *et al.,* 1970).

One of the most critical factors in immunohistological staining is proper fixation. Poorly or improperly fixed tissue will stain nonspecifically and allow diffusion of soluble antigens. Overfixation will destroy the antigen and underfixation causes loss of structure. Type and time of fixation seem to depend on the tissue being used and the antigen sought. We have tried a variety of fixatives, different concentrations of fixatives, and different fixation times. A fixative containing 4% paraformaldehyde, 0.1% glutaraldehyde in phosphate buffer, pH 7.2, is best for our work using the immunoperoxidase procedure. The added glutaraldehyde is not enough to destroy antigenicity but is sufficient to maintain ultrastructure. In addition we have used McLean's periodate–lysine–paraformaldehyde fixative (McLean and Nakane, 1974) as well as 4% paraformaldehyde. Following vascular perfusion with any of these fixatives, the tissue is removed, sliced at 1–2 mm, and placed in fresh cold fixative for 2½–4 hr. Tissue fixed by immersion only suffers greatly, especially the deep regions; it yields uneven fixation and allows leakage of antigens, two significant causes of nonspecific, background, or false positive staining.

7. IMMUNOHISTOLOGIC CONTROLS

Closer attention to controls as well as background staining in test slides has revealed that some of the nonpositive staining is not simply background or nonspecific. Rather, it appears that the control serum and the test serum are staining some specific structure(s) in the tissue in addition to the positively stained elements. This staining may be due to the Fc receptor site in brain tissue (Aarli *et al.*, 1975), poor fixation, and/or antigen leakage. When testing for the presence of a new antigen, or when using unfamiliar tissue, it is important to include in the experiment known tissue tested for a known antigen. In our case, glial fibrillary acidic (GFA) protein is routinely used as a positive control. A positive result here assures one that the experiment was conducted properly and aids in the evaluation of unknown material. When working with antigens which are presumed to be localized in a particular organ or organ system, control slides of various other organs should be tested. In our work with brain-specific antigens, sections of liver, heart, lung, kidney, and muscle are used as controls for the site specificity of these antigens. We currently use absorbed control sera and preimmunization control sera. Absorbed controls are immune sera which have been incubated with the specific antigen to remove the antibody. Absorbed controls assure us that the molecule which gives specific tissue staining is the same species that precipitates with the purified antigen. Results from preimmune and absorbed controls are comparable.

8. GENERAL IMMUNOHISTOCHEMICAL APPLICATION

The number of studies utilizing the peroxidase technique is increasing rapidly and to date its most widespread uses are the detection of immunoglobulins in various tissues (Taylor and Mason, 1974; Holubar *et al.*, 1975; Honigsmann *et al.*, 1975; Allen *et al.*, 1976; Stein and Drescher, 1973; Ueki *et al.*, 1974; Wolff-Schreiner and Wolf, 1973; Brown and Burns, 1973; Bosman and Feldman, 1970; Garvin *et el.*, 1974; Ishikawa *et al.*, 1975; Brown *et al.*, 1975), hormones (Sternberger and Petrali, 1975; Kraicer *et al.*, 1973; Ikonicoff and Cedard, 1973; Nakane, 1970, 1971, 1975; Hoffman and Hartroft, 1971; Tixier-Vidal *et al.*, 1975; Beaupain and Dieterlen-Li Evre, 1972; Osada, 1976; Bubenik *et al.*, 1975; Beauvillain *et al.*, 1975; Parsons *et al.*, 1974; Moriarty and Halmi, 1972; Hamanaka *et al.*, 1971; Robinson and Dawson, 1975; Parsons and Erlandsen, 1974; Phifer *et al.*, 1973; Baker and Drummond, 1972), viral and other pathogenic antigens (Burns, 1975*b*; Short and Walker, 1975; Patramanis *et al.*, 1973; Ruitenberg *et al.*, 1975; Herndon *et al.*, 1975; Hoshino *et al.*, 1972; Hashimoto *et al.*,

1973; Benjamin and Ray, 1975; Benjamin, 1974; Jenis *et al.*, 1973; Tabuchi *et al.*, 1976; Peterson *et al.*, 1972; Levaditi *et al.*, 1971, 1973; Hahon *et al.*, 1975; Lai *et al.*, 1975; Gerber *et al.*, 1974; Huang, 1975), enzymes (Nagatsu and Kondo, 1974; Vladutiu *et al.*, 1973; Daniels and Vogel, 1975; Mason and Taylor, 1975; Erlandsen *et al.*, 1974; Klockars and Osserman, 1974; Gould and Bernstein, 1975; Zeitoun *et al.*, 1972), renal tissue (Davies and Clark, 1975; Elias and Miller, 1975; Moroashi *et al.*, 1971; Bariety *et al.*, 1975; Mason *et al.*, 1975), blood cells (Mason *et al.*, 1975; Hinton *et al.*, 1973; Hirokawa *et al.*, 1973; Huhn *et al.*, 1974*a,b*; Bignon *et al.*, 1975), and cancer-related material (Primus *et al.*, 1975; Huitric, 1973; Taylor, 1974; Saunders and Wilder, 1974).

All of these immunohistological techniques are being employed and each has its advantages and disadvantages. Immunofluorescence and immunoperoxidases have been compared a number of times (Burns *et al.*, 1974; Asghar *et al.*, 1973; Bellon *et al.*, 1975; Boorsma *et al.*, 1975; Brown *et al.*, 1974; Barabino *et al.*, 1973; Dorling *et al.*, 1971; Fukuyama, 1971; Herrmann *et al.*, 1974; Nayak and Sachdeva, 1975; Wicker, 1971) in a variety of different systems. The choice to use one or another of these systems depends not only on the antigen(s) being studied but also on the level of localization (EM and/or LM), available equipment, and antisera. Despite claims that immunofluorescence is more sensitive and specific than immunoperoxidase, we have chosen the latter primarily for two reasons. First, ultrastructural localization is highly significant to our investigations and the immunoperoxidase technique combined with DAB is directly adaptable to electron microscopy. This allows close comparison between light and electron microscopic observations. Second, the permanency of the DAB deposit allows closer and more extended viewing time of the preparations. The problem of nonspecific staining occurs in all immunohistological techniques and being able to judge positive and negative staining is most critical. Since immunofluorescent preparations decrease in intensity after exposure to ultraviolet light, contemplative study of each preparation is not possible. The permanent DAB deposit affords this advantage.

Immunoperoxidase preparations can also be counterstained with most conventional histological stains as well as some histochemical procedures. Although immunofluorescent preparations can be counterstained (Cantella *et al.*, 1974; Schenk and Churukian, 1974), they are fewer in number and not as universally recognized.

We employ both immunoperoxidase and PAP procedures. Immunoperoxidase is most often used in conjuction with frozen sections or tissue culture for light microscopy and vibratome sections for electron microscopy. Although PAP is generally used for paraffin-embedded, formalin-fixed tissue sections, it can be used on frozen sections (Bigbee *et al.*, 1977) and tissue culture.

9.   NERVOUS SYSTEM ANTIGENS

9.1.   N-Acetyl Serotonin

The serotonin metabolite, N-acetyl serotonin, though not brain-specific, has been shown by immunofluorescence and immunoperoxidase to be localized in the retina, optic nerve and chiasma, suprachiasmatic nucleus, Harderian gland, cerebellum, spinal tract of the trigeminal nerve, reticular formation, and pineal gland (Bubenik et al., 1974, 1976a,b). Possible functions of N-acetyl serotonin and melatonin have been suggested based on these findings.

9.2.   Cyclic Adenosine 3',5'-Monophosphate

Bloom et al. (1972) have localized this nucleotide (AMP) by immunofluorescence to cells in the cerebellum, specifically the Purkinje cells. The response to noradrenergic stimulation by cyclic AMP in the Purkinje cells has also been studied (Siggins et al., 1973).

9.3.   Posterior Pituitary Hormones and Hypothalamic Regulatory Factors

Immunohistological localization of posterior pituitary hormones and their regulatory factors has been intensely studied using immunofluorescence and immunoperoxidase methods at the LM and EM levels.

Vasopressin (VP) and oxytocin (Ox) have been localized by immunofluorescence (Swaab et al., 1975) and immunoperoxidase (Zimmerman and Antunes, 1976) to the supraoptic nucleus (SON) and the paraventricular nucleus (PVN) of the hypothalamus. It has also been noted that VP is present but not Ox in the suprachiasmatic nucleus. Silverman (1976) has localized these hormones at the EM level.

Neurophysin (NP), a protein produced in the hypothalamus, is thought to be a carrier protein for VP and Ox (Vandesande et al., 1975). These hormones have been shown to be produced by different cells in the SON and PVN and it has been demonstrated that there exist at least two types of NP (Zimmerman et al., 1973), one specific for each hormone, NPII for VP and NPI for Ox (Vandesande et al., 1975). NP has been localized to neurons in the SON and PVN (Watkins, 1975a; Ellis and Watkins, 1975) as well as the suprachiasmatic nucleus (Zimmerman et al., 1975). NP is also found in the axons of the SON and PVN neurons (Watkins, 1975c; Zimmerman et al., 1973; Silverman and Zimmerman, 1975) as well as their terminals in the posterior pituitary and median eminence (Zimmerman et *al.*, 1973; Silverman and Zimmerman, 1975; Silverman *et al.*, 1975; Pelletier *et al.*, 1974*a*; Silverman, 1976), where the protein is localized as small granules. Watkins (1975*b*) has also studied the distribution of NP in non-mammalian vertebrates.

9.4. Anterior Pituitary Hormone Regulating Factors

Somatostatin or growth hormone release inhibiting factor (GHRIF) has been localized by immunofluorescence to the ventromedial and arcuate nuclei of the hypothalamus (Hökfelt *et al.*, 1974*a*) and by PAP to the preoptic and periventricular (especially anterior) areas of the hypothalamus (Alpert *et al.*, 1976; Parsons *et al.*, 1976) and lateral septal region and posterior hypothalamus (Parsons *et al.*, 1976). Axons from these areas containing somatostatin pass in the tuberoinfundibular tract (King *et al.*, 1975) caudal to those containing luteinizing hormone releasing hormone. These fibers appear to end exclusively in the external zone of the median eminence (Pelletier *et al.*, 1974*b*, 1975; Hökfelt *et al.*, 1974*a*) and organum vasculosum of the lamina terminalis (Pelletier *et al.*, 1976). Somatostatin has also been localized in extra hypothalamic/hypophyseal structures including the pineal gland (Pelletier *et al.*, 1975).

Luteinizing hormone releasing hormone (LHRH) has been shown to be present in neurons of the pre- and suprachiasmatic region and preoptic area of the hypothalamus (Barry *et al.*, 1974) and throughout the arcuate nucleus (King and Gerall, 1976). Axons containing LHRH pass in the tuberoinfundibular tract (King *et al.*, 1974). Some axons may end in the infundibular region near portal vessels (Barry *et al.*, 1974) while others end in the peripheral region of the median eminence (Baker *et al.*, 1974; Kordon *et al.*, 1974; Pelletier *et al.*, 1976). Secretory granules containing LHRH have been localized at the electron microscopic level in the median eminence (Pelletier *et al.*, 1974*c*), the first example of storage of a releasing factor in that region. Receptor sites for LHRH have been demonstrated in gonadotropic cells of the pituitary gland (Sternberger and Petrali, 1975).

9.5. Catecholamine Synthesizing Enzymes

The catecholamine neurotransmitters, dopamine (DA), norepinephrine (NE), and epinephrine (E), are synthesized from the aromatic amino acids phenylalanine and tyrosine (Tyr) in a series of reactions involving five enzymes. They are phenylalanine hydroxylase, tyrosine hydroxylase (TH), dopa decarboxylase (DDC), dopamine-β-hydroxylase (DBH), and phenylethanolamine-N-methyltransferase (PNMT) (Ganong, 1975). This is a stepwise reaction sequence producing all three neurotransmitters. TH catalyzes the formation of 3,4-dihydroxyphenylalanine (dopa) from Tyr and is the rate-limiting step for the entire reaction. DDC catalyzes the formation of DA from dopa, DBH the formation of NE from DA, and PNMT the formation of E from NE. Since any neuron utilizes only one of these transmitters, mapping their distribution provides chemical evidence for functional systems in the brain.

Localization of these transmitters was formerly restricted to formalde-hyde-condensed fluorescence (Falck *et al.,* 1962), formaldehyde in combi-nation with glyoxylic acid (Battenberg and Bloom, 1975), or glyoxylic acid alone (Watson and Barchas, 1977). The main problem here is that the fluorescence produced by these compounds is very similar and differentiat-ing them is difficult. The current trend is to localize immunohistochemically the synthesizing enzymes rather than the transmitters. By comparing the presence or absence of TH, DDC, DBH, or PNMT, the main transmitter of the neuron can be deduced. The ready accessibility of these enzymes in pure form, mainly from the adrenal medulla, permits the production of specific antibodies which then allow accurate localization of the enzymes in tissue.

9.5.1. Tyrosine Hydroxylase

Tyrosine hydroxylase (TH) has been localized in dopaminergic and noradrenergic neurons at both LM and EM levels by immunofluorescence and immunoperoxidase using mainly vibratome sections of aldehyde per-fused brain (Pickel *et al.,* 1975a,b, 1976a). In the noradrenergic system, TH was localized in the medulla and pons with particular reference to the locus ceruleus. At the LM level the reaction product was found in the cytoplasm of cell bodies and processes. At the EM level, the most intense reaction occurred in the membranes of endoplasmic reticulum and Golgi apparatus. TH was seen associated with neurotubules in the processes, but was not observed in axon terminals.

Staining of TH in the dopaminergic system was studied in the substan-tia nigra, arcuate nucleus of the hypothalamus, and nigrostriatal, mesolim-bic, and tuberoinfundibular tracts. TH localization was consistent in all areas studied, the nigrostriatal system being representative. Here, staining was visible in the cytoplasm of perikarya, proximal axons, and dendrites of moderately sized neurons, findings which correlate with previous histoflu-orescent data. The reaction product could be followed in processes to the caudate nucleus where they ended in association with myelinated axons. TH was associated with neurotubules in the processes and was granular or vesicular in the perikaryon. Staining in the dopaminergic system was more intense than in the noradrenergic system.

9.5.2. Dopa Decarboxylase

This enzyme, which catalyzes the decarboxylation of dopa to form dopamine, was first localized by Goldstein *et al.* (1971) by immunofluorescence. They reported that dopa decarboxylase (DDC) was present in both catecholamine- and serotonin-containing neurons (Goldstein *et al.*, 1972). The enzyme was further localized to neurons in the substantia nigra, hypothalamus, cerebral cortex, olfactory bulb, preoptic area, and limbic structures (Hökfelt *et al.*, 1973*b*, 1975*a*). Using ferritin-conjugated antibodies, Hökfelt *et al.* (1973*a*) demonstrated DDC in the cell bodies and dendrites of substantia nigra neurons. Because antibodies to DDC stain both catecholaminergic and serotonergic neurons, Hökfelt *et al.* (1973*b*) state that "antigenically indistinguishable enzymes decarboxylate dopa and 5-hydroxytryptophan."

9.5.3. Dopamine-β-hydroxylase

This enzyme has been the most extensively studied but mainly at the LM level with immunofluorescence. Tissue was most often prepared by removal and freezing without perfusion, cryostat sectioned, and fixed in chloroform–methanol or acetone.

Dopamine-β-hydroxylase (DBH) was first localized (Hartman and Udenfriend, 1970) near the cell body and processes of neurons in the supraotic nucleus of the hypothalamus; other brain areas gave ambiguous results. Fuxe *et al.* (1970) localized DBH in the medulla and pons, especially in the locus ceruleus. Expected positive cells in the midbrain and hypothalamus were negative and no nerve terminals or fiber staining was seen. The authors caution that the latter observation may be artifactual. From their results, they concluded that noradrenergic neurons are predominantly in the pons and medulla, while dopaminergic neurons are in the mesencephalon and hypothalamus. Hartman *et al.* (1972), using a purified antiglobulin fluorescein conjugate in place of the whole IgG fraction, found cell body staining similar to that reported by Fuxe *et al.* (1970), which agrees with previous histofluorescence data for norepinephrine. There was no staining in the midbrain raphe or substantia nigra and no cell body staining rostral to the pons. Axons from positive cells showed granular or beaded fluorescence and their terminals were most intense in the paraventricular and supraoptic nuclei of the hypothalamus and interstitial nucleus of the stria terminalis. Less intensely stained terminals were also seen in the anteroventral nucleus of the thalamus and the dentate gyrus of the hippocampus. Negative areas were considered to be composed of dopaminergic neurons.

DBH has also been localized in the area postrema (Torack *et al.*, 1973). This chemosensory area at the caudal end of the fourth ventricle receives a variety of norepinephrine terminals from the medulla, as well as containing norepinephrine neurons.

Recently, Pickel *et al.* (1976*a*) localized DBH at the LM and EM level by the PAP method in the locus ceruleus and its projections to the hypothalamus. The enzyme was localized as a granular reaction product throughout the cytoplasm with some selectivity in the Golgi apparatus, granules, and endoplasmic reticulum. In the proximal axons and dendrites the staining was associated with a reticulum of interconnecting membranes rather than with microtubules.

A review of techniques and applications for localization of DBH in tissue is available (Hartman, 1973) as well as a detailed atlas and discussion of the central adrenergic system as revealed by immunofluorescent labeling of DHB (Swanson and Hartman, 1975).

9.5.4. Phenylethanolamine-N-methyltransferase

Phenylethanolamine-*N*-methyltransferase (PNMT), the last of the five enzymes in the series, catalyzes the formation of epinephrine, the final product in the reaction sequence. Therefore, its presence indicates adrenergic neurons.

PNMT has been localized by immunofluorescence (Hökfelt *et al.*, 1974*b*) in multipolar neurons in two areas of the medulla. The first lies in the rostral medulla lateral to the olivary complex and caudal to the nucleus of the facial nerve, an area corresponding to the lateral reticular nucleus. The second group, also in the rostral medulla, lies close to the midline in the dorsal part of the reticular formation, ventral and medial to the vestibular nuclei.

A positive axon bundle was seen passing in the reticular formation of the pons–medulla. Positive nerve terminals were exhibited in visceral afferent and efferent nuclei of the brain and spinal cord, periventricular gray of the lower brainstem, and certain hypothalamic nuclei.

Since these four enzymes are closely related in the biochemistry of catecholamine synthesis, the most informative studies are those which investigate all or most of them in the same preparation. In this way, direct comparisons can be made and the dopaminergic, noradrenergic, and adrenergic pathways more clearly defined. Following is a list of such papers and the enzyme studied: Fuxe *et al.* (1971), DBH and PNMT; Hökfelt *et al.* (1973*a,b,c*), DDC, DBH, and PNMT; Goldstein *et al.* (1972), DDC, DBH, and PNMT; Hartman and Udenfriend (1972), DBH and monoamine oxidase; Goldstein *et al.* (1971), PNMT, DDC, and DBH; Pickel *et al.*

(1976*a*), TH, tryptophan hydroxylase, and DBH; Hökfelt *et al.* (1975*a*), TH, DDC, DBH, and PNMT. This last citation and Hökfelt *et al.* (1973*c*) also include discussions of techniques and methods used in the detection of catecholamine synthesizing enzymes as well as comparisons ·of various fixation and sectioning procedures.

9.6. Tryptophan Hydroxylase

As with the catecholamines, serotonin can be induced to fluoresce in order to localize serotoninergic neurons, but problems with interpretation have led investigators to localize immunohistochemically tryptophan hyroxylase (TrH), the enzyme catalyzing the first of two steps in the synthesis of serotonin from tryptophan. All immunohistochemical studies to date on TrH employ the PAP method on paraformaldehyde-perfused brain.

TrH has been localized at the LM level in the nuclei of the raphe, midbrain, pons, and medulla (Joh *et al.*, 1975; Pickel *et al.*, 1976*a*; Reis *et al.*, 1975). Labeled neurons are small and highly branched, and the enzyme is located in the cytoplasm of cell bodies and processes. Staining was often associated with heavily myelinated tracts, i.e., corticospinal tract, medial lemniscus, and medial longitudinal fasciculus. Positively stained bundles could be traced to the limbic forebrain area and specific hypothalamic nuclei. Axon terminals were seen in the cranial nerve motor nuclei, locus ceruleus, substantia nigra, nuclei of the raphe, floor of the fourth ventricle, and the suprachiasmatic nucleus of the hypothalamus.

At the EM level, cell body staining was associated with Golgi apparatus and rough endoplasmic reticulum as well as throughout the cytoplasm. In processes, TrH was associated with neurotubules.

9.7. Glutamic Acid Decarboxylase

The function of gamma-aminobutyric acid (GABA) in the central nervous system (CNS) is not fully understood, but it does appear to be an inhibitory transmitter. No satisfactory histochemical method exists to disclose GABA in tissue, but immunohistochemical localization of its synthesizing enzyme, glutamic acid decarboxylase (GAD), has been attempted several times. All of these studies employ the immunoperoxidase technique on aldehyde-perfused brain, mainly in the cerebellum (Saito *et al.*, 1974*a,b*; McLaughlin *et al.*, 1974; Wood *et al:*, 1974; Wood, 1976).

GAD is present in all layers of the cerebellum with significant punctate deposits around Purkinje cells and deep cerebellar nuclei. Basket cells, stellate cells, and Golgi II cell presynaptic terminals all showed strong positive staining. These synapses with Purkinje cells, Purkinje cell dendrites, and granule cells are thought to be inhibitory.

GAD has also been localized in the dorsal horn region of the spinal cord (Saito *et al.*, 1974*a*; Wood *et al.*, 1974), pyramidal cells of the hippocampus (Saito *et al.*, 1974*a*), retina, substantia nigra, and presynaptic terminals on anterior horn cells (Wood, 1976). All of these synapses are known to be inhibitory.

9.8. Choline *O*-Acetyltransferase

Acetylcholine (ACh), the neurotransmitter at the neuromuscular junction, is also involved with synaptic transmission in the CNS. Detection of ACh directly by histochemical means is not possible; however, methods are available to localize acetylcholinesterase (AChE) histochemically. Since AChE is present in nonnervous as well as nervous tissue, it is not a reliable marker for the localization of cholinergic neuronal elements. There is also a procedure by which choline *O*-acetyltransferase (ChAc), the synthesizing enzyme for ACh, can be localized as a lead mercaptide precipitate of coenzyme A which is released during the synthesis of ACh (Burt and Silver, 1973). This method is not specific because it depends on the presence of AChE inhibitor, and it cannot differentiate the coenzyme A produced by ChAc from that produced by other enzymes.

Recent use of immunohistochemical means to localize ChAc has provided the most specific demonstration of ChAc in the CNS. By immunofluorescence on spinal cord frozen sections, ChAc has been localized to the anterior horn cells (Eng *et al.*, 1974*b*; McGeer *et al.*, 1974). ChAc has also been shown in the cerebral cortex, subcortical white matter, and neostriatum (McGeer *et al.*, 1974). Using the PAP method on vibratome sections of aldehyde-perfused brain, ChAc has been localized in the cell body and processes of small interneurons of neostriatum (Hattori *et al.*, 1976). At the EM level, cell body deposits were associated with free and bound ribosomes and the outer membrane of mitochondria. In the processes, ChAc was associated with microtubules and vesicles. Synaptic boutons showed stained vesicles. Recently Kan *et al.* (1977, 1978) have confirmed the localization of ChAc in ventral horn motor neurons of the spinal cord by the PAP method and extended the study to the cerebellum. In cerebellum, ChAc was localized in mossy fibers, their synaptic terminals, and in glomeruli (Figure 1). These immunohistochemical findings are consistent with the distribution of ChAc in various layers of the cerebellum (McCaman and Hunt, 1965) and subfractionation studies of cerebellum (Israel and Whittaker, 1965; Fonnum, 1972; Balazs *et al.*, 1975) which suggested that mossy fibers are cholinergic.

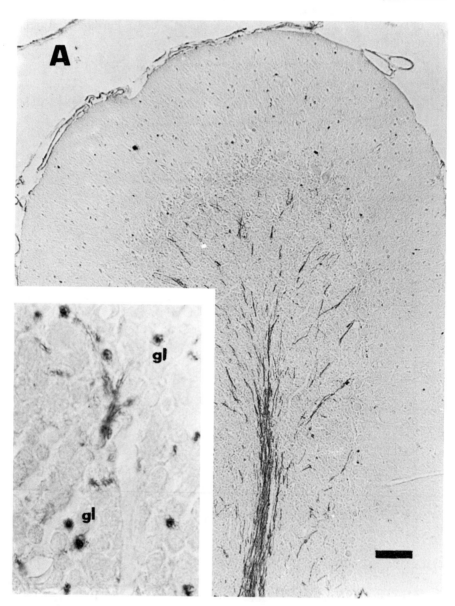

FIGURE 1. Paraffin sections of rabbit cerebellum stained for choline *O*-acetyltransferase (ChAc) by the PAP method. (A) Tissue treated with guinea pig anti-ChAc antiserum. (B) Tissue treated with this antiserum which has been repeatedly absorbed with purified ChAc. Positive staining is confined to afferent axons which pass in the medullary layer (me) of the

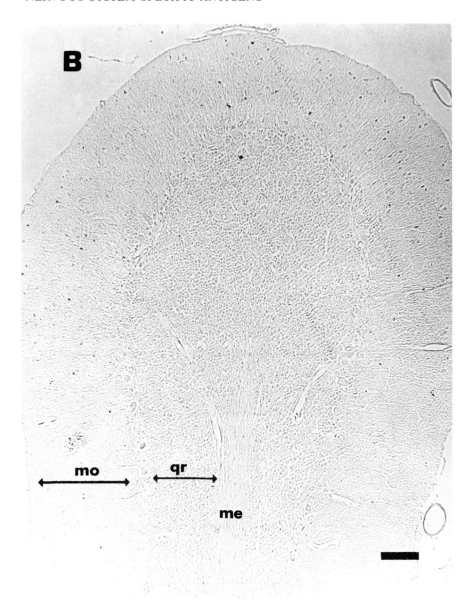

cerebellum, ascend, and end in the granular layer (gr) as mossy fibers. These mossy fibers form complex synaptic structures called glomeruli (gl) with cells and processes in the granular layer (insert). No positive staining occurs in the molecular layer (mo). Bar equals 100 μm.

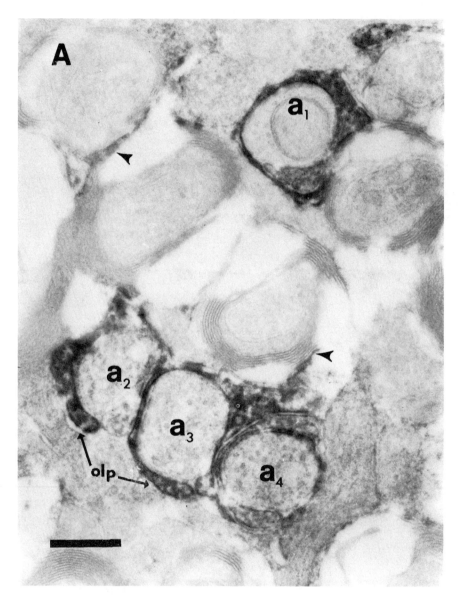

FIGURE 2. Electron micrographs of 15-day-old rat optic nerve illustrating the distribution of GFA protein and myelin basic protein. (A) Tissue stained for MBP shows cross sections of axons in various stages of myelination. Of particular interest are axons in the initial stages (a_1, a_2, a_3, a_4) where the oligodendroglia process (olp), filled with MBP, is just beginning to wrap around the axons. Inner and outer tongues of the processes are visible. Staining of intact, more

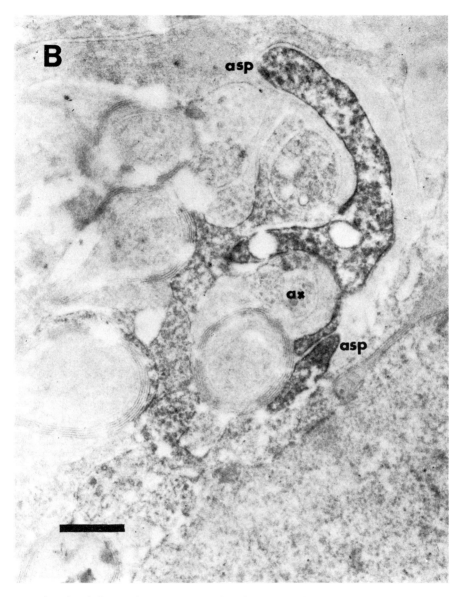

complete sheaths is poor; however, some staining is visible in disrupted ones (arrowheads). (B) Tissue stained for GFA protein showing that an unstained, presumably oligodendroglial process is interposed between the positively stained astrocyte process (asp) and the axon (ax). This indicates that myelinating and cuffing of axons are accomplished by different processes. Bar equals 0.5 μm.

9.9. Central Nervous System Myelin Proteins

The first attempt to localize CNS myelin basic protein (MBP) utilized the immunofluorescence technique applied to paraffin and frozen sections of spinal cord (Rauch and Raffel, 1964). Herndon *et al.* (1973), using the indirect immunoperoxidase technique (Nakane and Kawaoi, 1974), localized MBP to the major dense lines. It was quickly noted, however, that staining occurred only where the sheath was disrupted. Lack of staining of the intact sheath might be expected if the antigenic determinants of MBP are occluded within the intact sheath (Lennon *et al.*, 1971), or if the immunoreagents are unable to penetrate the sheath (Hirano *et al.*, 1969).

In an ongoing study of gliogenesis and myelination in the young rat optic nerve (Eng *et al.*, 1975), MBP was not detected by immunoperoxidase staining at the EM level until approximately 10 days postnatal. By 14 days postnatal, the amount of MBP was greatly increased and found in three places primarily. It is localized in the Golgi apparatus of oligodendroglia, in their processes, and also in disrupted and outer lamellae of myelin sheaths. The staining of oligodendroglia processes was amorphous and in greatest abundance in those processes wrapping around unmyelinated axons. These myelinating processes were stainable only during the very early stages of myelination for adjacent sheaths with more than a few wrappings were unstained.

Myelinating axons were wrapped by two types of processes. One, presumably an oligodendroglia process, which stained for MBP, was immediately adjacent to the axon. The second, presumably an astrocyte process external to the oligodendroglia process, stained for GFA protein. The inner process did not stain for GFA protein nor did the outer for MBP. These results indicate that the myelinating process and the cuffing process are from different cells (see Figure 2).

Staining of advanced myelin sheaths was confined to their outer edges or where the lamellae were disrupted. This could be due to the inability of the antiserum and HRPO conjugate molecules to penetrate the dense wrappings of the sheath. Explosion of the lamellae would provide a route by which the immunoglobulins could penetrate the tissue. In LM immunoperoxidase or PAP preparations, staining of the entire sheath is common (see Figure 3A). However, preparations for EM must be resectioned, thus removing the surface stain and exposing tissue deep in the section which was inaccessible to the immunoglobulins. Postembedding staining on ultrathin sections (Hardy *et al.*, 1970; Sternberger, 1974) might eliminate the problem of immunoglobulin penetration. Sternberger *et al.* (1977), in a preliminary report on postembedding staining of MBP in the optic nerve of *Xenopus*, have demonstrated the feasibility of this method.

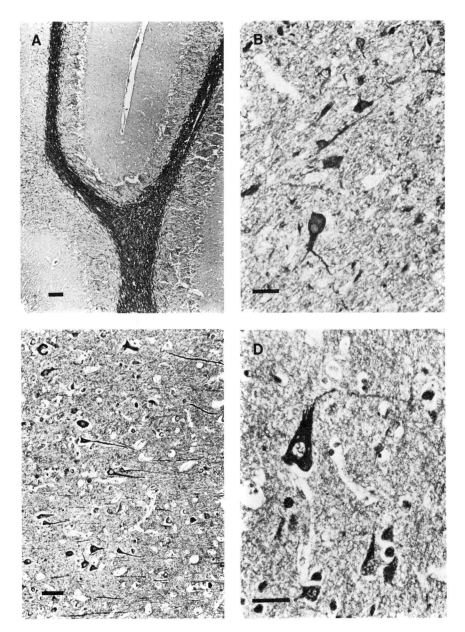

FIGURE 3. Paraffin sections stained for various antigens by the PAP method. (A) Guinea pig cerebellum stained for myelin basic protein. (B) Human cerebral cortex stained for antigen alpha (14-3-2). (C,D) Human cerebral cortex stained for neurotubules. Bar equals 100 μm.

Agrawal and co-workers (Agrawal *et al.*, 1977; Hartman *et al.*, 1976, 1977) have demonstrated the CNS myelin proteolipid protein (PLP) in the myelin sheath from various areas of the brain and during development by the indirect immunofluorescent technique.

Using an MBP–HRPO conjugate at the LM level, anti-MBP antibody has been demonstrated in lymph cells, plasma cells, and spinal cord infiltrates from rabbits injected with MBP and afflicted with experimental allergic encephalomyelitis (EAE) (Johnson *et al.*, 1971). This study was extended to the EM level where staining of anti-MBP antibody was confined in endoplasmic reticulum and the nuclear envelope of plasma cells (Johnson and Blum, 1972). With a similar LM method, Whitaker (1976) localized anti-MBP antibody in lymph nodes of EAE guinea pigs.

The LM immunoperoxidase or PAP staining pattern for cerebrosides (cerebroside antiserum kindly provided by M. W. Kies) was identical to that of MBP (see Figure 3A).

9.10. S-100 Protein

The most extensively studied soluble acidic protein found exclusively associated with the nervous system is the S-100 protein (Moore, 1965). Although its function remains unknown, theories about its role in learning have appeared (Hyden and Lange, 1970). Immunohistochemical localization of S-100 is a matter of controversy; its presence in glial cells is well accepted but its presence or absence in neurons is currently contested.

Chemical studies have produced data which suggest that S-100 is located in both glial and nerve cells (Perez *et al.*, 1970; Cicero *et al.*, 1970) and in the synaptosome fraction of guinea pig cerebral cortex (Donato and Michetti, 1974; Donato *et al.*, 1975).

The first attempt at S-100 localization in tissue (Hyden and McEwen, 1966) utilized indirect immunofluorescence on fresh frozen, acetone-fixed sections. Positive fluorescence was seen around the nuclei of oligodendroglia and within the nuclei of large neurons in the lateral vestibular nucleus (Deiter's nucleus). No staining was seen in neuronal cytoplasm or glial nuclei. Immunofluorescence staining of isolated nuclei (Michetti *et al.*, 1974) which were layered and air-dried on glass slides gave strong positive reaction with large nuclei and only a light reaction with small nuclei.

By free-hand dissection of neurons, Hyden and Rönnback (1975), using immunofluorescence on developing Purkinje cells and Deiter's nucleus cells, found membrane staining in undamaged cells and membrane and nuclear fluorescence in damaged cells. A similar technique employing the immunoperoxidase method (Hansson *et al.*, 1975) gave the same result.

The finding of S-100 in membranes of microdissected neurons could easily be the result of glial processes which are difficult to separate from the neurons. Sviridov *et al.* (1972) localized S-100 in nuclei of neurons, especially Purkinje cells, and glial cytoplasm using immunofluorescence on frozen and paraffin sections. Rapport *et al.* (1974) found S-100 in developing glia and neurons by immunofluorescence on chloroform–methanol-fixed frozen tissue sections. The S-100 was localized to Purkinje cells as early as 2 days postnatal, but not in glial cells until 5 days after birth. Positive S-100 staining was also seen in a variety of different types of neurons throughout the brain.

At the EM level, Haglid *et al.* (1974) demonstrated by immunoperoxidase the presence of S-100 in oligodendroglia membranes and all parts of astrocyte cytoplasm in the cerebral cortex. Neuronal staining was seen in nuclear and cell membranes, nucleoplasm, and pre- and post synaptic membranes. Staining was performed on vibratome sections with glutaraldehyde-linked HRPO conjugate. Tabuchi and Kirsch (1975) using immunoperoxidase on unperfused frozen sections reported finding S-100 in all layers of the cerebellum and Purkinje cells, but they noted that staining was predominantly glial with no glial nuclear staining.

Matus and Mughal (1975), using immunofluorescence and immunoperoxidase on frozen and vibratome sections of aldehyde-perfused brain, found S-100 staining restricted to glial cells. Some glial nuclei stained whereas others did not. No staining was visible in the pre- and postsynaptic membranes at the EM level. The authors stated that the electron dense material demonstrated in the presynaptic membranes by Haglid *et al.* (1975) was a natural feature of the synapse and did not represent specific S-100 immunoperoxidase activity. In a rebuttal to the findings of Matus and Mughal (1975), Haglid *et al.* (1975) stated that the addition of glutaraldehyde to the perfusate used by Matus and Mughal may have destroyed much of the S-100 and that the use of preimmunization serum as a control was inadequate.

Ludwin *et al.* (1976b), using indirect immunoperoxidase on frozen sections of McLean's fixative perfused rat brain, have also found S-100 in astrocytes, oligodendroglia, and some oligodendroglial nuclei. Boyd Hartman states that S-100 is most likely a glial-specific protein and that neuronal-associated S-100, if any, represents only a small fraction of the total brain content (personal communication).

Inconsistencies in reports of S-100 distribution may be due to technical aspects of the immunohistochemical procedures. Owing to the very high solubility of S-100, leakage or diffusion is quite possible if fixation is less than optimal. It is generally accepted that perfusion produces better fixation than either immersion or postfixation of fresh frozen tissue sections. Our own results (unpublished results) and those of Hartman (unpublished, personal communication) indicate that immunofluorescence staining of S-100 on fresh frozen sections produces excessive nonspecific staining and very poor localization. It appears that the method of tissue preparation determines where a soluble protein such as the S-100 protein is ultimately localized in the tissue and that excessive manipulation of the tissue prior to fixation and preparation of histologic sections may allow the S-100 to diffuse. We have obtained consistent and reproducible S-100 localization in agreement with those who have also used perfused animal brains (Hartman *et al.*, 1977; Matus and Mughal, 1975). We have found S-100 to be exclusively localized to glial elements in brain (Ludwin *et al.*, 1976*b*) (see Figure 4), Schwann cells in the peripheral nervous system, and satellite cells in sympathetic ganglia (Eng *et al.*, 1976*a*). Results are the same using paraffin or frozen sections of rabbit, rat, mouse, or human nervous tissue. We have seen no positive staining of neuronal structures.

In these studies, variation in fixation techniques, different immunohistologic techniques, different antisera, and different conjugation procedures have all contributed to varied results from the different laboratories. Careful studies in the future should resolve the present controversy.

9.11. Glial Fibrillary Acidic Protein

9.11.1. Chemistry of the GFA Protein

A water-soluble protein which has been designated glial fibrillary acidic (GFA) protein has been isolated from human pathologic tissue rich in fibrous astrocytes, i.e., old plaques from multiple sclerosis (MS) brains. The protein is isolated from MS plaques by ammonium sulfate precipitation and isoelectric precipitation (pH 5.7 by isoelectric focusing). The GFA protein contains high contents of aspartic and glutamic acid, alanine, and leucine; no cysteine; and negligible amounts of lipid and carbohydrate. The protein isolated from MS plaques migrates as two bands with molecular weights of 47,000 and 41,000 and that from normal brain 47,000 by sodium dodecyl sulfate (SDS) electrophoresis. Cyanogen bromide peptide maps of the protein analyzed on SDS gels show that 50% of the protein has degraded to a fraction with a molecular weight of 20,000–21,000 and the remaining in two fractions less than 13,000. The N-terminal amino acids of the two proteins from MS plaques as determined by dansylation are alanine and leucine (Eng *et al.*, 1970, 1971; Uyeda *et al.*, 1972; Bignami *et al.*, 1972; Eng, 1973). Isolation of water-soluble GFA protein from normal brain by conventional methods—ammonium sulfate fractionation, isoelectric precipitation, and column chromatography—has been hampered by its low solubility and tendency to self-aggregate and to coaggregate with other acidic proteins in the initial crude extract. In normal rat brain only about 15% of the total GFA protein immunologic activity can be extracted with phosphate buffer, pH 8. The majority of the GFA protein can be solubilized with solutions containing Sarkosyl, SDS, or 4 M urea (Lee et al., 1976). For this reason, recent published purification procedures for water-soluble GFA protein (Dahl and Bignami, 1973, 1974, 1975) and the unusual properties (Dahl, 1976a,b; Chan et al., 1975; Huston and Bignami, 1976) of such "purified" GFA protein must be verified by further work.

Bignami, Dahl, and co-workers (Chan et al., 1975; Dahl and Bignami, 1975, 1976; Dahl, 1976b) recently reported that the GFA protein isolated from bovine or rat brain has a molecular weight of 54,000 and an NH_2 terminal of methionine. The well-characterized neurotubule protein has these same properties and similar amino acid composition and cysteine content (Eng et al., 1974a; Bryan and Wilson, 1971; Lee et al., 1973; Luduena and Woodward, 1973; Eipper, 1974). Dahl (1976a) reported that "native" GFA protein was extremely susceptible to two types of proteolysis. At pH 8.0 proteolysis was not prevented by the addition of proteinase inhibitors. Careful inspection of her electrophoretic patterns reveals that the decrease in the 54,000 molecular weight native GFA protein is due mainly to aggregation as evidenced by a large amount of protein material which no longer enters the acrylamide gel following the various treatments of the native GFA protein (Dahl, 1976a, pp. 148–149, Figs. 2, 3). The fact that total GFA immunologic activity decreases and much of the native GFA protein is lost would suggest that the native GFA is a non-GFA protein such as neurotubules, which is coaggregating with a small amount of GFA protein present. The second type of proteolysis which Dahl reported is that which occurs at pH 6.0. In this case, there was also both a loss or decrease of native GFA protein and GFA protein immunologic activity. The loss of native GFA protein may be due to aggregation of neurotubules and the loss of immunologic activity of the GFA protein due also to aggregation, since the isoelectric point of GFA protein is pH 5.7–5.8 (Eng, 1973). This observation is consistent with the probability that Dahl's native GFA protein is a mixture of neurotubules or another yet unidentified protein such as neurofilaments and GFA protein.

The proteins of axons prepared from myelinated axons and isolated as myelin-free entities were separated by sodium dodecyl sulfate polyacrylamide gel electrophoresis (PAGE) (De Vries et al., 1971, 1976). A prominent protein fraction of molecular weight 47,000 (47K) had an amino acid composition that was similar to that of the GFA protein (Eng et al., 1971). Antibody prepared against the 47K fraction (obtained by PAGE) in the

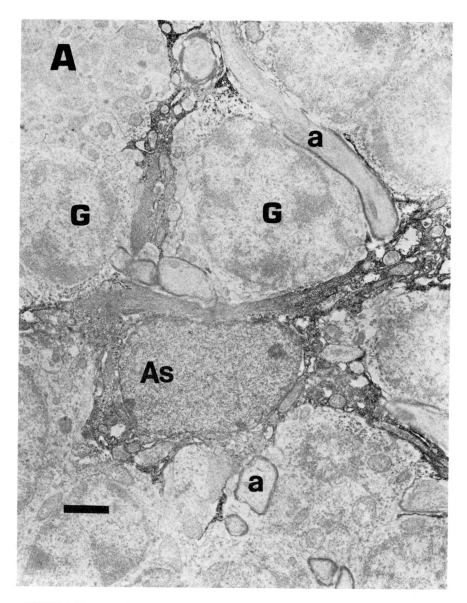

FIGURE 4. Electron micrographs of rat cerebellum stained for S-100 protein by the immuno-peroxidase method using vibratome sections. (A) Astrocyte (As) among numerous granule cells (G). Myelinated axons (a) are also present. Filaments in glial cell cytoplasm measure 100–

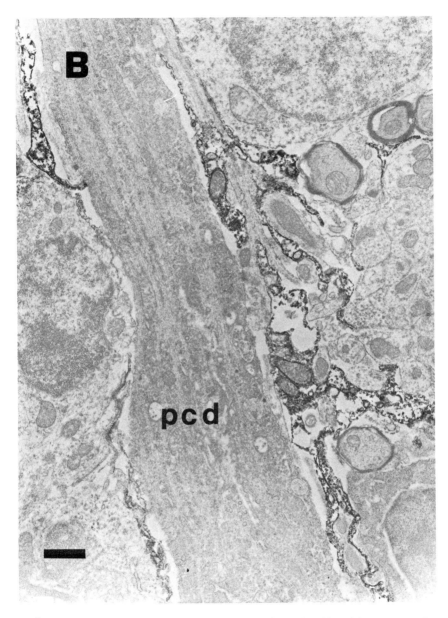

120 Å. (B) S-100 staining surrounding Purkinje cell dendrite (pcd). This staining corresponds to radial fibers of Bergmann glia seen at the LM level. Bar equals 1 μm.

guinea pig and rabbit formed immunoprecipitates with the GFA protein isolated from human and bovine nervous tissue. Using the Nakane method (1973) at the LM and EM levels, the GFA protein-specific antibody produced with the 47K fraction from myelin-free axons specifically stained only astroglial and not axonal elements. GFA protein and astrocytic processes containing GFA protein have been demonstrated in the myelinated axons, myelin-free axons, and crude myelin. These data suggest that the 47K protein fraction contains GFA protein derived from astroglia. While axon-specific proteins may be present in the 47K fraction, specific antibodies to axonal proteins could not be demonstrated with the 47K protein fraction in the present study (Eng *et al.*, 1976*b*). Starting with a myelin-free axonal preparation obtained from calf brain by a procedure very similar to that of De Vries *et al.* (1971) Shelanski and co-workers (Yen *et al.*, 1976) have isolated proteins of molecular weight 50,000 which they have called neurofilaments. These proteins have chemical and immunologic similarities to Dahl's GFA protein preparation. Our recent studies (Eng *et al.*, 1976*b*) suggest that the neurofilament preparation is substantially contaminated with glial filaments (GFA protein).

There are other proteins being studied which may be related to the GFA protein (Benda *et al.*, 1970; Bogoch, 1972; Delpech and Buffe, 1972; Mori and Morimoto, 1973, 1975; Delpech *et al.*, 1973, 1975; Johnson and Sinex, 1974; Cain *et al.*, 1974; Mori *et al.*, 1975; Delpech and Delpech, 1975).

9.11.2. Immunohistochemical Localization of the GFA Protein

Fine intracytoplasmic fibers differentially stained by special methods represent a distinctive feature of many astrocytes, especially in the white matter. Under the electron microscope these fibers appear as bundles of filaments 8–9 nm in diameter. These glial filaments are present only in small numbers within most astrocytes in the normal cerebral hemisphere; however, increased production of intracellular fibers in astrocytes (fibrous gliosis) is observed under a variety of pathological conditions, in aging, and under experimental conditions such as Wallerian degeneration of the central nervous system (Bignami and Eng, 1973). Chemical and immunohistological studies of the astrocytic fibers have shown its major constituent to be GFA protein (Figures 5 and 6). (Eng *et al.*, 1971; Bignami *et al.*, 1972; Eng and Kosek, 1974; Ludwin *et al.*, 1976*b*).

Using indirect immunofluorescence with GFA protein antiserum, Bignami and Dahl have studied GFA protein production during development (Bignami and Dahl, 1973, 1974*a*,*b*, 1975), in mutant mice (Bignami and Dahl, 1974*c*,*d*), and in response to trauma (Bignami *et al.*, 1974; Bignami

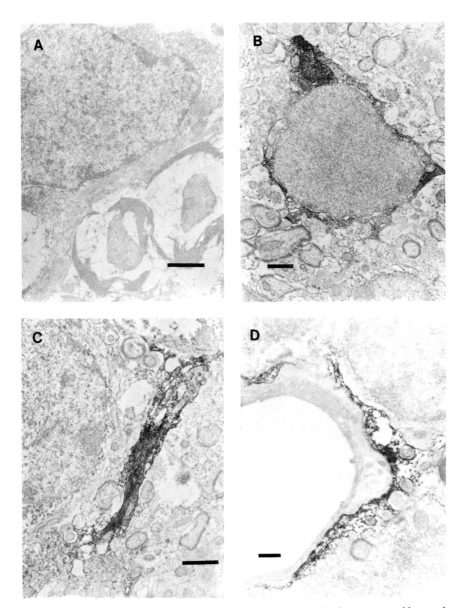

FIGURE 5. Electron micrographs of rat cerebellum stained by the immunoperoxidase technique using vibratome sections. (A) Control section treated with absorbed serum. Astrocyte nucleus in upper left is unstained as are the filaments in its cytoplasm. Unstained filaments measure 80–90 Å. Disrupted myelinated axons appear in the lower right. (B) Astrocyte whose cytoplasm is strongly stained for GFA protein using anti-GFA antiserum. Cross-sectional profiles of filaments in the cytoplasm measure 100–110 Å. (C) Astrocyte process positively stained for GFA protein. Filaments measure 100–120 Å. Golgi cell nucleus is in upper left. (D) Positively stained perivascular cuff surrounding blood vessel. Vessel structures and neuron (upper left) are unstained. Bar equals 1 μm.

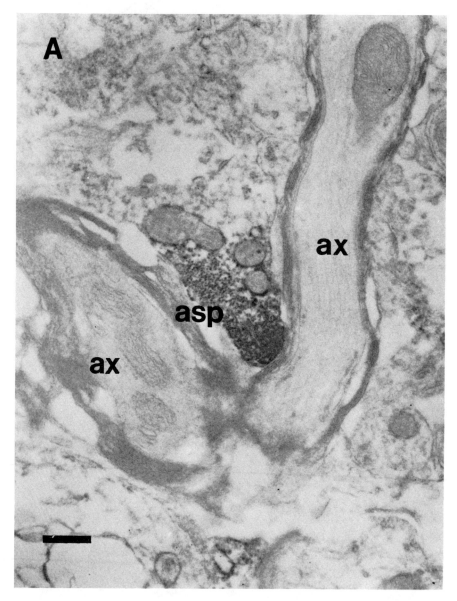

FIGURE 6. Electron micrographs of rat cerebellum stained for GFA protein by the immuno-peroxidase technique using vibratome sections. (A) Cross section of astrocyte process (asp) between two myelinated axons (ax). (B) Longitudinal section of astrocyte process filled with

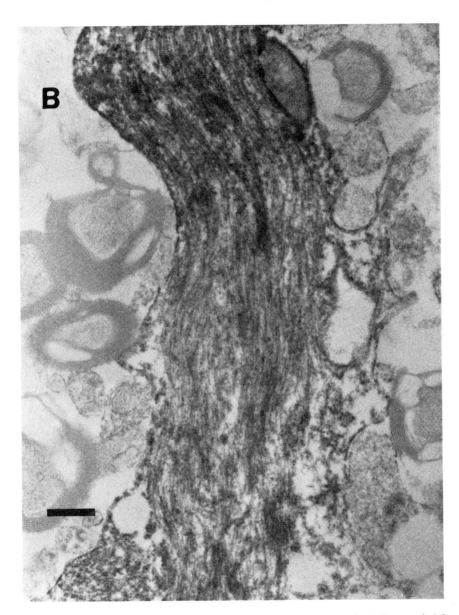

positively stained filaments. In both pictures, the axoplasm remains unstained. Bar equals 0.5 μm.

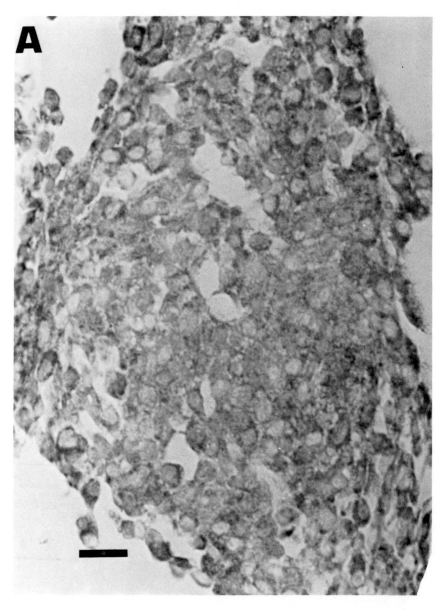

FIGURE 7. Photomicrographs of sections of C_6 glioma culture which was paraffin-embedded and stained for GFA protein by the PAP technique. (A) Control using absorbed serum. (B) Numerous cells positive for GFA protein which is localized only in their cytoplasm. Note that

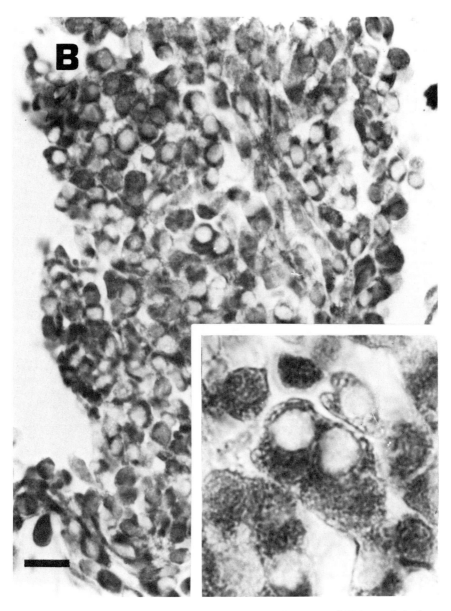

some stain more intensely than others, indicating a greater abundance of GFA protein in those cells. Inset, details of cytoplasmic staining. Bar equals 20 μm.

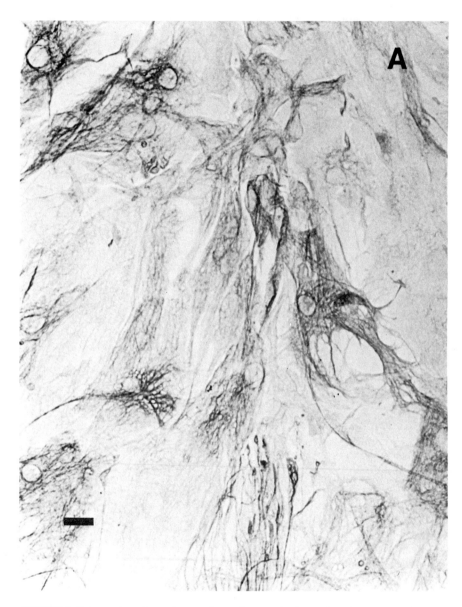

FIGURE 8. Primary monolayer tissue culture of mouse brain; 14-day-old culture stained for GFA protein by the PAP method. (A) Numerous astrocytes positively stained. (B) Details of

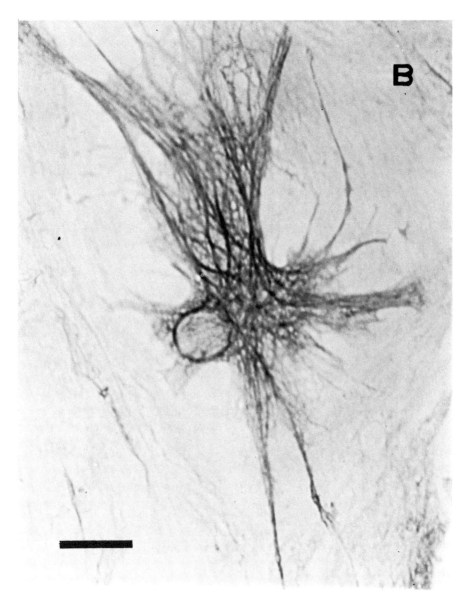

the staining. Bar equals 20 μm. (This study is being carried out in collaboration with Dr. M. Herman.)

and Dahl, 1976). GFA protein has been localized by immunofluorescence with GFA protein antiserum in glial cell culture from normal and abnormal brain tissue and brain tumors (Bissell *et al.*, 1974; Antanitus *et al.*, 1975, 1976; Vandenberg *et al.*, 1976; Gilden *et al.*, 1976).

GFA protein has also been localized by the PAP method in glial cells of the experimental mouse teratoma (Ludwin *et al.*, 1976*a*), in C-$_6$ glioma cells in culture (Figure 7) (Liao *et al.*, 1977, 1978), and in primary mouse brain tissue culture by the procedure described for the rat (Figure 8) (Bock *et al.*, 1975). The PAP method has permitted retrospective studies of formalin-fixed, paraffin-embedded pathologic human brain (Figures 3B– 3D, 9B–9D) (Eng *et al.*, 1976*a*) and tumors (Figure 9A) (Deck *et al.*, 1976).

9.12. 14-3-2 Protein, Antigen Alpha, and NSP-R

Moore's 14-3-2 protein from beef brain and antigen alpha from rat brain are considered to be acidic proteins specific to neurons (Moore and Perez, 1968; Bennett and Edelman, 1968). Bennett (1974) demonstrated by immunochemical and electrophoretic studies that antigen alpha and 14-3-2 are the same protein. More recently, 14-3-2 protein (NSP-R) has been isolated from rat brain by a different method and compared to 14-3-2 from beef brains (Marangos *et al.*, 1975). Both preparations had very similar amino acid compositions and identical antigenic properties. The enolase activity reported to be associated with 14-3-2 (Bock and Dissing, 1975) has been confirmed and shown to be a brain-specific isoenzyme (Zomzely-Neurath *et al.*, 1977).

Immunohistochemical localization of 14-3-2 was first attempted by Haglid *et al.* (1973) using immunofluorescence on fresh frozen human brain and a variety of human brain tumors. It was reported that 14-3-2 and S-100 proteins were present in neurons, 14-3-2 exhibiting a much stronger fluorescence. Utilizing the immunoperoxidase method of Nakane (1973), antigen alpha was localized to the cytoplasm of the cell body and processes of selective neurons in the rat brain (Kosek *et al.*, 1974) (see Figure 3B). Using the PAP method and NSP-R antiserum on paraffin sections of paraformaldehyde-perfused rat brain, NSP-R was demonstrated in neurons (Pickel *et al.*, 1976*b*). Immunofluorescence studies tracing 14-3-2 during development in the rat and chick have been reported (Hartman *et al.*, 1976, 1977).

9.13. Olfactory Bulb Protein

Following the identification of the olfactory bulb-specific protein (Margolis, 1972), it has been localized by immunofluorescence to the olfactory epithelium, olfactory nerves, and synaptic glomeruli in the bulb (Hartman

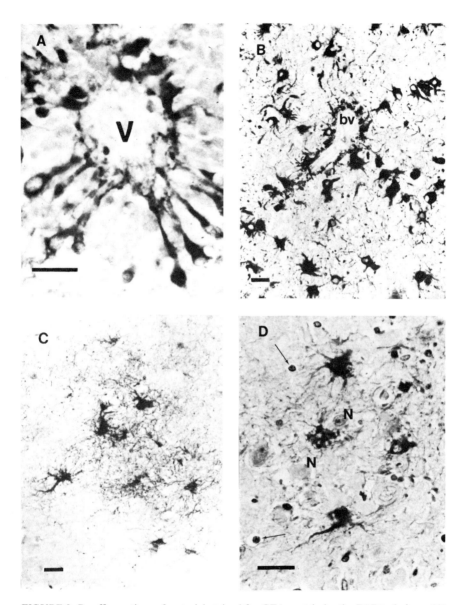

FIGURE 9. Paraffin sections of material stained for GFA protein by the PAP technique. (A) Astroblastoma tumor showing large reactive astroblasts surrounding and cuffing a blood vessel (V). Note the clear, unstained nuclei in some. (B) Alexander's disease characterized by extreme gliosis and intracytoplasmic inclusions. Here highly gliosed area, with large reactive astrocytes near and surrounding a small blood vessel (bv). (This study was done in collaboration with Dr. M. Norman.) (C) Multiple sclerosis plaque with dense astrocyte reaction and numerous fine processes. (D) Multiple sclerosis plaque which has been counterstained with hematoxylin and eosin to reveal detail of tissue elements not visible with PAP staining alone. In addition to the astrocytes, which are immunologically stained, other glial cells (arrows) and neurons (N) can be seen. Bar equals 20 μm.

and Margolis, 1975). These authors conclude that the protein is exclusively associated with the primary olfactory chemoreceptor neurons.

9.14. Substance P

Substance P, a neuron-specific polypeptide, has been localized by immunofluorescence to cell bodies in dorsal root ganglia and processes within the dorsal horn of the spinal cord (Hökfelt *et al.*, 1975*b*, 1976). Applying the PAP technique to paraffin sections of rat spinal cord, Pickel *et al.* (1977) confirmed the immunofluorescent findings and further localized substance P at the ultrastructural level using vibratome sections. They found substance P associated with large round vesicles in axon terminals.

ACKNOWLEDGMENTS

We thank Ms. Lorraine Macchello, Jeanne Kline, and Joan McFarland for their excellent assistance in the preparation of this manuscript. This chapter and our studies reported herein were supported by the Veterans Administration, MRIS 2390, and the National Institutes of Health.

10. REFERENCES

Aarli, J. A., Aparicio, S. R., Lumsden, C. E., and Tonder, O., 1975, Binding of normal human IgG to myelin sheaths, glia, and neurons, *Immunology* **28**:171–185.

Agrawal, H. C., Hartman, B. K., Fujimoto, K., Shearer, W. T., Kalmbach, S., and Margolis, F. L., 1977, Purification and immunohistochemical localization of rat brain myelin proteolipid protein, *J. Neurochem.* **28**:495–508.

Allen, W. D., Smith, C. G., and Porter, P., 1976, Evidence for the secretory transport mechanism of intestinal immunoglobulin. The ultrastructural distribution of IgM, *Immunology* **30(3)**:449–457.

Alpert, L. C., Brawer, J. R., Patel, Y. C., and Reichlin, S., 1976, Somatostatinergic neurons in anterior hypothalamus: Immunohistochemical localization, *Endocrinology* **98(1)**:255–258.

Antanitus, D. S., Choi, B. H., and Lapham, L. W., 1975, Immunofluorescence staining of astrocytes *in vitro* using antiserum to glial fibrillary acidic protein, *Brain Res.* **89**:363–367.

Antanitus, D. S., Choi, B. H., and Lapham, L. W., 1976, The demonstration of glial fibrillary acidic protein in the cerebrum of the human fetus by indirect immunofluorescence, *Brain Res.* **103**:613–616.

Asghar, S. S., Joost, T. Van, and Cormane, R. H., 1973, Comparison of immunofluorescence and immunoperoxidase techniques for detection of tissue antigen, *Arch. Dermatol. Forsch.* **248(2)**:99–108.

Avrameas, S., 1969*a*, Coupling of enzymes to proteins with glutaraldehyde. Use of the conjugates for the detection of antigens and antibodies, *Immunochemistry* **6(1)**:43–52.

Avrameas, S., 1969*b*, Indirect immunoenzyme techniques for the intracellular detection of antigens, *Immunochemistry* **6(6)**:825–831.

Avrameas, S., 1972, Enzyme markers: Their linkage with proteins and use in immunohistochemistry, *Histochem. J.* **4(4)**:321–330.

Avrameas, S., and Bouteille, M., 1968, Ultrastructural localization of antibody by antigen label with peroxidase, *Exp. Cell Res.* **53(1)**:166–176.

Avrameas, S., and Guilbert, B., 1971, A method for quantitative determination of cellular immunoglobulins by enzyme-labeled antibodies, *Eur. J. Immunol.* **1(5)**:394–396.

Avrameas, S., and Ternynck, T., 1971, Peroxidase-labelled antibody and Fab conjugates with enhanced intracellular penetration, *Immunochemistry* **8(12)**:1175–1179.

Aycock, E. K., 1973, Fluorescent antibody application in the diagnosis of fungal diseases, *J. Scand. Med. Assoc.* **69(3)**:88.

Baker, B. L., and Drummond, T., 1972, The cellular origins of corticotropin and melanotropin as revealed by immunochemical staining, *Am. J. Anat.* **134(4)**:395–409.

Baker, B. L., Dermody, W. C., and Reel, J. R., 1974, Localization of leuteinizing hormone releasing hormone in mammalian hypothalamus, *Am. J. Anat.* **139**:129–134.

Balazs, R., Hajos, F., Johnson, A. L., Reynierse, G. L. A., Tapia, R., and Wilkin, G. P., 1975, Subcellular fractionation of rat cerebellum: An electron microscopic and biochemical investigation. III. Isolation of large fragments of the cerebellar glomeruli, *Brain Res.* **86**:17–30.

Barabino, A., Di Benedetto, G., Villa, M. A., and Indiveri, F., 1973, Comparison of immunofluorescence with the enzyme-labeled antibody technic in the demonstration of antithyroid antibodies, *Boll. Soc. Ital. Biol. Sper.* **49(20)**:1186–1189.

Bariety, J., Druet, P., and Laliberte, F., 1975, Immunoperoxidase in glomerular pathology, *Pathol. Biol.* **23(6)**:485.

Barry, J., Dubois, M. P., and Carette, B., 1974, Immunofluorescence study of the preoptico-infundibular LRF neurosecretory pathway in the normal, castrated or testosterone-treated male guinea pig, *Endocrinology* **95(5)**:1416–1423.

Battenberg, E. L., and Bloom, F. E., 1975, A rapid, simple and more sensitive method for the demonstration of central catecholamine-containing neurons and axons by glyoxylic acid-induced fluorescence: I. Specificity, *Psychopharmacol. Commun.* **1(1)**:3–13.

Bauer, H., 1976, Diagnostic applications of the fluorescent antibody method, *Am. Fam. Physician* **13(2)**:74–80.

Beaupain, D., and Dieterlen-Li Evre, F., 1972, Immunohistologic demonstration of insulin in the chick embryonic pancreas, *C.R. Acad. Sci. [D] (Paris)* **275(3)**:413–415.

Beauvillain, J. C., Tramu, G., and Dubois, M. P., 1975, Characterization by different techniques of adrenocorticotropin and gonadotropin producing cells in Lerot pituitary (*Eliomys quercinus*), *Cell Tissue Res.* **158(3)**:301–317.

Bellon, B., Sapin, C., and Druet, P., 1975, The sensitivity of direct and indirect methods in immunofluorescence and immunoperoxidase techniques: A comparative study (author's transl.), *Ann. Immunol.* **126(1)**:15–22.

Benda, P., Mori, T., and Sweet, W. H., 1970, Demonstration of an astrocyte-specific cerebroprotein by an immunofluorescence study of human brain tumors, *J. Neurosurg.* **33**:281–286.

Benjamin, D. R., 1974, Rapid typing of herpes simplex virus strains using the indirect immunoperoxidase method, *Appl. Microbiol.* **28(4)**:568–571.

Benjamin, D. R., and Ray, C. G., 1975, Use of immunoperoxidase on brain tissue for the rapid diagnosis of herpes encephalitis, *Am. J. Clin. Pathol.* **64(4)**:472–476.

Bennett, G. S., 1974, Immunologic and electrophoretic identity between nervous system-specific proteins antigen alpha and 14-3-2, *Brain Res.* **68**:365–369.

Bennett, G. S., and Edelman, G. M., 1968, Isolation of an acidic protein from rat brain, *J. Biol. Chem.* **243**:6234–6241.

Bergquist, R., 1971, Manufacture of monospecific conjugates for fluorescent antibody work, *Acta Pathol. Microbiol. Scand. B* **79(3)**:444.

Beutner, E. H., 1961, Immunofluorescent staining: The fluorescent antibody method, *Bacterial Rev.* **25**:49–76.

Beutner, E. H., 1975, Uses for immunofluorescence tests of skin and sera. Utilization of immunofluorescence in the diagnosis of bullous diseases, lupus erythematosus, and certain other dermatoses, *Arch. Dermatol.* **111(3)**:371–381.

Bigbee, J. W., Kosek, J. C., and Eng, L. F., 1977, Effects of primary antiserum dilution on staining of "antigen rich" tissues with the peroxidase antiperoxidase technique, *J. Histochem. Cytochem.* **25**:443–447.

Bignami, A., and Dahl, D., 1973, Differentiation of astrocytes in the cerebellar cortex and the pyramidal tracts of the newborn rat. An immunofluorescence study with antibodies to a protein specific to astrocytes, *Brain Res.* **49**:393–402.

Bignami, A., and Dahl, D., 1974*a*, Astrocyte-specific protein and neuroglial differentiation. An immunofluorescence study with antibodies to the glial fibrillary acidic protein, *J. Comp. Neurol.* **153**:27–38.

Bignami, A., and Dahl, D., 1974*b,* Astrocyte-specific protein and radial glia in the cerebral cortex of newborn rat, *Nature* **252**:55–56.

Bignami, A., and Dahl, D., 1974*c,* Glial fibrillary acidic protein in mutant mice with deficiency of myelination: Quaking and Jimpy, *Acta Neuropathol. (Berlin)* **28**:269–272.

Bignami, A., and Dahl, D., 1974*d,* The development of Bergmann glia in mutant mice with cerebellar malformations: Reeler, staggerer and weaver. Immunofluorescence study with antibodies to the glial fibrillary acidic protein, *J. Comp. Neurol.* **155**:219–230.

Bignami, A., and Dahl, D., 1975, Astroglial protein in the developing spinal cord of the chick embryo, *Dev. Biol.* **44**:204–209.

Bignami, A., and Dahl, D., 1976, The astroglial response to stabbing. Immunofluorescence studies with antibodies to astrocyte-specific protein (GFA) in mammalian and submammalian vertebrates, *Neuropathol. Appl. Neurobiol.* **2**:99–111.

Bignami, A., and Eng, L. F., 1973, Biochemical studies of myelin in Wallerian degeneration of rat optic nerve, *J. Neurochem.* **20**:165–173.

Bignami, A., Eng, L. F., Dahl, D., and Uyeda, C. T., 1972, Localization of the glial fibrillary acidic protein in astrocytes by immunofluorescence, *Brain Res.* **43**:429–435.

Bignami, A., Forno, L., and Dahl, D., 1974, The neuroglial response to injury following spinal cord transection in the goldfish, *Exp. Neurol.* **44**:60–70.

Bignon, J., Chahinian, P., Feldmann, G., and Sapin, C., 1975, Ultrastructural immunoperoxidase demonstration of autologous albumin in the alveolar capillary membrane and in the alveolar lining material in normal rats, *J. Cell Biol.* **64(2)**:503–509.

Bissell, M. G., Rubinstein, L. J., Bignami, A., and Herman, M. M., 1974, Characteristics of the rat C-6 glioma maintained in organ culture systems. Production of glial fibrillary acidic protein in the absence of gliofibrillogenesis, *Brain Res.* **82**:77–89.

Bloom, F. E., Hoffer, B. J., Battenberg, E. R., and Siggins, G. R., 1972, Adenosine 3′,5′-monophosphate is localized in cerebellar neurons: Immunofluorescence evidence, *Science* **177**:436–438.

Blundell, G. P., 1970, Fluorescent antibody technics, *Prog. Clin. Pathol.* **3**:211–225.

Bock, E., and Dissing, J., 1975, Demonstration of enolase activity connected to the brain-specific protein 14-3-2, *Scand. J. Immunol. (Suppl. 4)* **2**:31–36.

Bock, E., Jorgensen, O. S., Dittmann, L., and Eng, L. F., 1975, Determination of brain-specific antigens in short-term cultivated rat astroglial cells and in rat synaptosomes, *J. Neurochem.* **25**:867–870.

Bocker, W., 1974, Use of a triple layer enzyme method as an alternative to immunofluorescence for the detection of tissue antigens, *Beitr. Pathol.* **153(4)**:410–414.

Bogoch, S., 1972, Brain glycoprotein 10B: Further evidence of the "signpost" role of brain glycoproteins in cell recognition, its change in brain tumor, and the presence of a "distance factor," in: *Functional and Structural Proteins of the Nervous System* (A. N. Davison, P. Mandel, and I. G. Morgan, eds.), pp. 39–52, Plenum Press, New York.

Boorsma, D. M., and Kalsbeek, G. L., 1975, A comparative study of horseradish peroxidase conjugates prepared with a one-step and a two-step method, *J. Histochem. Cytochem.* **23(3)**:200–207.

Boorsma, D. M., Nieboer, C., and Kalsbeek, G. L., 1975, Cutaneous immunohistochemistry. The direct immunoperoxidase and immunoglobulin-enzyme bridge methods compared with the immunofluorescence method in dermatology, *J. Cutan. Pathol.* **2(6)**:294–301.

Borek, F., 1961, The immunofluorescent antibody method in medical and biological research, *Bull. WHO* **24**:249–256.

Bosman, C., and Feldman, J. D., 1970, The proportion and structure of cells forming antibody, gamma G and gamma M immunoglobulins, and gamma G and gamma M antibodies, *Cell. Immunol.* **1(1)**:31–50.

Brandtzaeg, P., 1973, Two types of IgA immunocytes in man, *Nature New Biol.* **243**:142.

Brandtzaeg, P., 1975, Rhodamine conjugates: Specific and nonspecific binding properties in immunohistochemistry, *Ann. N.Y. Acad. Sci.* **254**:35–54.

Bretton, R., Ternynck, T., and Avrameas, S., 1972, Comparison of peroxidase and ferritin labelling of cell surface antigens, *Exp. Cell Res.* **71(1)**:145–155.

Brown, P. J., Bourne, F. J., and Steel, M., 1974, Immunoperoxidase and immunofluorescence techniques in pig tissues, *Histochemistry* **40(4)**:343–348.

Brown, P. J., Bourne, F. J., and Denny, H. R., 1975, Immunoglobulin-containing cells in pig mammary gland, *J. Anat.* **120(2)**:329–335.

Brown, W. R., and Burns, F. A., 1973, Application of peroxidase-labeled antibody methods to identification of immunoglobulin-containing cells in gastrointestinal tissues, *J. Immunol. Methods* **2(3)**:303–307.

Bryan, J., and Wilson, L., 1971, Are cytoplasmic microtubules heteropolymers? *Proc. Natl. Acad. Sci. U.S.A.* **68**:1762.

Bubenik, G. A., Brown, G. M., Uhlir, I., and Grota, L. J., 1974, Immunohistochemical localization of *N*-acetylindolealkylamine in pineal gland, retina and cerebellum, *Brain Res.* **81**:233–242.

Bubenik, G. A., Brown, G. M., and Grota, L. J., 1975, Localization of immunoreactive androgen in testicular tissue, *Endocrinology* **96(1)**:63–69.

Bubenik, G. A., Brown, G. M., and Grota, L. G., 1976*a,* Differential localization of *N*-acetylated indolealkylamines in CNS and the Harderian gland using immunohistology, *Brain Res.* **118**:417–427.

Bubenik, G. A., Brown, G. M., and Grota, L. J., 1976*b,* Immunohistochemical localization of melatonin in the rat Harderian gland, *J. Histochem. Cytochem.* **24(11)**:1173–1177.

Burns, J., 1975*a,* Background staining and sensitivity of the unlabelled antibody-enzyme (PAP) method. Comparison with the peroxidase-labelled antibody sandwich method using formalin-fixed paraffin embedded material, *Histochemistry* **43(3)**:291–294.

Burns, J., 1975*b,* Immunoperoxidase localisation of hepatitis B antigen (HB) in formalin-paraffin processed liver tissue, *Histochemistry* **44(2)**:133–135.

Burns, J., Hambridge, M., and Taylor, C. R., 1974, Intracellular immunoglobulins. A comparative study on three standard tissue processing methods using horseradish peroxidase and fluorochrome conjugates, *J. Clin. Pathol.* **27(7)**:548–557.

Burt, A. M., and Silver, A., 1973, Histochemistry of choline acetyltransferase: A critical analysis, *Brain Res.* **62**:509–516.

Cain, D. F., Ball, E. D., and Dekaban, A. S., 1974, Proteins of human brain tissue obtained during surgical procedures, *J. Neurochem.* **23**:561–568.

Cantella, R. A., Lopez, L. R., and Colichon, A. A., 1974, Improvement of specific fluorescence in the indirect fluorescent antibody method for detecting antinuclear antibodies using Evans blue dye as a counterstain, *Ann. Sclavo* **16(5)**:503–506.

Chan, P. H., Huston, J. S., Dahl, D., and Bignami, A., 1975, Purification and initial characterization of astroglial protein from bovine brain, *Fed. Proc.* **34**:224.

Chantler, S., 1975, Comparison of antihuman immunoglobulin and antihuman Fab conjugates for the detection of tissue autoantibodies by immunofluorescence, *Ann. N.Y. Acad. Sci.* **254**:66–68.

Cicero, T. J., Cowan, W. M., Moore, B. W., and Suntzeff, V., 1970, The cellular localization of the two brain-specific proteins, S-100 and 14-3-2, *Brain Res.* **18**:25–34.

Clayton, R. M., 1954, Localization of embryonic antigens by antisera labelled with fluorescent dyes, *Nature* **174**:1059.

Clyne, D. H., Norris, S. H., Modesto, R. R., Pesce, A. J., and Pollak, V. E., 1973, Antibody enzyme conjugates: The preparation of intermolecular conjugates of horseradish peroxidase and antibody and their use in immunohistology of renal cortex, *J. Histochem. Cytochem.* **21(3)**:233–240.

Coons, A. H., 1956, Histochemistry with labeled antibody, *Int. Rev. Cytol.* **5**:1–23.

Coons, A. H., 1958, *Fluorescent Antibody Methods* (J. F. Danielli, ed.), pp. 399–422, Academic Press, New York.

Coons, A. H., Creech, H. J., and Jones, R. N., 1941, Immunological properties of an antibody containing a fluorescent group, *Proc. Soc. Exp. Biol.* **47**:200–202.

Dahl, D., 1976*a*, Glial fibrillary acidic protein from bovine and rat brain. Degradation in tissues and homogenates, *Biochim. Biophys. Acta* **420**:142–154.

Dahl, D., 1976*b*, Isolation and initial characterization of glial fibrillary acidic protein from chicken, turtle, frog, and fish central nervous system, *Biochim. Biophys. Acta* **446**:41–50.

Dahl, D., and Bignami, A., 1973, Glial fibrillary acidic protein from normal human brain. Purification and properties, *Brain Res.* **57**:343–360.

Dahl, D., and Bignami, A., 1974, Heterogeneity of the glial fibrillary acidic protein in gliosed human brains, *J. Neurol. Sci.* **23**:551–563.

Dahl, D., and Bignami, A., 1975, Glial fibrillary acidic protein from normal and gliosed human brain. Demonstration of multiple related polypeptides, *Biochim. Biophys. Acta* **386**:41–51.

Dahl, D., and Bignami, A., 1976, Immunogenic properties of the glial fibrillary acidic protein, *Brain Res.* **116**:150–157.

Dal Canto, M. C., Blum, N. R., and Johnson, A. B., 1975, Immunofluorescence horseradish peroxidase-combined staining technique for demonstrating both immunoglobulin class and antigen-binding specificity of cellular antibody, *J. Histochem. Cytochem.* **23**:452.

Daniels, M. P., and Vogel, Z., 1975, Immunoperoxidase staining of alpha-bungarotoxin binding sites in muscle endplates shows distribution of acetylcholine receptors, *Nature* **254(5498)**:339–341.

Davies, D. R., and Clark, A. E., 1975, Demonstration of immunoglobulin containing deposits in glomerular basement membrane in experimental chronic serum sickness using horseradish peroxidase-labelled antiserum, *Br. J. Exp. Pathol.* **56(1)**:28–33.

Dayan, A. D., and Stokes, M. I., 1971, Immunofluorescent detection of measles-virus antigens in cerebrospinal-fluid cells in subacute sclerosing panencephalitis, *Lancet* **1(705)**:891–892.

Dayan, A. D., and Stokes, M. I., 1973, Rapid diagnosis of encephalitis by immunofluorescent examination of cerebrospinal-fluid cells, *Lancet* **1(796)**:177–179.

Deck, J. H., Eng, L. F., and Bigbee, J., 1976, A preliminary study of glioma morphology using the peroxidase-antiperoxidase immunohistological method for glial fibrillary acidic protein, *J. Neuropathol. Exp. Neurol.* **35**:362.

Delpech, B., and Buffe, D., 1972, Etude immunochimique des extraits salins du cerveau humain, *Ann. Inst. Pasteur* **122**:331–340.

Delpech, B., and Delpech, A., 1975, Caracterisation immunochimique d'un antigene neurospecifique non specifique d'espece. Etude quantitative et localisation histologique chez le rat, *Immunochemistry* **12**:691–697.

Delpech, B., Fidard, M. N., Schlosser, M., and Hernot, C., 1973, Quelques propriétés d'une glycoproteine antigeniquement spécifique du système nerveux, *C.R. Soc. Biol.* **167**:1029–1032.

Delpech, B., Chauzy, C., Delpech, A., and Maunoury, R., 1975, *Protides of the Biological Fluids,* 22nd Symposium (H. Peters, ed.), pp. 363–366, Pergamon Press, Oxford.

De Vries, G. H., Norton, W. T., and Raine, C. S., 1971, Axons: Isolation from mammalian central nervous system, *Science* **175**:1370–1372.

De Vries, G. H., Eng, L. F., Lewis, D. H., and Hadfield, M. G., 1976, The protein composition of bovine myelin-free axons, *Biochim. Biophys. Acta* **439**:133–145.

Dobzhanski, S. I., and Tabakova, L. S., 1974, Immunofluorescent method in dermatology (Review of the literature), *Vestn. Dermatol. Venerol.* **0(8)**:13–18.

Donato, R., and Michetti, F., 1974, S-100 protein in cerebral cortex synaptosomes, *Experientia* **30**:511–512.

Donato, R., Michetti, F., and Miani, N., 1975, Soluble and membrane-bound S-100 protein in cerebral cortex synaptosomes. Properties of the S-100 receptor, *Brain Res.* **98**:561–573.

Dorling, J., Johnson, G. D., Webb, J. A., and Smith, M. E., 1971, Use of peroxidase-conjugated antiglobulin as an alternative to immunofluorescence for the detection of antinuclear factor in serum, *J. Clin. Pathol.* **24(6)**:501–505.

Eipper, B. A., 1974, Properties of rat brain tubulin, *J. Biol. Chem.* **249**:1407–1416.

Elias, J. M., and Miller, F., 1975, A comparison of the unlabelled enzyme method with immunofluorescence for the evaluation of human immunologic renal disease, *Am. J. Clin. Pathol.* **64(4)**:464–471.

Ellis, H. K., and Watkins, W. B., 1975, Ontogeny of the pig hypothalamic neurosecretory system with particular reference to the distribution of neurophysin, *Cell Tissue Res.* **164(4)**:543–557.

Eng, L. F., 1973, Chemical characterization of the glial fibrillary acidic protein (GFAP), *Fed. Proc.* **32**:485.

Eng, L. F., and Kosek, J. C., 1974, Light and electron microscopic localization of the glial fibrillary acidic protein and S-100 protein by immunoenzymatic techniques, *Trans. Am. Soc. Neurochem.* **5**:160.

Eng, L. F., Gerstl, B., and Vanderhaeghen, J. J., 1970, A study of proteins in old multiple sclerosis plaques, *Trans. Am. Soc. Neurochem.* **1**:42.

Eng, L. F., Vanderhaeghen, J. J., Bignami, A., and Gerstl, B., 1971, An acidic protein isolated from fibrous astrocytes, *Brain Res.* **28**:351–354.

Eng, L. F., Pratt, D., and Wilson, L., 1974*a*, Biochemical and pharmacological comparison of microtubule protein from human and chick brain, *Neurobiology* **4**:301–308.

Eng, L. F., Uyeda, C. T., Chao, L. P., and Wolfgram, F., 1974*b*, Antibody to bovine choline acetyltransferase and immunofluorescent localization of the enzyme in neurons, *Nature* **250**:243–245.

Eng, L. F., Burkstaller, M., Bigbee, J., Kosek, J. C., and Kies, M. W., 1975, Immunohistologic comparison of the glial fibrillary acidic protein and myelin basic protein in the myelinating brain, 5th International Meeting of the International Society of Neurochemists, Barcelona, Spain, Abstract 41.

Eng, L. F., Kosek, J. C., Forno, L., Deck, J., and Bigbee, J., 1976*a*, Immunohistochemistry of brain proteins in fixed, paraffin-embedded tissue, *Trans. Am. Soc. Neurochem.* **7**:211.

Eng. L. F., DeVries, G. H., Lewis, D. L., and Bigbee, J., 1976*b*, Specific antibody to the major 47,000 MW protein fraction of bovine myelin-free axons, *Fed. Proc.* **35**:1766.

Erlandsen, S. L., Parsons, J. A., and Taylor, T. D., 1974, Ultrastructural immunocytochemical localization of lysozyme in the paneth cells of man, *J. Histochem. Cytochem.* **22(6)**:401–413.

Fagraeus, A., and Bergquist, N. R., 1975, The raison d'etre of standards in indirect immunofluorescence, *Ann. N.Y. Acad. Sci.* **254**:69–76.

Falck, B., Hillarp, N. A., Thieme, G., and Torp, A., 1962, Fluorescence of catecholamines and related compounds condensed with formaldehyde, *J. Histochem. Cytochem.* **10**:348–354.

Faulk, W. P., and Hijmans, W., 1972, Recent developments in immunofluorescence, *Prog. Allergy* **16**:9–39.

Fonnum, F., 1972, Application of microchemical analysis and subcellular fractionation techniques to the study of neurotransmitters in discrete areas of mammalian brain, *Adv. Biochem. Psychopharmacol.* **6**:75–88.

Fukuyama, K., 1971, The immunopathology of lupus erythematosus: A comparison of immunohistochemical techniques. II. Peroxidase method, *Adv. Biol. Skin* **11**:295–304.

Fuxe, K., Goldstein, M., Hökfelt, T., and Joh, T. H., 1970, Immunohistochemical localization of dopamine-β-hydroxylase in the peripheral and central nervous system, *Res. Commun. Chem. Pathol. Pharmacol.* **1(5)**:627–636.

Fuxe, K., Goldstein, M., Hökfelt, T., and Joh, T. H., 1971, Cellular localization of dopamine-β-hydroxylase and phenylethanolamine-*N*-methyl transferase as revealed by immunohistochemistry, *Prog. Brain Res.* **34**:127–138.

Ganong, W. F., 1975, Review of Medical Physiology, 7th ed., Lange, Los Altos, California, 587 pp.

Garvin, A. J., Spicer, S. S., Parmley, R. T., and Munster, A. M., 1974, Immunohistochemical demonstration of IgG in Reed-Sternberg and other cells in Hodgkin's disease, *J. Exp. Med.* **139(5)**:1077–1083.

Gerber, M. A., Hadziyannis, S., Vissoulis, C., Schaffner, F., Paronetto, F., and Popper, H., 1974, Electron microscopy and immunoelectronmicroscopy of cytoplasmic hepatitis B antigen in hepatocytes, *Am. J. Pathol.* **75(3)**:489–502.

Gilden, D. H., Wroblewska, Z., Eng, L. F., and Rorke, L. B., 1976, Identification of glial cells by immunofluorescence, *J. Neurol. Sci.* **29**:177–184.

Goldman, M., 1971, Introductory review: Immunofluorescence in parasitology, *Ann. N.Y. Acad. Sci.* **177**:130–133.

Goldstein, M., Fuxe, K., Hökfelt, T., and Joh, T. H., 1971, Immunohistochemical studies on phenylethanolamine-*N*-methyltransferase, dopa-decarboxylase and dopamine-β-hydroxylase, *Experientia* **27**:951–952.

Goldstein, M., Fuxe, K., and Hökfelt, T., 1972, Characterization and tissue localization of catecholamine synthesizing enzymes, *Pharmacol. Rev.* **24(2)**:293–309.

Gonatas, N. K., Stieber, A., Gonatas, J., Gambetti, P., Antoine, J. C., and Avrameas, S., 1974, Ultrastructural autoradiographic detection of intracellular immunoglobulins with iodinated Fab fragments of antibody. The combined use of ultrastructural autoradiography and peroxidase cytochemistry for the detection of two antigens (double labelling), *J. Histochem. Cytochem.* **22(11)**:999–1009.

Gordienko, V. M., and Kosmach, P. I., 1973, Method of enzyme labeling in immunohistochemistry, *Arkh. Patol.* **35(6)**:69–74.

Gould, S. F., and Bernstein, M. H., 1975, The localization of bovine sperm hyaluronidase, *Differentiation* **3(1–3)**:123–132.

Green, J. H., Gray, S. B., Jr., and Harrell, W. K., 1976, Stability of fluorescent antibody conjugates stored under various conditions, *J. Clin. Microbiol.* **3(1)**:1–4.

Haaijman, J. J., and Van Dalen, J. P., 1974, Quantification in immunofluorescence microscopy. A new standard for fluorescein and rhodamine emission measurement, *J. Immunol. Methods* **5(4)**:359–374.

Haglid, K., Carlsson, C. A., and Stavrou, D., 1973, An immunological study of human brain tumors concerning the brain specific proteins S-100 and 14-3-2, *Acta Neuropathol. (Berlin)* **24**:187–196.

Haglid, K., Hamberger, A., Hansson, H.-A., Hyden, H., Persson, L., and Rönnback, L., 1974, S-100 protein in synapses of the central nervous system, *Nature* **251**:532–534.

Haglid, K. G., Hamberger, A., Hansson, H.-A., Hyden, H., Persson, L., and Rönnback, L., 1975, Immunohistochemical localization of S-100 protein in brain, *Nature* **258**:748–749.

Hahon, N., Simpson, J., and Eckert, H. L., 1975, Assessment of virus infectivity by the immunofluorescent and immunoperoxidase techniques, *J. Clin. Microbiol.* **1(3)**:324–329.

Hamanaka, N., Tanizawa, O., Hashimoto, T., Yoshinare, S., and Okudaira, Y., 1971, Electron microscopic study on the localization of human chorionic gonadotropin (HCG) in the chorionic tissue by enzyme-labeled antibody technique, *J. Electron Microsc. (Tokyo)* **20(2)**:128–130.

Hansson, H.-A., Hyden, H., and Rönnback, L., 1975, Localization of S-100 protein in isolated nerve cells by immunoelectron microscopy, *Brain Res.* **93**:349–352.

Hardy, P. H., Petrali, J. P., and Sternberger, L. A., 1970, Postembedding staining for electron microscopy by the unlabeled antibody enzyme method, *J. Histochem. Cytochem.* **18**:678.

Hartman, B. K., 1973, Immunofluorescence of dopamine-*B*-hydroxylase. Application of improved methodology to the localization of the peripheral and central noradrenergic nervous system, *J. Histochem. Cytochem.* **21(4)**:312–332.

Hartman, B. K., and Margolis, F. L., 1975, Immunofluorescence localization of the olfactory marker protein, *Brain Res.* **96**:176–180.

Hartman, B. K., and Udenfriend, S., 1970, Immunofluorescent localization of dopamine-*B*-hydroxylase in tissues, *Mol. Pharmacol.* **6**:85–94.

Hartman, B. K., and Udenfriend, S., 1972, The application of immunological techniques to the study of enzymes regulating catecholamine synthesis and degradation, *Pharmacol. Rev.* **24(2)**:311–330.

Hartman, B. K., Zide, D., and Udenfriend, S., 1972, The use of dopamine-*B*-hydroxylase as a marker for the central noradrenergic nervous system in rat brain, *Proc. Natl. Acad. Sci. U.S.A.* **69(9)**:2722–2726.

Hartman, B. K., Moore, B. W., Shearers, W. T., Fujimoto, K., Kalmbach, S., and Agrawal, H. C., 1976, Biochemical differentiation of brain elements using nervous system specific proteins, *Trans. Am. Soc. Neurochem.* **7**:212.

Hartman, B. K., Cimino, M., Moore, B. W., and Agrawal, H. C., 1977, Immunohistochemical localization of brain specific proteins during development, *Trans. Am. Soc. Neurochem.* **8**:66.

Hashimoto, I., Seki, S., Ogura, H., and Oda, T., 1973, Electron microscopic examination of group-specific antigens in Rous sarcoma cells (mouse ascites) and in Rous sarcoma virus, *Gann* **64(1)**:41–46.

Hattori, T., Singh, V. K., McGeer, E. G., and McGeer, P. L., 1976, Immunohistochemical localization of choline acetyltransferase containing neostriatal neurons and their relationship with dopaminergic synapses, *Brain Res.* **102**:164–173.

Herndon, R. M., Rauch, H. C., and Einstein, E. R., 1973, Immunoelectron microscopic localization of the encephalitogenic basic protein in myelin, *Immunol. Commun.* **2(2)**:163–172.

Herndon, R. M., Rena-Descalzi, L., Griffin, D. E., and Coyle, P. K., 1975, Age dependence of viral expression. Electron microscopic and immunoperoxidase studies of measles virus replication in mice, *Lab. Invest.* **33(5)**:544–553.

Herrmann, J. E., Morse, S. A., and Collins, M. F., 1974, Comparison of techniques and immunoreagents used for indirect immunofluorescence and immunoperoxidase identification of enteroviruses, *Infect. Immun.* **10(1)**:220–226.

Hijams, W., and Schaeffer, M. (eds.), 1975, Fifth International Conference on Immunofluorescence and Related Staining Techniques, *Ann. N.Y. Acad. Sci.* **254.**

Hinton, D. M., Petrali, J. P., Meyer, H. G., and Sternberger, L. A., 1973, The unlabeled antibody enzyme method of immunohistochemistry. Molecular immunocytochemistry of antibodies on the erythrocyte surface, *J. Histochem. Cytochem.* **21(11)**:978–998.

Hirano, A., Becker, N. H., and Zimmerman, H. M., 1969, Isolation of the periaxonal space of the central myelinated nerve fiber with regard to the diffusion of peroxidase, *J. Histochem. Cytochem.* **17**:512–516.

Hirokawa, K., Esaki, Y., and Nariuchi, H., 1973, Role of germinal center in immune response enzyme immunohistochemical study using horseradish peroxidase, *Acta Pathol. Jap.* **23(4)**:739–753.

Hoffman, N. A., and Hartroft, P. M., 1971, Application of peroxidase-labeled antibodies to the localization of renin, *J. Histochem. Cytochem.* **19(12)**:811–813.

Hökfelt, T., Biberfeld, P., and Goldstein, M., 1973*a,* Attempts to trace amine neurons with immunohistochemistry, *J. Ultrastruct. Res.* **44**:437.

Hökfelt, T., Fuxe, K., and Goldstein, M., 1973*b,* Immunohistochemical studies on mono-amine-containing cell systems, *Brain Res.* **62**:461–469.

Hökfelt, T., Fuxe, K., Goldstein, M., and Joh, T. H., 1973*c,* Immunohistochemical localization of three catecholamine synthesizing enzymes: Aspects on methodology, *Histochemie* **33**:231–254.

Hökfelt, T., Efendic, S., Johansson, O., Luft, R., and Arimura, A., 1974*a,* Immunohistochemical localization of somatostatin (growth hormone release-inhibiting factor) in the guinea pig brain, *Brain Res.* **80(1)**:165–169.

Hökfelt, T., Fuxe, K., Goldstein, M., and Johansson, O., 1974*b,* Immunohistochemical evidence for the existence of adrenalin neurons in the rat brain, *Brain Res.* **66**:235–251.

Hökfelt, T., Fuxe, K., and Goldstein, M., 1975*a,* Applications of immunohistochemistry to studies on monoamine cell systems with special reference to nervous tissue, *Ann. N.Y. Acad. Sci.* **254**:407–432.

Hökfelt, T., Kellerth, J.-O., Nilsson, G., and Pernow, B., 1975*b,* Experimental immunohisto-chemical studies on the localization and distribution of substance P in cat primary sensory neurons, *Brain Res.* **100**:235–252.

Hökfelt, T., Elde, R., Johansson, O., Luft, R., Nilsson, G., and Arimura, A., 1976, Immuno-histochemical evidence for separate populations of somatostatin-containing and substance P-containing primary afferent neurons in the rat, *Neuroscience* **1**:131–136.

Holubar, K., Wolff, K., Konrad, K., and Beutner, E. H., 1975, Ultrastructural localization of immunoglobulins in bullous pemphigoid skin. Employment of a new peroxidase–anti-peroxidase multistep method, *J. Invest. Dermatol.* **64(4)**:220–227.

Holubar, K., Stingle, G., and Albini, B., 1976, Letter: Practice and methodology of defined immunofluorescence technic. Concise instructions for the clinical laboratory or medical practice, respectively, *Hautarzt* **27(2)**:78–89.

Honigsmann, H., Holobar, K., Wolff, K., and Beutner, E. H., 1975, Immunochemical localization of *in vivo* bound immunoglobulins in pemphigus vulgaris epidermis. Employ-ment of a peroxidase–antiperoxidase multistep technique for light and electron micros-copy, *Arch. Dermatol. Res.* **254(2)**:113–120.

Hoshino, M., Maeno, K., and Iinuma, M., 1972, Ultrastructural localization of Newcastle disease virus surface antigen in infected HeLa cells as revealed by an enzyme-labelled antibody method, *Experientia* **28(5)**:611–613.

Huang, S. N., 1975, Immunohistochemical demonstration of hepatitis B core and surface antigens in paraffin sections, *Lab. Invest.* **33(1)**:88–95.

Huhn, D., Rodt, H., and Thierfelder, S., 1974*a,* Immunohistochemical investigations in T-lymphocytes of the mouse, *Blut* **28(6)**:415–429.

Huhn, D., Rodt, H., and Thierfelder, S., 1974*b,* Immunohistochemical studies on mouse lymphocytes. Labeling with anti-T and anti-B-cell globulin, *Blut* **29(5)**:332–343.

Huitric, E., 1973, An ultrastructural study of the localization of the carcinoembryonic antigen in adenocarcinomas of the human colon, *Ann. Immunol. (Paris)* **124(4)**:603–608.

Humair, L. M., 1969, Immunohistologic studies of kidney diseases, *J. Urol. Nephrol. (Paris)* **75(4)**:282–284.

Hunter, E. F., 1975, The fluorescent treponemal antibody-absorption (FTA-ABS) test for syphilis, *CRC Crit. Rev. Clin. Lab. Sci.* **5(3)**:315–330.

Huston, J. S., and Bignami, A., 1976, Structural properties of GFA protein from bovine brain, *Fed. Proc.* **35**:1482.

Hyden, H., and Lange, P. W., 1970, S-100 brain protein: Correlation with behavior, *Proc. Natl. Acad. Sci. U.S.A.* **67**:1959–1966.

Hyden, H., and McEwen, B., 1966, A glial protein specific for the nervous system, *Proc. Natl. Acad. Sci. U.S.A.* **55**:354–358.

Hyden, H., and Rönnback, L., 1975, S-100 on isolated neurons and glial cells from rat, rabbit, and guinea pig during early postnatal development, *Neurobiology* **5**:291–302.

Iakovleva, N. I., 1975, Quantitative method for the immunofluorescence reaction with the cerebrospinal fluid of patients with various forms of syphilis, *Vestn. Dermatol. Venerol.* **(2)**:31–36.

Ikonicoff, L. D., and Cedard, L., 1973, Localization of human chorionic gonadotropic and somatomammotropic hormones by the peroxidase immunohistoenzymologic method in villi and amniotic epithelium of human placentas (from 6 weeks to term), *Am. J. Obstet. Gynecol.* **116(8)**:1124–1132.

Ishikawa, H., Smiley, J. D., and Ziff, M., 1975, Electron microscopic demonstration of immunoglobulin deposition in rheumatoid cartilage, *Arthritis Rheum.* **18(6)**:563–576.

Israel, M., and Whittaker, V. P., 1965, Isolation of giant mossy fiber endings from the cerebella from different species, *Experientia* **21**:325–326.

Jenis, E. H., Knieser, M. R., Rothouse, P. A., Jensen, G. E., and Scott, R. M., 1973, Subacute sclerosing panencephalitis. Immunoultrastructural localization of measles-virus antigen, *Arch. Pathol.* **95(2)**:81–89.

Joh, T. H., Shikimi, T., Pickel, V. M., and Rees, D. J., 1975, Brain tryptophan hydroxylase: Purification and production of antibodies to, and cellular and ultrastructural localization in, serotonergic neurons of rat midbrain, *Proc. Natl. Acad. Sci. U.S.A.* **72**:3575.

Johnson, A. B., and Blum, N. R., 1972, Peroxidase-labeled antigens in light and electron immunohistochemistry and the utilization in studies of experimental allergic encephalomyelitis, *Abstr. Histochem. Soc.* **7**:841.

Johnson, A. B., Wisniewski, H. M., Raine, C. S., Eylar, E. H., and Terry, R. D., 1971, Specific binding of peroxidase-labeled myelin basic protein in allergic encephalomyelitis, *Proc. Natl. Acad. Sci. U.S.A.* **68(11)**:2694–2698.

Johnson, L., and Sinex, F. M., 1974, On the relationship of brain filaments to microtubules, *J. Neurochem.* **22**:321–326.

Joncas, J. H., Gilker, J. C., and Chagnon, A., 1974, Limitations of immunofluorescence tests in the diagnosis of infectious mononucleosis, *Can. Med. Assoc. J.* **110(7)**:793–794.

Kalis, J. M., Burgess, A. C., and Balfour, H. H., Jr., 1975, Serological diagnosis of California (La Crosse) encephalitis by immunofluorescence, *J. Clin. Microbiol.* **1(5)**:448–450.

Kan, K.-S. K., Chao, L.-P., and Eng, L. F., 1977, Immunohistochemical localization of choline acetyltransferase in CNS, *Trans. Am. Soc. Neurochem.* **8**:171.

Kan, K.-S. K., Chao, L.-P., and Eng, L. F., 1978, Immunohistochemical localization of choline acetyltransferase in the rabbit cerebellum, *Brain Res.*, **146**:221–229.

Kawaoi, A., 1975, Application of immunofluorescence technique to the endocrine research (author's transl.), *Protein Nucleic Acid Enzyme (Tokyo)* **20(11)**:1014–1020.

Kawarai, Y., and Nakane, P. K., 1970, Localization of tissue antigens on the ultrathin sections with peroxidase-labeled antibody method, *J. Histochem. Cytochem.* **18(3)**:161–166.

King, J. C., and Gerall, A. A., 1976, Localization of luteinizing hormone-releasing hormone, *J. Histochem. Cytochem.* **24(7)**:829–845.

King, J. C., Parsons, J. A., Erlandsen, S. L., and Williams, T. H., 1974, Luteinizing hormone-releasing hormone (LH-RH) pathway of the rat hypothalamus revealed by the unlabeled antibody peroxidase–antiperoxidase method, *Cell Tissue Res.*, **153(2)**:211–217.

King, J. C., Gerall, A. A., Fishback, J. B., and Elkind, K. E., 1975, Growth hormone-release inhibiting hormone (GH-RIH) pathway of the rat hypothalamus revealed by the unlabeled antibody peroxidase–antiperoxidase method, *Cell Tissue Res.* **160(4)**:423–430.

Klein, G., Gergely, L., and Goldstein, G., 1971, Two-color immunofluorescence studies on EBV-determined antigens, *Clin. Exp. Immunol.* **8**:593.

Klockars, M., and Osserman, E. F., 1974, Localization of lysozyme in normal rat tissues by an immunoperoxidase method, *J. Histochem. Cytochem.* **22(3)**:139–146.

Knight, V., Brasier, F., Greenberg, S. B., and Jones, D. B., 1975, Immunofluorescent diagnosis of acute viral infection, *South. Med. J.* **68(6)**:764–766.

Kordon, C., Kerdelhu, E. B., Pattou, E., Jutisz, M., and Sawyer, C. H., 1974, Immunocyto-chemical localization of LH-RH in axons and nerve terminals of the rat median eminence, *Proc. Soc. Exp. Biol. Med.* **147(1)**:122–127.

Kosek, J. C., Bennett, G. S., and Eng, L. F., 1974, Light and electron microscopic localization of antigen alpha by immunoenzymatic techniques, *Trans. Am. Soc. Neurochem.* **5**:167.

Koshi, G., and Chacko, J., 1971, Rapid diagnosis of bacterial meningitis by the fluorescent-antibody (FA) technique, *Indian J. Med. Res.* **59(7)**:996–1001.

Kraehenbuhl, J. P., and Jamieson, J. D., 1974, Localization of intracellular antigens by immunoelectron microscopy, *Int. Rev. Exp. Pathol.* **13(0)**:1–53.

Kraehenbuhl, J. P., De Grandi, P. B., and Campiche, M. A., 1971, Ultrastructural localization of intracellular antigen using enzyme-labeled antibody fragments, *J. Cell Biol.* **50(2)**:432–445.

Kraicer, J., Gosbee, J. L., and Bencosme, S. A., 1973, Pars intermedia and pars distalis: Two sites of ACTH production in the rat hypophysis, *Neuroendocrinology* **11(3)**:156–176.

Kuhlmann, W. D., and Miller, H. R., 1971, A comparative study of the techniques for ultrastructural localization of antienzyme antibodies, *J. Ultrastruct. Res.* **35(3)**:370–385.

Kuhlmann, W. D., Avrameas, S., and Ternynck, T., 1974, A comparative study for ultrastruc-tural localization of intracellular immunoglobulins using peroxidase conjugates, *J. Immunol. Methods* **5(1)**:33–48.

Lai, C. H., Listgarten, M. A., and Rosan, B., 1975, Immunoelectron microscopic identification and localization of *Streptococcus sanguis* with peroxidase-labeled antibody: Localization of *Streptococcus sanguis* in intact dental plaque, *Infect. Immun.* **11(1)**:200–210.

Lee, J. C., Frigon, R. P., and Timasheff, S. N., 1973, The chemical characterization of calf brain microtubule protein subunits, *J. Biol. Chem.* **248**:7253–7262.

Lee, Y.-L., Eng, L. F., and Miles, L. E. M., 1976, Extraction and immunologic identity of "soluble" and "insoluble" GFA protein, *Trans. Am. Soc. Neurochem.* **7**:240.

Lennon, V. R., Wittingham, J., Carnegie, P. R., McPherson, T. A., and Mackay, I. R., 1971, Detection of antibodies to the basic protein of human myelin by radioimmunoassay and immunofluorescence, *J. Immunol.* **107**:56–62.

Levaditi, J. C., Atanasio, P., Gamet, A., and Guillon, J. C., 1971, Diagnosis of rabies. Problems arising from the immunofluorescence and immunoperoxidase methods, *Arch. Inst. Pasteur Alger.* **49**:75–83.

Levaditi, J. C., Atanasio, P., Gamet, A., and Guillon, J. C., 1973, Diagnosis of rabies by the immunofluorescence and immunoperoxidase methods, *Bull. Soc. Pathol. Exot.* **66(1)**:12–20.

Liao, C. L., Herman, M. M., Bensch, K. G., and Eng, L. F., 1977, Glial fibrillary acidic protein content in rat C-6 glioma cells *in vitro*, *Trans. Am. Soc. Neurochem.* **8**:141.

Liao, C. L., Eng, L. F., Herman, M. M., and Bensch, K. G., 1978, Localization and solubility of glial fibrillary acidic protein in rat C-6 glioma cells. An immunohistologic and immuno-radiometric study, *J. Neurochem.*, in press.

Linthicum, D. S., and Sell, S., 1975, Topography of lymphocyte surface immunoglobulin using scanning immunoelectron microscopy, *J. Ultrastruct. Res.* **51(1)**:55–68.

Liu, C., 1975, Rapid diagnosis of viral infections, *South. Med. J.* **68(6)**:679–680.

Luders, G., and Adam, W., 1972, Current applications and results of immunofluorescence technic in dermatology, venereology, and andrology, *Z. Haut. Geschlechtskr.* **47(10)**:479–490.

Luduena, R. F., and Woodward, D., 1973, Isolation and partial characterization of alpha and beta tubulin from outer doublets of sea urchin sperm and microtubules of chick embryo brain, *Proc. Natl. Acad. Sci. U.S.A.* **70**:3594–3598.

Ludwin, S. K., Eng, L. F., Vandenberg, S. R., Kosek, J. C., and Herman, M. M., 1976a, Glial differentiation in an experimental mouse teratoma, *J. Neuropathol. Exp. Neurol.* **35**:102.

Ludwin, S. K., Kosek, J. C., and Eng, L. F., 1976b, The topographical distribution of S-100 and GFA proteins in the adult rat brain: An immunohistochemical study using horseradish peroxidase-labeled antibodies, *J. Comp. Neurol.* **165**:197–208.

Mannik, M., and Downey, W., 1973, Studies on the conjugation of horseradish peroxidase to Fab fragments, *J. Immunol. Methods* **3(3)**:233–241.

Marangos, P. J., Zomzely-Neurath, C., Luk, C. M., and York, C., 1975, Isolation and characterization of the nervous system-specific protein 14-3-2 from rat brain, *J. Biol. Chem.* **250**:1884–1891.

Margolis, F. L., 1972, A brain protein unique to the olfactory bulb, *Proc. Natl. Acad. Sci. U.S.A.* **69(5)**:1221–1224.

Marucci, A. A., and Dougherty, R. M., 1975, Use of the unlabeled antibody immunohistochemical technique for the detection of human antibody, *J. Histochem. Cytochem.* **23(8)**:618–623.

Marucci, A. A., Di Stefano, H. S., and Dougherty, R. M., 1974, Preparation and use of soluble ferritin–antiferritin complexes as a specific marker for immunoelectron microscopy, *J. Histochem. Cytochem.* **22(1)**:35–39.

Mason, D. Y., and Taylor, C. R., 1975, The distribution of muramidase (lysozyme) in human tissues, *J. Clin. Pathol.* **28(2)**:124–132.

Mason, D. Y., Farrell, C., and Taylor, C. R., 1975, The detection of intracellular antigens in human leucocytes by immunoperoxidase staining, *Br. J. Haematol.* **31(3)**:361–370.

Matus, A., and Mughal, S., 1975, Immunohistochemical localisation of S-100 protein in brain, *Nature* **258**:746–748.

McCaman, R. E., and Hunt, J. M., 1965, Microdetermination of choline acetylase in nervous tissue, *J. Neurochem.* **12**:253–259.

McCloskey, R. T., 1971, The value of immunofluorescence in the study of human renal disease, *J. Exp. Med.* **134(3)**:Suppl. 242S+.

McGeer, P. L., McGeer, E. G., Singh, V. K., and Chase, W. H., 1974, Choline acetyltransferase localization in the central nervous system by immunohistochemistry, *Brain Res.* **81**:373–379.

McKinney, R. M., and Spillane, J. T., 1975, An approach to quantitation in rhodamine isothiocyanate labeling, *Ann. N.Y. Acad. Sci.* **254**:55–64.

McKinney, R., Thacker, L., and Hebert, G. A., 1976, Conjugation methods in immunofluorescence, *J. Dent. Res.* **55**:A38–A44.

McLaughlin, B. J., Wood, J. G., Saito, K., Barker, R., Vaughn, J. E., Roberts, E., and Wu, J.-Y., 1974, The fine structural localization of glutamate decarboxylase in synaptic terminals of rodent cerebellum, *Brain Res.* **76**:377–391.

McLean, I. W., and Nakane, P. K., 1974, Periodate-lysine-paraformaldehyde fixative. A new fixation for immunoelectron microscopy, *J. Histochem. Cytochem.* **22(12)**:1077–1083.

Michetti, F., Miani, N., De Renzis, G., Caniglia, A., and Correr, S., 1974, Nuclear localization of S-100 protein, *J. Neurochem.* **22**:239–244.

Miller, H. R., 1972, Fixation and tissue preservation for antibody studies, *Histochem. J.* **4(4)**:305–320.

Modesto, R. R., and Pesce, A. J., 1973, Use of toluene diisocyanate for the preparation of a peroxidase-labelled antibody conjugate. Quantitation of the amount of diisocyanate bound, *Biochim. Biophys. Acta* **295(1)**:283–295.

Moore, B. W., 1965, A soluble protein characteristic of the nervous system, *Biochem. Biophys. Res. Commun.* **19**:739–744.

Moore, B. W., and Perez, V. J., 1968, Specific acidic proteins of the nervous system, in: *Physiological and Biochemical Aspects of Nervous Integration* (F. D. Carlson, ed.), pp. 343–360, Prentice-Hall, Englewood Cliffs, N.J.

Morgan, C., Hsu, K. C., Rifkind, R. A., Knox, A. W., and Rose, H. M., 1961, The application of ferritin-conjugated antibody to electron microscopic studies of influenza virus in infected cells. II. The interior of the cell, *J. Exp. Med.* **114**:833.

Mori, T., and Morimoto, K., 1973, Astroprotein, an astrocyte-specific cerebroprotein, in normal brain and glioma, Fourth International Meeting of the International Society for Neurochemistry, Tokyo, Abstract, p. 174.

Mori, T., and Morimoto, K., 1975, Studies on the identity of astroprotein, *Igaku-no-ayumi* **92**:16–17.

Mori, T., Morimoto, K., Ushio, Y., Hayakawa, T., and Mogami, H., 1975, Radioimmunoassay of astroprotein (an astrocyte-specific cerebroprotein) in cerebrospinal fluid from patients with glioma: A preliminary study, *Neurol. Med. Chir.* **15**:23–25.

Moriarty, G. C., and Halmi, N. S., 1972, Electron microscopic study of the adrenocorticotropin-producing cell with the use of unlabeled antibody and the soluble peroxidase–antiperoxidase complex, *J. Histochem. Cytochem.* **20(8)**:590–603.

Moriarty, G. C., Moriarty, C. M., and Sternberger, L. A., 1973, Ultrastructural immunocytochemistry with unlabeled antibodies and the peroxidase–antiperoxidase complex. A technique more sensitive than radioimmunoassay, *J. Histochem. Cytochem.* **21(9)**:825–833.

Moroashi, I., Kinoshita, Y., and Kujima, K., 1971, Application of enzyme-labeled antibody technic to the renal tissue—Observation of the light microscopy level and comparison with findings in fluorescent antibody technic, *Jap. J. Allergy* **20(5)**:353–360.

Nagatsu, I., and Kondo, Y., 1974, Immunoelectronmicroscopic localization of phenylethanolamine-*N*-methyltransferase in the bovine adrenal medulla, *Histochemie* **42(4)**:351–358.

Nairn, R. C., and Morrack, J. R., 1969, *Fluorescent Protein Tracing,* Williams & Wilkins, Baltimore.

Nairn, R. C., Rolland, J. M., Ward, H. A., Matthews, N., and Chalmers, P. J., 1975, Immunofluorescence in cancer investigation and research, *Ann. N.Y. Acad. Sci.* **254**:523–527.

Nakane, P. K., 1968, Simultaneous localization of multiple tissue antigens using the peroxidase-labeled antibody method: A study on pituitary glands of the rat, *J. Histochem. Cytochem.* **16(9)**:557–560.

Nakane, P. K., 1970, Classifications of anterior pituitary cell types with immunoenzyme histochemistry, *J. Histochem. Cytochem.* **18(1)**:9–20.

Nakane, P. K., 1971, Application of peroxidase-labelled antibodies to the intracellular localization of hormones, *Acta Endocrinol. (Copenhagen), Suppl.* **153**:190–204.

Nakane, P. K., 1973, *Electron Microscopy and Cytochemistry* (E. Wisse, W. T. Daems, I. Molenaar, and P. van Duijn, eds.), pp. 129–143, North-Holland, Amsterdam.

Nakane, P. K., 1975, Localization of hormones with the peroxidase-labeled antibody method, *Methods Enzymol.* **37** Pt.B:133–144.

Nakane, P. K., and Kawaoi, A., 1974, Peroxidase-labeled antibody. A new method of conjugation, *J. Histochem. Cytochem.* **22(12)**:1084–1091.

Nakane, P. K., and Pierce, G. B., Jr., 1966, Enzyme-labeled antibodies: Preparation and application for localization of antigens, *J. Histochem. Cytochem.* **14**:929.

Nakane, P. K., and Pierce, G. B., Jr., 1967, Enzyme-labeled antibodies for the light and electron microscopic localization of tissue antigens, *J. Cell Biol.* **33(2)**:307–318.

Nayak, N. C., and Sachdeva, R., 1975, Localization of hepatitis B surface antigen in conventional paraffin sections of the liver. Comparison of immunofluorescence, immunoperoxidase, and orcein staining methods with regard to their specificity and reliability as antigen marker, *Am. J. Pathol.* **81(3)**:479–492.

Osada, H., 1976, Further purification and immunohistological localization of human placental lactogen in syncytiotrophoblasts (author's transl.), *Folia Endocrinol. Jpn.* **52(1)**:36–53.

Parsons, J. A., and Erlandsen, S. L., 1974, Ultrastructural immunocytochemical localization of prolactin in rat anterior pituitary by use of the unlabeled antibody enzyme method, *J. Histochem. Cytochem.* **22(5)**:340–351.

Parsons, J. A., Erlandsen, S. L., and Debault, L. E., 1974, Identification of prolactin cells in a mammosomatotropic tumor by the unlabeled-antibody peroxidase–antiperoxidase method, *Proc. Soc. Exp. Biol. Med.* **145(2)**:524–527.

Parsons, J. A., Erlandsen, S. L., Hegre, O. D., McEvoy, R. C., and Elde, R. P., 1976, Central and peripheral localization of somatostatin immunoenzyme immunocytochemical studies, *J. Histochem. Cytochem.* **24(7)**:872–882.

Patramanis, I., Marketakis, J., Kaklamanis, E., Tzamouranis, N., and Pavlatos, M., 1973, The application of the immunoenzyme method in microbiology, *J. Immunol. Methods* **2(3)**:251–260.

Pearse, A. F. E., 1968, *Histochemistry,* Little, Brown, Boston, Mass.

Pelletier, G., Leclerc, R., Labrie, F., and Puviani, R., 1974a, Electron microscopic immunohistochemical localization of neurophysin in the rat hypothalamus and median eminence, *Mol. Cell. Endocrinol.* **1**:157–166.

Pelletier, G., Labrie, F., Arimura, A., and Schally, A. V., 1974b, Electron microscopic immunohistochemical localization of growth hormone-release inhibitor hormone (somatostatin) in the rat median eminence, *Am. J. Anat.* **140**:445–450.

Pelletier, G., Labrie, F., Puviani, R., Arimura, A., and Schally, A. V., 1974c, Immunohistochemical localization of luteinizing hormone-release hormone in the rat median eminence, *Endocrinology* **95**:314–317.

Pelletier, G., Leclerc, R., Dube, D., Labrie, F., Puviani, R., Arimura, A., and Schally, A. V., 1975, Localization of growth hormone release-inhibiting hormone (somatostatin) in the rat brain, *Am. J. Anat.* **142(3)**:397–401.

Pelletier, G., Leclerc, R., and Dube, D., 1976, Immunohistochemical localization of hypothalamic hormones, *J. Histochem. Cytochem.* **24(7)**:864–871.

Perez, V. J., Olney, J. W., Cicero, T. J., Moore, B. W., and Bahn, B. A., 1970, Wallerian degeneration in rabbit optic nerve: Cellular localization in the central nervous system of the S-100 and 14-3-2 proteins, *J. Neurochem.* **17**:511–519.

Pernis, B., Forni, L., and Amant, L., 1970, Immunoglobulin spots on the surface of rabbit lymphocytes, *J. Exp. Med.* **132**:1001.

Peterson, J. W., Lospalloto, J. J., and Finkelstein, R. A., 1972, Localization of cholera toxin *in vivo, J. Infect. Dis.* **126(6)**:617–628.

Petrali, J. P., Hinton, D. M., Moriarty, G. C., and Sternberger, L. A., 1974, The unlabeled antibody enzyme method of immunocytochemistry. Quantitative comparison of sensitivities with and without peroxidase–antiperoxidase complex, *J. Histochem. Cytochem.* **22(8)**:782–801.

Petrusz, P., Dimeo, P., Ordronneau, P., Weaver, C., and Keefer, D. A., 1975, Improved immunoglobulin–enzyme bridge method for light microscopic demonstration of hormone-containing cells of the rat adenohypophysis, *Hisp. Med.* **46(1)**:9–26.

Phifer, R. F., Midgley, A. R., and Spicer, S. S., 1973, Immunohistologic and histologic evidence that follicle-stimulating hormone and leuteinizing hormone are present in the same cell type in the human pars distalis, *J. Clin. Endocrinol. Metab.* **36(1)**:125–141.

Pickel, V. M., Joh, T. H., and Reis, D. J., 1975a, Ultrastructural localization of tyrosine hydroxylase in noradrenergic neurons of brain, *Proc. Natl. Acad. Sci. U.S.A.* **72(2)**:659–663.

Pickel, V. M., Joh, T. H., Field, P. M., Becker, C. G., and Reis, D. J., 1975b, Cellular localization of tyrosine hydroxylase by immunohistochemistry, *J. Histochem. Cytochem.* **23(1)**:1–12.

Pickel, V. M., Joh, T. H., and Reis, D. J., 1976a, Monoamine-synthesizing enzymes in central dopaminergic noradrenergic and serotonergic neurons. Immunocytochemical localization by light and electron microscopy, *J. Histochem. Cytochem.* **24(7)**:792–806.

Pickel, V. M., Reis, D. J., Marangos, P. J., and Zomzely-Neurath, C., 1976b, Immunocytochemical localization of nervous system specific protein (NSP-R) in rat brain, *Brain Res.* **105**:184–187.

Pickel, V. M., Reis, D. J., and Leeman, S. E., 1977, Ultrastructural localization of substance P in neurons of rat spinal cord, *Brain Res.* **122**:534–540.

Primus, F. J., Wang, R. H., Sharkey, R. M., and Goldenberg, D. M., 1975, Detection of carcinoembryonic antigen in tissue section by immunoperoxidase, *Immunol. Methods* **8(3)**:267–275.

Rapport, M. M., Laer, H., Mahadik, S., and Graf, L., 1974, Immunohistological appearance of the S-100 protein in developing rat brain, *Trans. Am. Soc. Neurochem.* **5**:58.

Rauch, H. C., and Raffel, S., 1964, Immunofluorescent localization of encephalitogenic protein in myelin, *J. Immunol.* **92**:452–455.

Reis, D. J., Pickel, V. M., Shikimi, T., and Joh, T. H., 1975, Rat brain tryptophan hydroxylase: Immunohistochemical localization by light and electron microscopy, *Trans. Am. Soc. Neurochem.* **6(1)**:155.

Riggs, J. L., Loh, P. C., and Eveland, W. C., 1960, A simple fractionation method for preparation of fluorescein-labelled gamma globulin, *Proc. Soc. Exp. Biol.* **105**:655–658.

Robinson, G., and Dawson, I., 1975, Immunochemical studies of the endocrine cells of the gastrointestinal tract. II. An immunoperoxidase technique for the localization of secretin-containing cells in human duodenum, *J. Clin. Pathol.* **28(8)**:631–635.

Rojas-Espinosa, O., Dannenberg, J., Sternberger, L. A., and Tsuda, T., 1974, The role of cathepsin D in the pathogenesis of tuberculosis, *Am. J. Pathol.* **74(1)**:1–12.

Rombert, P. C., 1974, Contribution of immunofluorescence to the diagnosis of helminthiasis, *An. Inst. Hig. Med. Trop. (Lisb.)* **2(1–4)**:201–310.

Rothbarth, P. H., Olthof, J., and Mul, N. A. J., 1975, Experience with a new fluorochrome, in: "Fifth International Conference on Immunofluorescence and Related Staining Techniques," *Ann. N.Y. Acad. Sci.* **254**:65.

Ruitenberg, E. J., Ljungstr, O. M., Steerenberg, P. A., and Buys, J., 1975, Application of immunofluorescence and immunoenzyme methods in the serodiagnosis of trichinella spiralis infection, *Ann. N.Y. Acad. Sci.* **254**:296–303.

Saito, K., Barber, R., Wu, J.-Y., Vaughn, J. E., and Roberts, E., 1974a, Immunohistochemical localization of glutamic acid decarboxylase in rat central nervous system at light microscopic level, *Trans. Am. Soc. Neurochem.* **5(1)**:113.

Saito, K., Barber, R., Wu, J.-Y., Matsuda, T., and Vaughn, J. E., 1974b, Immunohistochemical localization of glutamate decarboxylase in rat cerebellum, *Proc. Natl. Acad. Sci. U.S.A.* **71(2)**:269–273.

Saunders, G. C., and Wilder, M. E., 1974, Disease screening with enzyme-labeled antibodies, *J. Infect. Dis.* **129(3)**:362–364.

Schenk, E. A., and Churukian, C. J., 1974, Immunofluorescence counterstains, *J. Histochem. Cytochem.* **22(10)**:962–966.

Shinski, G. E., and Rusina, L. I., 1975, Value of the immunofluorescence reaction in the diagnosis of syphilis by study of the cerebrospinal fluid, *Lab. Delo* **11**:694–695.

Short, J. A., and Walker, P. D., 1975, The location of bacterial antigens on sections of *Bacillus cereus* by use of the soluble peroxidase–antiperoxidase complex and unlabelled antibody, *J. Gen. Microbiol.* **89(1)**:93–101.

Siggins, G. R., Battenberg, E. F., Hoffer, B. J., and Bloom, F. E., 1973, Noradrenergic stimulation of cyclic adenosine monophosphate in rat Purkinje neurons: An immunocytochemical study, *Science* **177**:585–588.

Silverman, A. J., 1976, Ultrastructural studies on the localization of neurohypophyseal hormones and their carrier proteins, *J. Histochem. Cytochem.* **24(7)**:816–827.

Silverman, A. J., and Zimmerman, E. A., 1975, Ultrastructural immunocytochemical localization of neurophysin and vasopressin in the median eminence and posterior pituitary of the guinea pig, *Cell Tissue Res.* **159(3)**:291–301.

Silverman, A. J., Koyolowski, G. P., and Zimmerman, E. A., 1975, Ultrastructural immunocytochemical localization of neurophysin (NP) and vasopressin (VP) in the neural lobe and median eminence of guinea pig, *Anat. Rec.* **181**:479–480.

Singer, S. J., 1975, Present capabilities and future prospects of high resolution immunoelectron microscopy, *Immunochemistry* **12(6–7)**:615–616.

Smit, J. W., Meijer, C. J., Decary, F., and Feltkamp-Vroom, T. M., 1974, Paraformaldehyde fixation in immunofluorescence and immunoelectron microscopy. Preservation of tissue and cell surface membrane antigens, *J. Immunol. Methods* **6(1–2)**:93–98.

Springer, E. L., Riggs, J. L., and Hackett, A. J., 1974, Viral identification by scanning electron microscopy of preparations stained with fluorescein-labelled antibody, *J. Virol.* **14(6)**:1623–1626.

Stauffer, L. R., Hill, E. D., Holland, J. W., and Altemeier, W. A., 1975, Indirect fluorescent antibody procedure for the rapid detection and identification of bacteroides and fusobacterium in clinical specimens, *J. Clin. Microbiol.* **2(4)**:337–344.

Stein, H., and Drescher, S., 1973, Demonstration of surface IgM in blood lymphocytes using the immunoperoxidase method, *Blut* **26(1)**:35–42.

Sternberger, L. A., 1969, Some new developments in immunocytochemistry, *Mikroscopie* **25**:346–361.

Sternberger, L. A., 1974, *Immunocytochemistry*, Prentice-Hall, Englewood Cliffs, N.J.

Sternberger, L. A., and Petrali, J. P., 1975, Quantitative immunocytochemistry of pituitary receptors for leutenizing hormone-releasing hormone, *Cell Tissue Res.* **162(2)**:141–176.

Sternberger, L. A., Hanker, J. S., Donati, E. J., Petrali, J. P., and Seligman, A. M., 1966, Method for enchancement of electron microscopic visualization of embedded antigen by bridging osmium to uranium antibody with thiocarbohydrazide, *J. Histochem. Cytochem.* **14(10)**:711–718.

Sternberger, L. A., Hardy, P. H., Jr., Cuculis, J. J., and Meyer, H. G., 1970, The unlabelled antibody enzyme method of immunohistochemistry: Preparation and properties of soluble antigen–antibody complex (horseradish peroxidase–antihorseradish peroxidase) and its use in identification of spirochetes, *J. Histochem. Cytochem.* **18(5)**:315–333.

Sternberger, N., Tabira, T., Kies, M. W., and Webster, H., 1977, Immunocytochemical staining of basic protein in CNS myelin, *Trans. Am. Soc. Neurochem.* **8(2)**:157 (Abstract 180).

Storch, H., 1972, Immune enzyme technic, *Z. Gesamte Inn. Med.* **27(14)**:589–594.

Straus, W., 1972, Improved staining for peroxidase with benzidine and improved double staining immunoperoxidase procedures, *J. Histochem. Cytochem.* **20(4)**:272–278.

Striker, G. E., Donati, E. J., Petrali, J. P., and Sternberger, L. A., 1966, Post-embedding staining for electron microscopy with ferritin–antibody conjugates, *Exp. Mol. Pathol. Suppl.* **3**:52–58.

Sviridov, S. M., Dorochkin, L. I., Ivano, V. N., Maletskaya, E. I., and Bakhtina, T. K., 1972, Immunohistochemical studies of S-100 protein during postnatal ontogenesis of the brain of two strains of rats, *J. Neurochem.* **19**:713–718.

Swaab, D. F., Pool, C. W., and Nijveldt, F., 1975, Immunofluorescence of vasopressin and oxytocin in the rat hypothalamo-neurohypophyseal system, *J. Neural Transm.* **36**(3–4):195–215.

Swanson, L. W., and Hartman, B. K., 1975, The central adrenergic system; an immunofluorescence study of the location of cell bodies and their efferent connections in the rat utilizing dopamine-β-hydroxylase as a marker, *J. Comp. Neurol.* **163**:467.

Tabuchi, K., and Kirsch, W. M., 1975, Immunocytochemical localization of S-100 in neurons and glia of hamster cerebellum, *Brain Res.* **92**:175–180.

Tabuchi, K., Lehman, J. M., and Kirsch, W. M., 1976, Immunocytochemical localization of simian virus 40 T antigen with peroxidase-labelled antibody fragments, *J. Virol.* **17**(2):668–671.

Taylor, C. E., 1975, Quantitative immunofluorescence studies: A contribution towards standardization, in: *Current Studies on Standardization Problems in Clinical Pathology, Haematology, and Radiotherapy in Hodgkin's Disease* (G. Astaldi, ed.), pp. 73–77, Excerpta Medica, Amsterdam.

Taylor, C. E., and Heimer, G. V., 1974, Measuring immunofluorescence emission in terms of standard international physical units, *J. Biol. Stand.* **2**(1):11–20.

Taylor, C. R., 1974, The nature of Reed-Sternberg cells and other malignant reticulum cells, *Lancet* **2**(7884):802–807.

Taylor, C. R., and Burns, J., 1974, The demonstration of plasma cells and other immunoglobulin-containing cells in formalin-fixed, paraffin-embedded tissues using peroxidase-labelled antibody, *J. Clin. Pathol.* **27**(1):14–20.

Taylor, C. R., and Mason, D. Y., 1974, The immunohistological detection of intracellular immunoglobulin in formalin-paraffin sections from multiple myeloma and related conditions using the immunoperoxidase technique, *Clin. Exp. Immunol.* **18**(3):417–429.

Thomason, B. M., and Herbert, G. A., 1974, Evaluation of commercial conjugates for fluorescent antibody detection of salmonellae, *Appl. Microbiol.* **27**(5):862–869.

Tixier-Vidal, A., Tougard, C., Kerdelhue, B., and Jutisz, M., 1975, Light and electron microscopic studies on immunocytochemical localization of gonadotropic hormones in the rat pituitary gland with antisera against bovine FSH, LH, LH alpha, and LH beta, *Ann. N.Y. Acad. Sci.* **254**:433–461.

Torack, R. M., Stranahan, P., and Hartman, B. K., 1973, The role of norepinephrine in the function of the area postrema. I. Immunofluorescent localization of dopamine-B-hydroxylase and electron microscopy, *Brain Res.* **61**:235–252.

Ueki, H., Wolff, H. H., and Braun-Falco, O., 1974, Cutaneous localization of human gamma-globulins in lupus erythematosus. An electron-microscopical study using the peroxidase-labeled antibody technique, *Arch. Dermatol. Forsch.* **248**(4):297–314.

Uyeda, C. T., Eng, L. F., and Bignami, A., 1972, Immunological study of the glial fibrillary acidic protein, *Brain Res.* **37**:81–89.

Vandenberg, S. R., Ludwin, S. K., Herman, M. M., and Bignami, A., 1976, *In vitro* astrocytic differentiation from embryoid bodies of an experimental mouse testicular teratoma, *Am. J. Pathol.* **83**:197–212.

Vandesande, F., Dierickx, K., and Demey, J., 1975, Identification of the vasopressin-neurophysin II and the oxytocin-neurophysin I producing neurons in the bovine hypothalamus, *Cell Tissue Res.* **156**(2):189–200.

Vinogradov, V. I. A., 1974, Method of controlled conjugation of fluorescein isothiocyanate with anti-influenza horse gamma globulin, *Lab. Delo* **7**(9):403–405.

Vladutio, G. D., Bigazzi, P. E., and Rose, N. R., 1973, Localization of a primate-specific esterase using immunofluorescence and immunoperoxidase techniques, *J. Histochem. Cytochem.* **21(6)**:559–567.

Wagner, B., and Wagner, M., 1972, Immunoelectron microscopic localization of cell wall antigens in streptococci. I. Comparative demonstration of M protein of *Streptococcus pyogenes* with ferritin-, peroxidase-, and ferrocin-labelled antibodies, *Zentralbl. Bakteriol. [Orig. A]* **222(4)**:468–483.

Wajgt, A., 1971, Immunofluorescence: Its use in neurological diagnostics and neuropathological studies, *Neurol. Neurochir. Pol.* **5(6)**:881–887.

Watkins, W. B., 1975a, Presence of neurophysin and vasopressin in the hypothalamic magnocellular nuclei of rats homozygous and heterozygous for diabetes insipidus (Brattleboro strain) as revealed by immunoperoxidase history, *Cell Tissue Res.* **157(1)**:101–113.

Watkins, W. B., 1975b, Immunocytochemical identification of neurophysin-secreting neurons in the hypothalamo-neurohypophyseal system of some non-mammalian vertebrates, *Cell Tissue Res.* **162(4)**:511–521.

Watkins, W. B., 1975c, Time of fixation and the localization of Gomori-positive and neurophysin-containing structures in the rat hypothalamus, *Cell Tissue Res.* **162(4)**:523–530.

Watson, S. J., and Barchas, J. D., 1977, Catecholamine histofluorescence using cryostat and glyoxylic acid on unperfused frozen brain: A detailed description of the technique, *Histochem. J.* **9(2)**:183–195.

Whitaker, J. N., 1976, The effects of glutaraldehyde treatment and horseradish peroxidase conjugation on the immunoreactivity of bovine myelin encephalitogenic protein, *J. Histochem. Cytochem.* **24(5)**:652–655.

Wicker, R., 1971, Comparison of immunofluorescent and immunoenzymatic techniques applied to the study of viral antigens, *Ann. N.Y. Acad. Sci.* **177**:490–500.

Wilkinson, A. E., 1973, Fluorescent treponemal antibody tests on cerebrospinal fluid, *Br. J. Vener. Dis.* **49(4)**:346–349.

Wilson, C. B., 1975, Immunofluorescence in differentiating the immunopathogenesis of renal disease, *Ariz. Med.* **32(4)**:283–289.

Wilson, C. E., Donati, E. J., Petrali, J. P., Voicich, J. V., and Sternberger, L. A., 1966, Cytochemical timing of ultrastructural events: Formation of bacterial flagella studied by immunouranium technique, *Exp. Mol. Pathol. Suppl.* **3**:44–51.

Wolff-Schreiner, E., and Wolff, K., 1973, Immunoglobulins at the dermal–epidermal junction in lupus erythematosus: Ultrastructural investigations, *Arch. Dermatol. Forsch.* **246(3)**:193–210.

Wood, J. G., 1976, Recent results in the electron microscopic localization of enzymes associated with the GABA system, *Trans. Am. Soc. Neurochem.* **7(1)**:210 (Abstract 273).

Wood, J. G., McLaughlin, B. J., Saito, K., Roberts, E., and Wu, J.-Y., 1974, Fine structural localization of glutamic acid decarboxylase in rodent cerebellum and spinal cord, *Trans. Am. Soc. Neurochem.* **5(1)**:114.

Yen, S.-H., Dahl, D., Schachner, M., and Shelanski, M. L., 1976, Biochemistry of the filaments of brain, *Proc. Natl. Acad. Sci. U.S.A.* **73**:529–533.

Yokota, S., and Nagata, T., 1974, Ultrastructural localization of catalase on ultracryotomic sections of mouse liver by ferritin-conjugated antibody technique, *Histochemistry* **40(2)**:165–174.

Zeitoun, P., Duclert, N., Liautaud, F., Potet, F., and Zylberberg, L., 1972, Intracellular localization of pepsinogen in guinea pig pyloric mucosa by immunohistochemistry: Histochemical and electron microscopic correlated structures, *Lab. Invest.* **27(2)**:218–225.

Zimmerman, E. A., and Antunes, J. L., 1976, Organization of the hypothalamic-pituitary system: Current concepts from immunohistochemical studies, *J. Histochem. Cytochem.* **24**(7):807–815.

Zimmerman, E. A., Hsu, K. C., Robinson, A. G., Carmel, P. W., Frantz, A. G., and Tannenbaum, M., 1973, Studies of neurophysin-secreting neurons with immunoperoxidase techniques employing antibody to bovine neurophysin. I. Light microscopic findings in monkey and bovine tissues, *Endocrinology* **92**(3):931–940.

Zomzely-Neurath, C., Marangos, P., and Keller, A., 1977, Nervous system-specific proteins and cerebral function, *Trans. Am. Soc. Neurochem.* **8**:65.

CHAPTER 3

MACROMOLECULAR COMPOSITION AND FUNCTIONAL ORGANIZATION OF SYNAPTIC STRUCTURES

SAHEBARAO P. MAHADIK, HADASSAH TAMIR, AND MAURICE M. RAPPORT

Division of Neuroscience
New York State Psychiatric Institute
and
Department of Biochemistry
Columbia University College of Physicians and Surgeons
New York, New York

1. INTRODUCTION

There is general agreement that what makes the nervous system so special has its highest form of expression in synaptic connections. These minute regions located either between nerve cells or at neuromuscular junctions present a great challenge to neurochemists because of the formidable obstacles that must be overcome to determine their structure and functional organization. Although we have made tremendous advances over the past

99

20 years in delineating mechanisms concerned with chemical neurotrans-mitters—mechanisms of biosynthesis, catabolism, storage, release, agonist action, and reuptake—we have learned precious little about the chemical composition and molecular organization of the synaptic structures them-selves, of the axon terminals, postsynaptic differentiations, and intersynap-tic material where all the activity of chemical transmission is taking place. Demand for this information is increasing, since investigators in the more biological disciplines now recognize that molecular organization contains the key for solving many of the enigmas associated with synaptogenesis, neural plasticity, and learning.

It would be sufficiently challenging if there were only a single type of synapse whose neurochemical aspects we had to explore, but morpholo-gists can now clearly distinguish at least two distinct types: one, asymmet-rical, with well-defined synaptic thickenings and spherical vesicles, such as those found on the dendritic spines of pyramidal cells; and the other, symmetrical, with poorly defined thickenings and flattened vesicles, most often found on cell bodies. It is reasonable to expect that with careful examination of different brain regions, with the sorting out of excitatory and inhibitory functions and the assignment of specific neurotransmitter systems to them, more elaborate distinctions between different types of synapses will be made.

The feasibility of examining the chemical composition of such minute structures is a tribute to the pioneering studies of Gray and Whittaker (1962) and of De Robertis *et al.* (1962) who showed, about 15 years ago, that pinched-off axon terminals could be obtained as subcellular fractions after careful disruption of brain tissue. With ultracentrifugation as the basic tool for preparing subcellular fractions, neurochemists have been able to study an ever increasing number of the molecular constituents of synaptic structures, adopting such additional techniques as tissue culture, autora-diography, electron microscopy, histochemistry, microdissection, immu-nochemistry, and electrophoresis.

In this chapter we, for the most part, restrict our attention to synaptic structures from the mammalian central nervous system (CNS). Studies of nonmammalian nervous tissues are still limited, whereas the characteriza-tion of neuromuscular junctions is a chapter in itself. The task of reviewing this area was made simpler but much more challenging by the critical and scholarly examination of synapses published by Jones (1975), the summary of Mahler *et al.* (1975) of their studies on synaptic membranes, and the thoughtful review presented by Barondes (1974).

We are mainly concerned here with the preparation and characteriza-tion of synaptic structures, with macromolecules which appear or become enriched as synaptic structures are prepared, and with topographical localization of such molecules, their transport and degradation, and their potential functions. Macromolecules involved in the biosynthesis, storage, and release of neurotransmitters and other biogenic amines are touched on only briefly, since a full discussion of this subject has been presented elsewhere (Hall, 1972; Berl *et al.*, 1973; Berl and Nicklas, 1975; Van der Kloot and Kita, 1974).

2. PREPARATION OF SYNAPTIC STRUCTURES

2.1. Methodology

Axon terminals (synaptosomes) and their postsynaptic connections contain a number of elements that are susceptible to separation and discrete analysis. These include mitochondria, vesicles, cytoplasm, presynaptic plasma membrane, synaptic junctions (comprised of elements of both pre- and postsynaptic material), and "postsynaptic densities" (fragments corresponding to densely staining material in the postsynaptic region). Efforts to separate these elements in order to identify their molecular components represent one of the most challenging areas of neurochemical experimentation since procedural improvements are introduced without objective criteria of achievement, and success can only be judged by later developments and experience in depth.

The two most important steps in securing subcellular fractions of high quality are (1) disruption of the tissue and (2) separation of particles based on differences in size, shape, density, charge, or ability to bind specific chemical groups. Disruption of brain tissue is a function of shearing forces during homogenization that are markedly affected by the clearance between mortar and pestle, the number of vertical strokes of the pestle, the speed of rotation of the pestle, and the viscosity of the medium. In addition, pH and concentrations of divalent cations are important. These factors have been discussed by Appel *et al.* (1972). Pretreatment with collagenase and hyaluronidase have been used to assist disruption, e.g., of superior cervical ganglion (Wilson and Cooper, 1972). The experiences of many workers have been summarized by Jones (1975). The nature of the tissue with which one starts frequently influences the degree of homogeneity or purity obtainable in subfractions. For example, when preparing rat brain synaptosomes, cortex yields a cleaner product than whole cerebral hemispheres, and synaptosome fractions from 15-day-old rat brain are much less contaminated by myelin and lysosomes than those from brains of older rats. It is not unreasonable to suggest that the present state of the art requires optimization of the isolation procedure for each species, age, and region of brain with which one starts and for each subcellular component for which one looks.

The most widely used procedures for particle separation are based on two steps: first, differential centrifugation; and second, gradient centrifugation in different media using either sedimentation or flotation. Sucrose is the most commonly used medium, despite its recognized limitations: it causes synaptosome shrinkage and possibly nonspecific association between membranes (Day *et al.*, 1971). Other media such as Ficoll–sucrose (Kurokawa *et al.*, 1965; Abdel-Latif, 1966; De Robertis *et al.*, 1967*a*), cesium chloride (Kornguth *et al.*, 1967; Levitan *et al.*, 1972), silica (Lagercrantz and Pertoft, 1972), and sodium diatrizoate (Tamir *et al.*, 1974) have also been used. Both differential (or velocity) centrifugation and isopycnic (also called equilibrium or buoyant density) centrifugation (for physicochemical discussion see Spanner, 1972) are required, since neither method alone suffices to separate particles having very similar isopycnic banding densities (Cotman, 1972).

Other methods for separating subcellular particles that have been reported but have not yet been used widely enough to permit evaluation are electrophoretic separation (Hanning, 1967; Vos *et al.*, 1968; Sellinger and Borens, 1969; Ryan *et al.*, 1971; Tkachenko, 1972), DEAE Sephadex column chromatography (Kadota and Kanaseki, 1969), Millipore filter filtration (Baldessarini and Vogt, 1971; Morgan *et al.*, 1973*a*), affinity binding to concanavalin A (Con A)–Sepharose (Bittiger, 1975), and molecular sieving (Richter and Marchbanks, 1971; Whittaker *et al.*, 1972; Morris, 1973).

2.2. Synaptosomes

Inasmuch as isolated synaptosomes display certain properties associated with intact cells such as glycolysis, uptake and release of neurotransmitters, and uptake of amino acids, one needs to evaluate the quality of preparations of synaptosomes in relation to the preservation of such properties as well as by the degree of contamination with other subcellular particles such as myelin, mitochondria, microsomes, and various membrane fragments derived from sources other than axon terminals. One then faces compromise between the more extensive treatments necessary to secure greater purity (homogeneity is a more realistic criterion) and the attendant loss of functional properties that such treatments produce through alterations both in the integrity of membranes and in the conformations of biologically active labile proteins. Furthermore, extensive treatments lead to an increasing degree of selection since the yield decreases and the losses are not uniform.*

A common denominator in some half a dozen procedures described for the preparation of synaptosomes is the use of a 10% homogenate of brain tissue in 0.32 M sucrose. Additions of EDTA and phosphate greatly enhance the specific ATPase activity in membranes obtained from such synaptosomes, whereas addition of Ca^{2+} is essential if synaptosome preparations are to be used for obtaining synaptic junctions and postsynaptic densities. The various procedures have been compared in satisfying detail by Jones (1975) who has indicated variations employed by different investigators to reduce contaminants. For example, Morgan et al. (1971) and Gurd et al. (1974) removed microsomal contaminants by repeated washing, whereas Tamir et al. (1974) achieved a comparable result in a different medium by reducing the centrifugal force and the time of centrifugation. In this novel method of preparing synaptosomes, Tamir et al. (1974) utilized for the isopycnic centrifugation step a medium of high density which had a lower viscosity than sucrose or Ficoll–sucrose. The medium contained high concentrations of sodium diatrizoate (3,5-diacetamido-2,4,6-triiodobenzoate), a nontoxic substance used clinically for its radioopacity, and previously employed to separate spores from bacteria (Tamir and Gilvarg, 1966), competent from noncompetent cells (Cahn and Fox, 1968), and lymphocytes from blood and spleen (Perper et al., 1968). Tamir et al. (1974) found that by centrifugation of the P_2 fraction (crude synaptosomes plus mitochondria) on a linear gradient of 10–18% diatrizoate, synaptosomes could be obtained in twice the yield obtainable with sucrose. Synaptosomes prepared by the two methods showed very similar properties with respect

---

*It is clear that one can only approach such compromises with a degree of confidence that depends on the magnitude of the biological activity or the concentration of a particular component used as a criterion. When these quantities are small, as is the natural consequence of increasingly sophisticated attempts to acquire additional fine detail, the risk that any particular attribute may eventually have to be assigned to some contaminant becomes progressively greater. We need only to consider that at least 90% of the neuronal volume of most neurons is attributable to axoplasm to appreciate how small a portion of the total brain matter is really an essential part of the synaptic regions, despite their very large numbers. What constitutes a "good preparation" of synaptosomes therefore depends on what it is to be used for, just as the concept of "purity" of any chemical is inseparable from the purpose for which one requires the particular restriction of properties that is attained with increasing purity. For these reasons, when the properties of synaptosomes were first investigated, demands were not as severe as in the present period, in which much greater emphasis is placed on characterization of synaptosomal subfractions such as vesicles, membranes, and synaptic junctions.

to Na,K-ATPase, acetylcholinesterase, lactic acid dehydrogenase, glucose utilization, serotonin uptake, β-glucuronidase, RNA polymerase, and $2',3'$-cyclic nucleotide phosphohydrolase. The increased yield resulted from the improved separation of synaptosomes from the denser mitochondria: since their shrinkage in diatrizoate was much less than in sucrose, synaptosomes could be collected at a density of 1.073 g/ml (in diatrizoate) instead of 1.161 g/ml (in sucrose). The diatrizoate medium also permitted isolation of a morphologically homogeneous preparation of vesicles (see later).

Evidence has been presented to show that nerve endings utilizing different chemical transmitters exhibit some differences in density. When De Robertis *et al.* (1962) prepared synaptosomes on a five-step gradient, two fractions, C and D, showed high concentrations of synaptosomes by electron microscopy, but the C fraction contained much higher levels than the D fraction of bound acetylcholine, acetylcholinesterase, and choline acetyltransferase. Thus fraction C was enriched in cholinergic nerve terminals relative to fraction D. Shortly thereafter it was found (Salganicoff and De Robertis, 1963) that fraction D was enriched in glutamic acid decarboxylase and contained γ-aminobutyric acid (GABA). Supporting observations were reported by Fonnum (1968*a*) in studies of two synaptosome fractions obtained from step gradients of sucrose. Fractions B and C but not fraction D were found to contain other biogenic amines such as serotonin (Zieher and De Robertis, 1963), histamine (Kataoka and De Robertis, 1967), and catecholamines (De Robertis, 1964*a*). Michaelson and Whittaker (1963) found that nerve endings containing serotonin had a higher density than those containing acetylcholine. These observations led to a reconsideration of the physiological basis for the differences in density: less dense terminals (fraction C) were thought to represent enrichment in excitatory elements, whereas the more dense terminals (fraction D) represented enrichment in the inhibitory type. However, Whittaker (1968) attributed these separations of synaptosomal populations to differential losses of mitochondria and to shrinkage of synaptosomes in the higher density bands.

Direct evidence for two or more kinds of synaptosomes was provided by McGovern *et al.* (1973) who were able to separate the P_2B (synaptosome) fraction obtained by flotation on Ficoll–sucrose into lighter (P_2B_2) and heavier (P_2B_3) bands, the former containing adrenergic transmitters and their associated enzymes, and the latter containing acetylcholine and acetylcholinesterase. The separation of synaptosomes mediating the action of different neurotransmitters has been studied after incubating brain slices from different regions with labeled neurotransmitters (Iversen and Snyder, 1968; Green *et al.*, 1969; Kuhar *et al.*, 1970; Gfeller *et al.*, 1971). A very slight degree of separation on continuous sucrose gradients was obtainable.

Bretz *et al.* (1974) obtained three nerve ending fractions from rat brain using zonal isopycnic centrifugation through a continuous sucrose gradient with densities of 1.11–1.20 g/ml. These three fractions differed in ability to accumulate selectively exogenous neurotransmitters *in vitro*. Those with lowest density (1.137 g/ml) showed preferential uptake of choline; those with intermediate density (1.149 g/ml) showed a preferential uptake of GABA; and those with highest density (1.165 g/ml) showed preferential uptake of norepinephrine and dopamine.

Two types of synaptosomes were detected in preparations from rat forebrain differing in morphology and distribution of Con A binding sites (Matus and Walters, 1976). Those with prominent postsynaptic densities (corresponding to type 1 synapses) showed separation of the postsynaptic elements on incubation at 37°C for 30 min, whereas those without prominent postsynaptic attachments (corresponding to type 2 synapses) were not altered.

2.3. Components Derived from Synaptosomes

Disruption of synaptosomes, usually by hypoosmotic shock either in water (De Robertis *et al.*, 1962; Whittaker *et al.*, 1964) or in slightly alkaline buffers (Cotman and Mathews, 1971), produces a number of particles of different types in addition to components of the synaptosomal cytosol: synaptic vesicles, mitochondria, membrane fragments, and synaptic junctions composed of bits of pre- and postsynaptic membrane and intervening material. Of these particles, membranes present the greatest difficulty in purification and characterization for several reasons. One is that fragments may coalesce after disruption of the particles from which they originate, and then appear as artifacts in a variety of sizes. Another is that they may arise from many different sources, e.g., axons, glial cells, smooth and rough endoplasmic reticulum, Golgi apparatus, mitochondria, myelin, lysosomes, and nuclei.

Initial efforts to fractionate subsynaptic particles (Whittaker *et al.*, 1964) on step gradients of sucrose produced seven fractions designated as 0 (cytosol) and D, E, F, G, H, and I. D was composed of small vesicular structures about 500 Å in diameter; E consisted of membrane fragments, occasional large synaptic vesicles, and fragments of myelin; F contained membrane fragments of various sizes extending from the "dimensions of microsomes" to those of intact synaptosomes, as well as thick nonvesicular membranes resembling the postsynaptic region; G was similar but without the thick membranes; H contained intact synaptosomes, and I was composed of small mitochondria with a few shrunken synaptosomes. The morphological and biochemical properties of these fractions showed considerable overlap, and many procedures (Cotman and Mathews, 1971;

Morgan *et al.,* 1971; Gurd *et al.,* 1974; Tamir *et al.,* 1976*a*) have since been described which produced fractions of greater homogeneity. It should be noted that although there is much evidence for heterogeneity in axon terminals and their synaptic connections, synaptosomes are too often regarded, in studies concerned with derived fragments, as a homogeneous entity.

2.3.1. Synaptic Membranes

Although much effort has been devoted to the purification of synaptic plasma membranes as the main focus of attention in synaptosome structure, investigators have recognized that the total membrane fraction resulting from hypoosmotic lysis of synaptosome preparations contains both identifiable and unidentifiable membrane fragments. Since the buoyant densities of many membranes are very similar, the list of possible contaminants is extensive and includes endoplasmic reticulum, Golgi apparatus, lysosomes, dendritic membranes, perikaryal and axonal membranes, glial membranes, myelin, and lysosomal and mitochondrial membrane fragments. As has been repeatedly stressed, the quality of the synaptosome preparation, the method used for its disruption, and the conditions employed for subsequent fractionation by isopycnic centrifugation are all of considerable importance in determining the character of the final product. This is especially important since morphological, chemical, or enzymatic markers that are truly specific for only one type of membrane are still rare. For example, gangliosides appear to be particularly enriched in neuronal plasma membranes (Lapetina *et al.,* 1967; Derry and Wolfe, 1968; Morgan *et al.,* 1971; Breckenridge *et al.,* 1972), but they are probably also present in dendritic and perikaryal membranes and in myelin (Suzuki, 1970) and glial elements (Norton and Poduslo, 1971; Hamberger and Svennerholm, 1971).

Evidence obtained by several groups of investigators indicates that synaptic membranes are less dense than the bulk of the particulate material obtained after disruption of synaptosomes. Recent attempts to take advantage of this lesser density to prepare such membranes rapidly have shown some success (Jones and Matus, 1974). Although these membrane preparations remain contaminated with substantial amounts of myelin, fragments of axons, dendrites, and glia, as well as other vesicular elements (judging by electron micrographic evidence), they may be very useful as a source of synaptic junctions (see later).

In these rapid methods, the crude synaptosomal–mitochondrial fraction (P_2) is lysed and the fragments are then fractionated on sucrose gradients either by flotation–sedimentation on step gradients (Jones and

Matus, 1974) or by zonal centrifugation on linear gradients (Cotman *et al.*, 1968a; McBride *et al.*, 1970).

The longer methods start with purified synaptosomes. Low yields of synaptic membranes obtained from synaptosomes prepared with Ficoll–sucrose (Autilio *et al.*, 1968) are probably due to incomplete disruption (Cotman and Mathews, 1971), and make it difficult to rule out contamination by substantial amounts of other types of membranes. Such contamination is even greater starting with synaptosomes prepared with sucrose, since such preparations contain large quantities of membranes derived either from axons (Lemkey-Johnston and Dekermenjian, 1970) or from unidentifiable sources. Cotman *et al.* (1971a) showed that glial membranes sediment in the P_2 fraction and have isopycnic banding properties on sucrose gradients that are very similar to those of synaptic plasma membranes and "synaptosomes." Other methods of preparing synaptic plasma membranes from purified synaptosomes claim one advantage or another that may or may not be of great importance depending on what the membranes are to be used for. McBride *et al.* (1970) used zonal centrifugation on an exponential (15–45%) gradient of sucrose to obtain membranes in a single operation from the osmotically shocked P_2 fraction of cortex, and claimed advantages in shortened time of preparation, improved yield, and simplicity in gradient preparation. Cotman and Mathews (1971) prepared synaptic membranes (from synaptosomes obtained on Ficoll–sucrose gradients) that were believed to be "60 to 80% pure." They reported that osmotic lysis of synaptosomes at alkaline pH (8.1) was more effective than that at neutral pH (7.4) and improved the separation of synaptic membranes from mitochondria. In this way 1.5–2.0 mg of synaptic plasma membrane of "very high purity" was obtained per gram of brain tissue. Morgan *et al.* (1971) also prepared synaptic plasma membranes from synaptosomes isolated on Ficoll–sucrose gradients. They emphasized the use of ethylene diamine tetraacetic acid phosphate (EDTA-phosphate) for homogenization, and the need to wash the P_2 fraction thoroughly in order to reduce contamination by microsomes and membranes enriched in acetylcholinesterase. Following shock, the bulk of the particulate material was sedimented at 11,500 $\times$ g for 15 min, and synaptic plasma membranes were subsequently isolated from the supernatant. Although the yield was greatly diminished, the advantage claimed was in elimination of material whose sedimentation properties were not altered significantly by osmotic shock. They believed their synaptic plasma membrane preparation to be "85 to 90% pure" judged by an extensive enzyme profile to estimate contaminants as well as to define intrinsic properties of the plasma membrane.

In the procedure of Levitan *et al.* (1972) microsomal contamination was reduced by collecting the P_2 fraction at lower centrifugal force (7000 $\times$

g for 30 min.). Mitochondria were eliminated by two steps of gradient centrifugation: one on sucrose, the other on cesium chloride. The procedure was more rapid and resulted in a better yield than that of Morgan *et al.* (1971). Gurd *et al.* (1974) also improved the yield; crude synaptosomes were first subjected to differential flotation on gradients of Ficoll–sucrose and then the conditions of Cotman and Mathews (1971) were employed for shock.

The use of diatrizoate for isopycnic centrifugation was recently applied to the preparation of synaptic membranes from synaptosomes obtained with diatrizoate (Tamir *et al.,* 1976*a*). The procedure was short, maintained physiological pH during disruption, and gave a high yield of synaptic plasma membranes in two fractions (A and B) having the same high quality as those previously reported. In this procedure, the P_2B fraction of cortical tissue (trimmed from the hemispheres) was disrupted in the presence of 0.32 M sucrose–0.1 mM EDTA–1 mM phosphate at pH 7.5. The total membrane fragments were then collected and separated into five fractions on a step gradient of sodium diatrizoate (in half-strength Krebs–Ringer without calcium) using concentrations of 22, 18, 16, 14, and 10%. Membrane protein was divided among the fractions as follows (in order of increasing buoyant density): A, 3% (2–5%), B, 5% (3–8%), C, 8% (6–11%), D, 73% (65–81%), and E, a mitochondrial pellet, 11% (7–18%). Fractions A and B were judged to be highly purified synaptic plasma membranes by electron microscopic appearance and enzyme profile, showing high intrinsic activities (Na,K-ATPase, acetylcholinesterase, neuraminidase) and very little contamination (endoplasmic reticulum, lysosomes, mitochondrial membranes). Slab gel analysis of the polypeptide components of these fractions revealed several polypeptides not found in microsomal membranes, indicating that microsomal contamination was not significant and that synaptic plasma membranes have distinctive proteins which may serve for further characterization. For example, subcellular fractions of brain contain over 70 polypeptides detectable by one-dimensional gradient slab gel analysis (Figure 1) (Mahadik *et al.,* 1976). Four of these polypeptides— two with molecular weights below 19,000, one in the range 30,000–50,000, and one close to 50,000, possibly a microtubule peptide (Bhattacharyya and Wolf, 1975)—were not seen in either mitochondrial or microsomal fractions.

2.3.2. Synaptic Vesicles

As has been pointed out (Jones, 1975) the vesicles in axon terminals can be divided morphologically into at least three types on the basis of size, electron density, and shape. Most of these vesicles are assumed to store

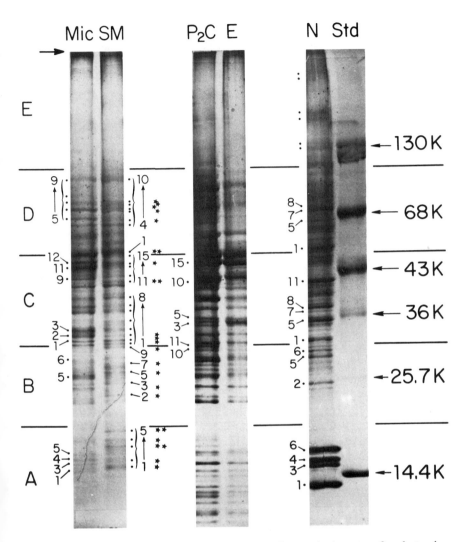

FIGURE 1. Polypeptide patterns of subcellular fractions from rat brain cortex after electrophoresis on a 25-cm-gradient slab gel of 9–25% acrylamide at pH 8.8. Mic, microsomes; SM, synaptic membrane fraction A; P₂C, mitochondria from brain homogenate; E, mitochondria from synaptosomes; N, nuclear fraction; Std, standard proteins. The zones indicated on the left represent molecular weight ranges: A, <19,000; B, 19,000–30,000; C, 30,000–50,000; D, 50,000–100,000; E, >100,000. Numbers within a zone indicate particular polypeptide bands. Single star indicates bands not present in microsomes; double star indicates bands seen only in synaptic membranes.

chemical transmitters. The isolation and properties of synaptic vesicles which are released when synaptosomes are disrupted have been discussed in considerable detail by Marchbanks (1974). When the disruption is brought about by osmotic shock, the vesicles probably lose their transmitter since they are sensitive to the osmolarity of the medium (Marchbanks, 1967, 1968; Marchbanks and Israel, 1971) or, alternatively, as suggested by Marchbanks and Israel (1972), there may be exchange of transmitter between the core of the vesicle and its surface. It therefore appears that maintenance of isotonicity of the medium is necessary in order to obtain vesicles preserving their original content of transmitter (Israel *et al.,* 1970). Coated vesicles (also called basket or complex vesicles, since they are surrounded by radiating spikes) were isolated by Kadota and Kadota (1973) who also obtained plain (hollow) vesicles and some flocculent material from a crude synaptosome fraction of guinea pig brain. Careful morphological analysis of the coated vesicles revealed clear differences in sizes and shapes.

A very good preparation of cholinergic synaptic vesicles was obtained from bovine superior cervical ganglion (Wilson *et al.,* 1973). The disrupted P_2 fraction was placed on a continuous sucrose gradient (0.3–0.6 M with a 2 M cushion). The fraction collecting between 0.36 and 0.41 M was enriched in vesicles based on electron microscopic appearance and high acetylcholine content, representing a recovery of 40–60% of that present in the P_2 fraction. Dopamine and norepinephrine were not detected, suggesting the absence of contamination by noncholinergic vesicles.

A simple and rapid method of preparing coated vesicles from pig brain without isolation of synaptosomes has been developed by Pearse (1975). The particulate material collecting between 20,000 × g for 30 min and 55,000 × g for 60 min in the presence of 1 mM ethylene glycol tetraacetic acid (EGTA) and 0.5 mM guanosine triphosphate (GTP) was further fractionated on a continuous sucrose gradient of 5–60%. The middle band was collected, concentrated, and refractionated on a 20–60% gradient. The coated vesicles, banding at a sucrose concentration of 50–55%, were obtained in a yield of 4 mg from 100 g of brain. The vesicles, 600 Å in diameter, had a networklike appearance and contained only one protein species with a molecular weight of 180,000 daltons on electrophoresis [pH 6.7, 7.5% sodium dodecyl sulfate (SDS) slab gel]. Digestion with proteases showed that this protein, called clathrin, is on the external surface of the vesicles. No mention was made of the presence of neurotransmitters in these vesicles.

Passage of synaptic vesicles through Millipore filters of appropriate pore size has been used to remove contaminating membranes (Morgan *et al.,* 1973a).

Synaptosomes prepared by the diatrizoate method (Tamir *et al.*, 1974) showed better ultrastructural preservation of vesicles than synaptosomes prepared with sucrose. Following osmotic lysis of the synaptosomes in water, synaptic vesicles were collected by centrifugation of the supernatant remaining after removal of the membrane fraction. When the resuspended pellet was layered over 10% sodium diatrizoate and centrifuged at 50,000 × g for 60 min, two distinct bands were obtained, one below and the other above the interface. The vesicles were then collected by centrifugation at 100,000 × g for 30 min. The less dense fraction contained small vesicles, was homogeneous morphologically, was free of myelin and mitochondria, exhibited very low acetylcholinesterase activity, and contained almost all (97%) of its total ATPase as Mg-ATPase. The heavier vesicle fraction contained larger vesicles, was less homogeneous, exhibited five times greater acetylcholinesterase activity, and had its ATPase activity distributed almost equally between Mg-ATPase and Na,K-ATPase. Significant differences between the two fractions in their protein or lipid components have not yet been detected.

A very homogeneous preparation of synaptic vesicles from guinea pig cortex synaptosomes has been described (Nagy *et al.,* 1976). It contained only Mg-ATPase and Ca-ATPase and was estimated to contain 13–56% cholinergic vesicles based on acetylcholine content.

It would certainly appear that the preparation of synaptic vesicles with minimal alteration of properties requires the development of rapid procedures with maintenance of physiological conditions during synaptosomal disruption. One method might involve the use of lysolecithin for disruption. Since the lysolecithin would probably remain bound to the synaptosomal membrane, it should be possible to adjust the concentration to secure lysis of synaptosomes without altering the vesicular membrane. Another possibility is immune lysis, using antibodies directed against constituents of the plasma membrane that are not present in vesicles, e.g., gangliosides.

2.3.3. Mitochondria

Cytochemical evidence has indicated differences between presynaptic and other neuronal mitochondria (Hajos and Kerpel-Fronius, 1973). Since mitochondria have a higher density than other synaptosomal components (Whittaker and Barker, 1972) it has been relatively simple to obtain almost pure preparations of synaptosomal mitochondria after disruption of synaptosomes. However, if the synaptosomes are not first carefully purified, the fraction will also contain mitochondria originating in neuronal cell bodies and glia. Common contaminants of mitochondrial pellets obtained from synaptosomes are large membrane fragments and undisrupted synapto-somes. Improved separations are obtainable by increasing the density of the mitochondria through accumulation of a product of mitochondrial oxidation (Davis and Bloom, 1970; Cotman and Taylor, 1972) but whether such accumulation leaves the physiological state of the mitochondria unaltered has not yet been established. Mitochondria with well-preserved cristae and good capacity for ATP synthesis were obtained by fractionation on sodium diatrizoate (Tamir *et al.*, 1975). They differed from mitochondria of the P_2C fraction (originating in neuronal and glial cell bodies) in having a much larger number of electron-lucent rather than electron-dense cristae, lower Mg-ATPase activity, lower capacity for ATP synthesis [dinitro-phenol- (DNP) and Ca^{2+}-sensitive], and higher monoamine oxidase (MAO) activity (type A). The MAO was also insensitive to pargyline (10^{-5} M). Only minor differences were detectable in the polypeptide components of the two populations of mitochondria (Mahadik *et al.*, 1976). Isolation of distinct populations of mitochondria was also reported by Lai *et al.* (1975). Lai and Clark (1976) have shown that synaptic mitochondria differ from nonsynaptic mitochondria in their densities, oxidation rates of different substrates, and levels of various enzymes.

2.3.4. Synaptic Junctional Complexes

Synaptic junctional complexes contain fragments of pre- and postsyn-aptic plasma membrane plus the densely staining material seen both in synaptic clefts and in close proximity to the intracellular surfaces of pre- and postsynaptic membranes. Electron microscopic examination of the earliest preparations of synaptosomes (De Robertis *et al.*, 1962; Gray and Whittaker, 1962) revealed the presence of these synaptic junctional complexes, and they were subsequently found together with synaptic plasma membranes when these were separated from other subcellular elements. By solubilizing the membranes with detergent (0.1% Triton X-100) Fiszer and De Robertis (1967) showed that the insoluble material, after purification by isopycnic centrifugation on a sucrose gradient (De Robertis *et al.*, 1967*a*), was composed of a pair of synaptic membranes joined by intersyn-aptic filaments and material corresponding to the subsynaptic web of the postsynaptic membrane (De Robertis, 1964*b*). The most important advance leading to the isolation of junctional complexes was the development of selective staining techniques, such as ethanol–phosphotungstic acid (Bloom and Aghajanian, 1966, 1968) and bismuth iodide–uranyl–lead (Pfenninger, 1971).

Two independently developed methods of preparing synaptic junc-tional complexes (Cotman and Taylor, 1972; Davis and Bloom, 1973*a*) had many features in common. Synaptic membranes were first obtained directly from the crude synaptosomal–mitochondrial fraction (P_2). The membrane pellet was then incubated with sodium succinate and iodonitro-tetrazolium violet (INT) (Davis and Bloom, 1970, 1973b) to reduce mito-chondrial contamination. After rebanding, such contamination was esti-mated to be less than 5% based on cytochrome oxidase activity. Membranes were solubilized with Triton X-100, and insoluble synaptic junctional complexes were then isolated by centrifugation on sucrose gra-dients in the presence of 50 μM $CaCl_2$.*

Earlier Kornguth et al. (1969) described conditions in which synaptic junctional complexes† were very well preserved despite centrifugation for 72 hr. The tissue was homogenized in 0.32 M sucrose containing 1 mM $MgCl_2$ and potassium phosphate buffer, isolating "synaptic complexes" by centrifugation first on sucrose gradients containing 10 mM $MgCl_2$, and then for 72 hr on gradients of 0.14 M sucrose in cesium chloride. Separation of synaptic junctional complexes from synaptosomes in the final fraction was not attempted.

Jones and Matus (1974) reported that their preparation of synaptic plasma membranes contained large numbers of well-preserved synaptic junctional complexes. Although these were not further purified, their ultra-structure was compared with such complexes in intact tissue (Matus et al., 1975a) providing useful morphological information.

2.3.5. Postsynaptic Densities

Different types of synapses have different specializations of postsyn-aptic dense material. In the asymmetric type this material is prominent (Gray, 1959a, 1969; Walberg, 1968) whereas in the symmetric type it is sparse or absent. This dense material has been referred to as postsynaptic density (Akert et al., 1969; Bloom, 1970a), subsynaptic web (De Robertis, 1964b), or postsynaptic thickening (Palay, 1956; Gray, 1959b).

Postsynaptic densities are enriched in preparations of synaptic junc-tional complexes. Cotman et al. (1974) used either such preparations or synaptic plasma membranes as a source of postsynaptic densities. By treatment with N-lauroyl sarcosinate (lauroyl N-methylglycine) followed by density gradient centrifugation, postsynaptic densities in good yield

---

*The essential differences between the two methods were that Cotman and Taylor prepared a 30% homogenate of brain tissue in 0.32 M sucrose containing 1 mM $MgCl_2$, diluted the homogenate to 10% with sucrose, and neutralized all solutions to pH 7.0, whereas Davis and Bloom prepared a 10% homogenate at pH 7.0 in 0.32 M sucrose containing 1 mM $MgCl_2$ and 0.05 mM $CaCl_2$.

†As pointed out by Cotman, this is essentially a synaptosome preparation.

(almost 0.5 mg protein from 20 g of rat forebrain) and high purity were obtained at the interface of 1.4 and 2.2 M sucrose.

Walters and Matus (1975a) obtained postsynaptic densities from synaptic plasma membranes prepared according to Jones and Matus (1974) by solubilizing the limit membrane with sodium deoxycholate. The insoluble material was collected at 100,000 × g for 60 min, and, without further purification, was subjected to a detailed ultrastructural study, revealing the close relationship between postsynaptic densities and the synaptic lattice (Matus and Walters, 1975). The only enzyme activity recovered in postsynaptic densities was 3′,5′-cyclic nucleotide phosphodiesterase (Cotman *et al.*, 1974). Only very low levels of Na,K-ATPase, cytochrome c oxidase, acid phosphatase, and 5′-nucleotidase were detected, suggesting the essential absence of membrane contaminants. However, since the need to use detergents to isolate this fraction resulted in activities that were both low and variable, this criterion remains ambiguous.

2.3.6. Cerebellar Glomerular Complexes

The cerebellar glomerular complex contains the mossy fiber rosette, granule cell dendrites, Golgi cell dendrites and axons, and remnants of the glial capsule. Methods for the isolation of such complexes have been described (Hajos *et al.*, 1974; Balazs *et al.*, 1975; Hamberger *et al.*, 1975, 1976). Hajos and co-workers (1974) isolated a fraction from rat cerebellum by differential centrifugation on sucrose gradients, both step and linear. This preparation was found to have high relative specific activity (RSA) for glutamic acid decarboxylase and low RSA for choline acetyltransferase. In the method of Hamberger's group (1975, 1976), slices of rabbit cerebellum were incubated at 37°C for 30 min in a medium containing Tris and phosphate buffers at pH 7.6, NaCl, KCl, MgCl₂, glucose, and Ficoll. The tissue was then disrupted by passage through nylon mesh, diluted with medium containing sucrose, NaCl, Tris buffer, EDTA, and Ficoll, and sieved through nylon of progressively decreasing pore size (500, 200, 100, 50 μm). The pellet obtained by centrifugation at 150 × g for 5 min was fractionated further, first on a Ficoll gradient (where it banded at the interface of 15.7/19% Ficoll) and then on a step gradient of sucrose (where it was recovered between 1.2 and 1.4 M sucrose). The fraction could not be isolated from very young rabbits. From the 40-day-old rabbit, 0.15 mg of protein per cerebellum was obtained in the final glomerular complex fraction. Wilson *et al.* (1976) have shown that these glomerular complexes exhibit high-affinity uptake of GABA, glutamate, aspartate, and glycine, by utilizing glucose as a source of energy. These preparations of glomerular complexes may serve to identify the neurotransmitter(s) in mossy fiber terminals.

2.3.7. Receptors

Binding is such a common phenomenon that the introduction of radioactively labeled ligands has led to the detection of receptors in the CNS for almost everything looked for. In order to select systems of biological importance, certain criteria of ligand binding usually need to be considered, such as high affinity, stereospecificity, temperature dependence, and inhibition of binding by specific antagonists.

Most of the work describing the partial purification of receptors for biogenic amines and other neurotransmitters has been reviewed by De Robertis (1975*a,b*). Acetylcholine receptors in isolated nerve endings were first reported by De Robertis *et al.* (1967*a*). They found that treatment of isolated synaptic junctional complexes with Triton X-100 did not affect binding of two cholinergic blocking agents, D-tubocurarine and methyl hexamethonium, whereas acetylcholinesterase and ATPase were completely solubilized. These results suggested that acetylcholine receptors were localized in the synaptic junctional complex, whereas the enzymes were more widely distributed. The instability of receptors after separation from synaptic plasma membranes, reflected in the great loss of binding activity for both agonists and antagonists, has severely hampered extensive purification.

The most successful isolation efforts have attended studies of nicotinic-type acetylcholine receptors found in electroplax of eel and torpedo electric organs (Eldefrawi and Eldefrawi, 1973; Chang, 1974; Heilbronn and Mattson, 1974; Raftery *et al.*, 1974; Karlin, 1975; Maelicke and Reich, 1976). Very high concentrations of receptor protein are present in these tissues.

In the mammalian CNS, acetylcholine receptors, which represent only a very small amount of protein, are of two types: muscarinic and nicotinic. Most cholinergic synapses in brain are thought to be muscarinic (Snyder *et al.*, 1975; Lowy *et al.*, 1976). However, partial solubilization and characterization of cholinergic receptors from brain that bind α-bungarotoxin (and are therefore nicotinic receptors) have been achieved (Salvaterra *et al.*, 1975; Lowy *et al.*, 1976). The aggregate weight of the receptor complex including detergent (Triton X-100), purified by affinity chromatography, was calculated from its hydrodynamic properties to be 357,000 daltons

(Salvaterra and Mahler, 1976). The α-bungarotoxin binding sites are found mainly in brainstem and spinal cord.

Neurophysiological studies indicate that several amino acids have transmitter properties in the CNS, the most prominent being GABA, glutamic acid, aspartic acid, glycine, and taurine (Snyder *et al.*, 1973). Glycine is an inhibitory transmitter in spinal cord and brainstem (see Chapter 5 of this volume). Receptors in these areas have not been characterized.

Michaelis *et al.* (1974) found that the high-affinity binding of glutamic acid in synaptic membranes was stereospecific for L-glutamate and completely reversible. The binding was inhibited by both neuroexcitatory and neuroinhibitory amino acids, but not by amino acids devoid of such pharmacological activity. Binding activity was solubilized with Triton X-100, suggesting the presence of receptors.

Enna and Snyder (1975) reported the Na^+-independent binding of labeled GABA to synaptic membrane fractions of rat brain. This binding is evidence for a neuronal GABA receptor since it can be distinguished from the Na^+-dependent binding which they suggest is involved in the GABA-accumulating system of glia.

Orrego and Valdes (1973) reported that glycine receptors in the cerebral cortex are probably involved in transport. Functional interpretation of the binding of some amino acids therefore presents a special problem since such binding may represent either receptors (postsynaptic) for amino acid transmitters or carriers involved in amino acid transport.

Receptors have also been used as markers for the isolation and characterization of membranes. Various techniques for receptor identification, characterization, and measurement have been reviewed by Cuatrecasas (1974). Chang *et al.* (1975) have used ^{125}I-labeled lectins, insulin, cholera toxin, and other receptor ligands to label plasma membranes as an aid to their isolation.

3. CHARACTERIZATION OF SYNAPTIC STRUCTURES

3.1. Morphology

Identification of subcellular particles isolated for biochemical analysis with structures seen in intact tissue has relied heavily on histological staining (for an extensive discussion, see Pfenninger, 1973) and cytochemical techniques. Morphological features of subsynaptic structures as seen by electron microscopy have been discussed in considerable detail by Jones (1975). Alterations in morphology occur during isolation of subcellular particles, and therefore gentle conditions and rapid procedures are needed to minimize such changes. Isolated synaptosomes have a complex fine structure which is revealed by electron microscopy using positive staining of thin sections (Whittaker and Gray, 1962) or negative staining (Horne and Whittaker, 1962). They correspond to axon terminals earlier described as thin-walled bags containing cytoplasm packed with synaptic vesicles and a number of mitochondria (Palay and Palade, 1954; De Robertis and Bennett, 1955); some have attached a thickened portion of postsynaptic membrane. Although isolated synaptic plasma membranes show the trilamellar structure, they vary too much in size and shape for morphological characterization. Synaptic junctional complexes can be identified because of their specific staining properties (Pfenninger, 1973) which also facilitate comparisons with similar structures in intact tissue (Matus *et al.,* 1975*a*).

The morphology of synaptic vesicles has received a great deal of attention, and at least three types have been distinguished: dense-cored, plain (or hollow), and coated. Plain vesicles have a mean diameter of 470 ± 110 Å (Whittaker *et al.,* 1964). Coated vesicles (Kanaseki and Kadota, 1969) are characterized by a surrounding latticelike network giving them a diameter of about 600 Å. The possible artifactual nature of the coats has been brought to attention (Gray, 1972), but there are implications (Matus, 1976*a,b*) for a relation of the coats to a supramolecular structure (cytonet).

Mitochondria are much larger than vesicles, and because of their size, assessment of the uniformity of isolated fractions requires determination of particle size distribution in random samples. A negative staining technique may be useful for quantitative estimation of the number of mitochondria by electron microscopy (Gregson and Williams, 1969).

3.2. Enzyme Profiles

The highly organized structures of the synapse and its numerous subsynaptic components suggest that these components should contain distinctive sets of enzymes in order to carry out their specialized functions. A number of enzymes and other substances that can serve as markers have been reported by Whittaker and Barker (1972). In order to establish whether a given enzyme is characteristic of a particular subsynaptic structure, it is necessary to study its distribution in subcellular fractions, its relative enrichment during fractionation, its recovery, and its specific activity. In addition some consideration must be given to (1) the presence and removal of endogenous inhibitors or activators, (2) accessibility of the exogenous substrate to membrane-bound enzyme, (3) dilution of radioactive substrate by endogenous substrate in the membrane, and (4) the nature of the interaction of the enzyme with other membrane components (alterations in the membrane during isolation caused by exposure to unphysiological media such as sucrose may extract or inactivate enzymes or cause changes in conformation that introduce steric problems) (De Robertis *et al.*, 1967*b*; Reijnierse *et al.*, 1976). It has been calculated (Morgan *et al.*, 1971) that based on physiological data (Harvey and McIlwain, 1969) a specific marker enzyme for neuronal plasma membrane should show at least a 10- to 15-fold enrichment in the pure fraction relative to the homogenate.

3.2.1. Synaptosomes

Enzymes that represent intrinsic activities of synaptosomes are Na,K-ATPase (Skou, 1957; Hosie, 1965), acetylcholinesterase (Gray and Whittaker, 1962; De Robertis *et al.*, 1962; Sellinger and Borens, 1969), 5'-nucleotidase (Steck and Wallach, 1970), neuraminidase (Schengrund and Rosenberg, 1970), and glutamic acid decarboxylase (Salganicoff and De Robertis, 1963; Weinstein *et al.*, 1963). Although these enzymes may show elevated specific activities in synaptosomes and derived synaptosomal fragments, this does not mean that they are specific markers for synaptic structures, since they may also be present in other subcellular organelles. For characterizing the intactness of synaptosomes by their retention of cytosol, lactic acid dehydrogenase (Johnson and Whittaker, 1963) and the enzymes of glycolysis (Tamir *et al.*, 1974) have been most useful, whereas to detect mitochondrial contamination, the activities of succinic acid dehydrogenase, cytochrome oxidase, and MAO have been used (Sottocasa *et al.*, 1967; Smoley *et al.*, 1970).

3.2.2. Synaptic Membranes

Synaptic plasma membranes have been studied extensively both for intrinsic enzyme activities and for enzymes indicating contamination by other subcellular fractions such as mitochondria, microsomes, lysosomes, and myelin. Na,K-ATPase has been of particular interest since its presence in peripheral nerve was established (Skou, 1957), where it presumably functions in the active extrusion of Na^+ from nerve tissue (Bonting *et al.*, 1962). Morgan *et al.* (1971) believed their synaptic plasma membrane preparation to be almost 90% pure, based on a 10- to 15-fold enrichment of Na,K-ATPase with respect to the homogenate compared with only a fivefold enrichment found by others (Hosie, 1965; Cotman and Mathews, 1971). However, since a soluble, dialyzable inhibitor of this enzyme has been found in brain (Schaffer *et al.*, 1974), one may question the advisability of using the activity of this enzyme in homogenates for reference purposes. The inhibitor, which acts like ascorbic acid, can be neutralized by chelators such as EDTA, EGTA, *o*-phenanthroline, and α,α'-dipyridyl.

The specific activity of Na,K-ATPase in synaptic plasma membrane fractions prepared with EDTA in the homogenizing medium is much higher than when EDTA is omitted (Morgan *et al.*, 1971; Gurd *et al.*, 1974; Tamir *et al.*, 1976a). This would suggest that either the soluble inhibitor or heavy metals interfere with ATPase activity in such particulates. Rodriguez de Lores Arnaiz *et al.* (1967) showed that membranes from cholinergic nerve endings were enriched in acetylcholinesterase, whereas Na,K-ATPase was enriched in membranes from both cholinergic and noncholinergic terminals. Na,K-ATPase has been demonstrated histochemically (Daniel and Guth, 1975) in both synaptosomes and their plasma membranes.

Several other enzymes, such as 5'-nucleotidase (Steck and Wallach, 1970) and alkaline phosphatase, which have been used to characterize plasma membranes from cells in liver (Emmelot and Bos, 1966) and other tissues (Bosman *et al.*, 1968), have been used to study synaptic plasma membranes. Cotman and Mathews (1971) found that alkaline phosphatase paralleled Na,K-ATPase for enrichment and increase in RSA in the most concentrated synaptic plasma membrane fractions (fractions 2 and 3) whereas 5'-nucleotidase and acetylcholinesterase showed only slight enrichment, with lower RSAs than fraction 1. A possible explanation is that particles in fraction 1 may be derived from axonal and dendritic membranes and endoplasmic reticulum, which have been shown by histochemical analysis (Kokko *et al.*, 1965; Shute and Lewis, 1966; Novikoff, 1967) to contain acetylcholinesterase. This enzyme is also associated with small neuronal elements in neuropil (Kokko *et al.*, 1965) and with thin axons (Shute and Lewis, 1966). Histochemical analysis has also shown 5'-nucleotidase to be present in glial cells (Torack and Barrnett, 1964).

In their best synaptic plasma membrane fraction (F), Morgan *et al.* (1971) found that although the specific activities of acetylcholinesterase, 5'-nucleotidase, and Na,K-ATPase were high, the enrichments referred to the homogenate were nil, slight, and 12-fold, respectively. A very low activity of NADPH-cytochrome *c* reductase and a low content of RNA ruled out contamination by smooth and rough endoplasmic reticulum as contaminants responsible for acetylcholinesterase activity. The high acetylcholinesterase activity was thought (based on histochemical evidence) (Darin de Lorenzo *et al.*, 1969; Teravainen, 1969; Westrum and Boderson, 1976) to indicate the presynaptic origin of the membranes in this fraction. However, in an extensive review of acetylcholinesterase, Rosenberry (1975) has pointed out that the particulate form of the enzyme is localized in both pre- and postsynaptic sites of excitable membranes.

The synaptic plasma membrane fractions prepared by Tamir *et al.* (1976a) and Jones and Matus (1974) also contained high specific activities of acetylcholinesterase. Tamir *et al.* (1976a) ruled out microsomal contaminants on the basis of RNA content (below detectable levels), low activity of NADPH-cytochrome c reductase (one-fourth of that present in purified microsomes), and polypeptide composition. These observations, enzyme stability, and the absence of endogenous inhibitors would all support acetylcholinesterase as an enzyme marker for synaptic plasma membranes that may be preferable to Na,K-ATPase, provided microsomal contamination is controlled.

A number of enzyme markers have been used to indicate contamination of synaptic structures by elements of myelin, mitochondria, lysosomes, and the various components of microsomes, particularly smooth and rough endoplasmic reticulum. Morgan et al. (1971) estimated less than 1% mitochondrial contamination of their synaptic membrane fractions E and F, and 3% contamination of fraction G, using cytochrome oxidase and succinic acid dehydrogenase (SDH) as markers for inner mitochondrial membranes (Sottocasa et al., 1967). Cotman and Mathews (1971) estimated less than 5% mitochondrial contamination of their synaptic membrane fraction based on cytochrome oxidase, whereas Gurd et al. (1974) reported insignificant SDH activity in their best fraction. Markers for outer mitochondrial membrane include monoamine oxidase (Smoley et al., 1970) and antimycin- or rotenone-insensitive NADH-cytochrome c reductase (Sottocasa et al., 1967), but the latter enzyme is also present in microsomes (Heidrich et al., 1970) and in nuclear membranes (Kashnig and Kasper, 1969). Cotman and Mathews (1971) reported that cytochrome oxidase and NADH-cytochrome c reductase showed parallel patterns. Since the outer mitochondrial membrane is believed to account for less than 10% of total mitochondrial protein (Brunner and Bucher, 1970), the upper limit for gross contamination by intact mitochondria is only 19% using these outer membrane markers. Morgan et al. (1971) observed very high MAO activity in synaptic plasma membranes, comparable to that present in mitochondria and greater than would be expected from contamination with fragments of mitochondrial outer membrane as estimated from NADH-cytochrome c reductase activity. The suggestion of Morgan et al. (1971) that this observation might indicate the presence of MAO in some structure other than mitochondrial outer membrane, e.g., other membranes (De Champlain et al., 1969) or the synaptic membranes themselves (Arora et al., 1974), would depend on MAO and NADH-cytochrome c reductase having comparable stability. Tamir et al. (1976a) have also found higher MAO activity than expected in the purest synaptic plasma membrane fraction. The nonmitochondrial origin of MAO in synaptic membranes is supported by the observations (Arora et al., 1974) of differences in the enzyme's extractability and response to specific inhibitors.

For microsomal contamination, NADPH-cytochrome c reductase of smooth endoplasmic reticulum is a more specific marker than NADH-cytochrome c reductase, since the latter is also present in mitochondria (Smoley *et al.*, 1970). Although Morgan *et al.* (1971) did not detect this activity in their synaptic membrane fractions, Gurd *et al.* (1974) reported high specific activity for this enzyme in such membrane preparations. In the best fraction obtained by Tamir *et al.* (1976*a*) this enzyme was present with a specific activity about 25% of that in purified microsomes. Correcting for the absence of rough endoplasmic reticulum on the basis of undetectable RNA, the contamination of the synaptic membrane fraction by elements of smooth endoplasmic reticulum was estimated to be no more than 5%.

Acid phosphatase, β-N-acetylglucosaminidase, and β-glucuronidase have all been used to indicate lysosomal contamination. Although the acid phosphatase activity in the synaptic plasma membrane preparation of Morgan *et al.* (1971) was almost insignificant, it was higher in the preparations of Cotman and Mathews (1971), Gurd *et al.* (1974), and Verity *et al.* (1973). Osmotic shock at alkaline pH may disrupt lysosomes into fragments that band with synaptic membranes. Cotman and Mathews (1971) found that acid phosphatase and β-N-acetylglucosaminidase cannot be removed from synaptic membranes by washing, but can be removed by Triton X-100 (0.05%) under conditions in which the membrane itself is resistant (Cotman *et al.*, 1971*c*). Synaptic membranes prepared by Tamir *et al.* (1976*a*) were free of β-glucuronidase.

The activity of lactic acid dehydrogenase, a marker for cytosol (Johnson and Whittaker, 1963), is very low in all synaptic membrane preparations. However, the presence of all cytoplasmic constituents cannot be excluded because of the type of binding described for choline acetyltransferase (Tucek, 1966; Fonnum, 1967, 1968*b*) and pyruvate kinase (Tamir *et al.*, 1972). The binding of some proteins (enzymes) to membrane preparations is markedly influenced by pH, ionic strength, and divalent metals, suggesting regulatory mechanisms that may be functionally involved in the distribution of such proteins between soluble and particulate phases.

The very high activity of 2',3'-cyclic AMP-phosphohydrolase (CNPH; see Chapter 1 of this volume) in myelin makes this enzyme the preferred marker for myelin contamination (Kurihara and Tsukada, 1967). Morgan *et al.* (1971) found significant activity of this enzyme in their synaptic membrane preparation, whereas the activity reported by Tamir *et al.* (1976*a*) indicated myelin contamination to be less than 0.5%. This low contamination was attributed both to careful trimming of cortical tissue to remove white matter and to the use of diatrizoate instead of sucrose, thereby minimizing the "interactions" between synaptic membranes and myelin noted by Day *et al.* (1971), or "cosedimentation" as interpreted by Doyle and Cotman (1972).

Cotman *et al.* (1971*b*) have studied a number of enzymes involved in lipid metabolism as possible markers for subcellular fractions and concluded that inositol-CMP-phosphatidyl (CDP-diglyceride) transferase is predominantly microsomal, that carnitine acetyltransferase and "phosphatidic acid cytidyl" transferase are localized principally in mitochondria, and that β-galactosidase, although it is considered to be a lysosomal enzyme, had its highest RSA in synaptic membranes. It has been reported, however, that this enzyme often sediments with mitochondria, and Morgan *et al.* (1971) observed high specific activities for both β-galactosidase and β-glucosidase in their mitochondrial fraction.

Neuraminidase, which was shown to be present in synaptic membranes (Schengrund and Rosenberg, 1970; Tettamanti *et al.*, 1972), was found to have the highest specific activity in synaptic membrane fractions A and B by Tamir *et al.* (1976*a*), to be barely detectable in fraction D, and undetectable in fraction E (mitochondrial pellet). This enzyme is potentially very useful for characterization of synaptic plasma membranes since it shows the largest differential between fractions A and D, but more sensitive methods for its measurement are required to overcome the low activity. The presence of neuraminidase in synaptic membranes, which are known to contain high concentrations of bound neuraminic acid (Tettamanti *et al.*, 1973), suggests that the molecules involved participate in some dynamic process related to neuronal function.

A number of studies have been reported which are concerned with glycosylation both *in vivo* and *in vitro* of proteins at nerve endings (for references, see Barondes, 1974). There is considerable evidence that glycoproteins are synthesized in the cell body and reach the nerve endings by axonal transport. However, kinetic studies indicate that glucosamine can be incorporated directly at axon terminals (Barondes, 1968; Barondes and Dutton, 1969; Zatz and Barondes, 1971), pointing to the presence of glycosyl transferases.* The presence of such transferases in synaptosomal membranes was difficult to establish with certainty because of the very high level of such enzyme activity in the Golgi components of microsomes and in mitochondria. Using highly purified preparations of synaptic membranes, Reith *et al.* (1972) showed that these membranes contained about half as much galactosyl transferase activity as microsomes and one-eighth as much as Golgi apparatus, indicating that this enzyme is an intrinsic membrane property. Dutton *et al.* (1973) showed that the synaptosome fraction incorporated glucosamine more actively than either mitochondria or microsomes. Louisot and Broquet (1975) studied the glycosyl transferases of synaptosomes and mitochondria of rat brain. Transferases for mannose, galactose, fucose, N-acetylglucosamine, and N-acetylgalactosa-

---

*Incorporation of glucosamine may result from biosynthesis of neuraminic acid by pathways not requiring glycosyl transferases.

mine were all present in synaptosomes. Mannosyl transferase was also present in synaptic vesicles and mitochondria. The biosynthesis of glycoproteins and gangliosides involves glycosyl transferases that are probably different. The activities of enzymes that mediate ganglioside synthesis change rapidly during development. Studies of the subcellular distribution of such enzymes in rat brain (Di Cesare and Dain, 1972) showed that UDP-N-acetylgalactosamine:$G_{M3}N$-acetylgalactosaminyl transferase and UDP-galactose:G_{M2} galactosyl transferase were present in synaptic membranes 7 days after birth. In adult rats these activities decrease to very low levels. The glycosyl transferases are more tightly bound to the membrane than acetylcholinesterase, and remain associated with gangliosides when acetylcholinesterase is solubilized with Triton X-100 (0.1%). The subcellular distribution of glycosyl transferases from embryonic chick brain involved in glycoprotein, ganglioside, and chondroitin sulfate synthesis has been reported in two independent studies (Brandt *et al.,* 1975; Den *et al.,* 1975). Developmental patterns for three enzymes enriched in synaptosomes (prepared according to Gray and Whittaker, 1962) and required for glycoprotein synthesis showed that activities were maximal between 7 and 21 days (day of hatching) and then fell suddenly (Brandt *et al.,* 1975). In the studies of Den *et al.* (1975) six of seven glycosyl transferases were present in particulates. The exception, UDP-galactose-glycoprotein galactosyl transferase, was in both soluble and particulate compartments in young animals but became entirely particulate in older animals.

3.2.3. Synaptic Mitochondria

Synaptic mitochondria are readily characterized by the capacity to synthesize ATP or by individual enzyme markers present in inner or outer membranes as discussed earlier: MAO, Mg-ATPase, antimycin- or rotenone-insensitive NADH-cytochrome c reductase, cytochrome oxidase, and succinic acid dehydrogenase. Succinic acid dehydrogenase may have some limitations since Neidle *et al.* (1969) detected a population of mitochondria devoid of this enzyme activity. The relatively high density of mitochondria permits them to be purified easily, the major contaminant being undisrupted synaptosomes. Synaptosomal contamination may be detected from the presence of Na,K-ATPase, lactic acid dehydrogenase, or glycolytic activity.

3.2.4. Synaptic Vesicles

Enzymes useful in the characterization of synaptic vesicles of brain are Mg-ATPase and Mg,Ca-ATPase (Kadota *et al.,* 1967), acetylcholinesterase

(De Robertis *et al.*, 1963), 3',5'-cyclic nucleotide phosphodiesterase (De Robertis *et al.*, 1967*b;* Johnson *et al.*, 1973), tyrosine hydroxylase (Fahn *et al.*, 1969), dopamine-β-hydroxylase (Pollard *et al.*, 1973), and protein kinases (Maeno *et al.*, 1971). The presence of Na,K-ATPase in vesicles from CNS is not established. Tamir *et al.* (1974) found little of this enzyme in their small vesicle preparation but substantial amounts in their large vesicle preparation. Tanaka (1974) found that the ATPase of plain synaptic vesicles was Mg,Ca-ATPase, indicating an actomyosinlike enzyme, whereas the ATPase of coated vesicles was more dependent on Ca^{2+}. ATPase of plain vesicles was stimulated by reserpine at low concentration whereas the enzyme of coated vesicles was unaffected.

Higher specific activity for a "nucleoside diphosphate phosphohydrolase" was found in coated vesicles compared with plain vesicles ("synaptic vesicles") (Kadota and Kadota, 1973). In the two vesicle preparations of Tamir *et al.* (1974) acetylcholinesterase activity was almost five times higher in the large vesicles than in the small vesicles. The dopamine-β-hydroxylase activity of both fractions was high (L. Friedman, H. Tamir, and M. Goldstein, unpublished studies). Synaptic vesicles from bovine caudate nucleus were found to have the highest RSA values for tyrosine hydroxylase, acetylcholinesterase, and acetylcholine by Fahn *et al.* (1969).

3.3.   Proteins and Polypeptides

Proteins of subsynaptic particles may be grouped into three categories for purposes of discussion: proteins with known biological activity, fibrous proteins, and proteins whose biological roles are still not established.

3.3.1.   Biologically Active Proteins

These proteins are comprised of several types: enzymes involved in the metabolism (biosynthesis and breakdown) of neurotransmitters; proteins involved in the storage, release, and uptake of neurotransmitters; receptor proteins; a group of protein kinases, some activated by neurotransmitters either directly or indirectly (via cAMP or cGMP) and the phosphoproteins, phosphatases, and phosphodiesterases belonging to this system; proteins involved in energy metabolism; and a large number of enzymes involved in turnover of synaptic components. We will not consider mitochondrial proteins involved in protein and nucleic acid synthesis.

Proteins involved in neurotransmitter metabolism, storage, and release have been discussed in detail (Hall, 1972; Costa and Meek, 1974) and protein receptors have been given a full presentation (De Robertis, 1975*b;*

Cohen and Changeux, 1975). A review of protein phosphorylation in the central nervous system has recently appeared (Williams and Rodnight, 1977) and a more general review was presented earlier (Rubin and Rosen, 1975).

Protein phosphorylating systems, several of which are dependent on cyclic nucleotides, are present in both presynaptic and postsynaptic regions. Five proteins involved in phosphorylation are adenylate cyclase (De Robertis *et al.*, 1967*b*), phosphodiesterase (De Robertis *et al.*, 1967*b*; Cheung and Salganicoff, 1967; Florendo *et al.*, 1971), protein kinase (Maeno *et al.*, 1971), the substrate for protein kinase (Johnson *et al.*, 1971), and phosphoprotein phosphatases (Maeno and Greengard, 1972).

Two protein substrates, proteins I and II, for endogenous protein kinase have been found in synaptic membranes (Ueda *et al.*, 1973). Protein I (molecular weight 86,000) is unique for nervous tissue, whereas protein II (molecular weight 48,000) is present in both membranes and cytosol of a number of different tissues. The complex of "protein II kinase–protein II–protein II phosphatase" in synaptic membranes has been solubilized (Ueda *et al.*, 1975) showing the close physical association of the components in the membrane. Adenylate cyclase and cyclic nucleotide phosphodiesterase were found to be associated with synaptic membranes (De Robertis *et al.*, 1967*b*; Cheung and Salganicoff, 1967), but were also present in other subcellular fractions such as microsomes.

All these proteins are potentially involved in mediating the effects of neurotransmitters in the *postsynaptic* region of certain types of synapses. The sequence of postsynaptic events in the hypothetical model has been discussed by Greengard (1976). The mechanism proposed for neurotransmitter effects on phosphorylation is by activation of adenylate or guanylate cyclases (Krueger *et al.*, 1975). Such effects are especially marked for dopamine and norepinephrine in the caudate nucleus and dopamine in the superior cervical ganglion. Dopamine-sensitive adenylate cyclase in various dopaminergic tracts of the CNS is receiving considerable attention as a possible site of action of antipsychotic drugs (Carlsson and Lindqvist, 1963; Kebabian *et al.*, 1972; Matthysse, 1973; Snyder *et al.*, 1974; Iversen, 1975).

In *presynaptic* regions cAMP-dependent protein kinases appear to be involved in the regulation of neurotransmitter synthesis. cAMP activates tyrosine hydroxylase (Goldstein *et al.*, 1973; Harris *et al.*, 1974), the rate-controlling enzyme for dopamine and norepinephrine synthesis, and this activation is almost certainly mediated by a protein kinase: it requires both ATP and Mg^{2+} (Mergenroth *et al.*, 1975; Lovenberg *et al.*, 1975; Lloyd and Kaufman, 1975), it occurs with purified protein kinase (Mergenroth *et al.*, 1975), and it is abolished by various inhibitors, both specific and nonspecific, of brain protein kinases (Mergenroth *et al.*, 1975).

The best-established functional component of synaptic membranes is a polypeptide of 95,000 daltons, a subunit of Na,K-ATPase, which can be identified by its phosphorylation (Welsh, 1972) according to the accepted mechanism for Na,K-ATPase (Uesugi *et al.*, 1971).

3.3.2. Fibrous Proteins

Four morphologically distinct types of intracellular fibrous structures that differ in diameter and in location have been described in mammalian nervous tissue: microtubules (200–260 Å), neurofilaments (90–100 Å), microfilaments (50 Å), and astrocytic filaments that are still smaller and exist in bundles rather than as single fibers (Peters *et al.*, 1970; Wuerker, 1970). Gray (1975*a*) has established through novel conditions of fixation that axonal microtubules in rat and frog brain extend through the terminal to the presynaptic membrane and are coated with synaptic vesicles. Connections between synaptic vesicles and microtubules in the spinal cord of lamprey ammocoete were earlier seen by Smith (1971). Axon terminals also contain neurofilaments (Gray and Guillery, 1966; Metuzals and Mushynski, 1974).

Fibrous structures are all composed of arrays of protein units, e.g., the unit protein of microtubules is tubulin which has a molecular weight of 110,000 daltons and a sedimentation coefficient of 6 S for the dimer (Shelanski and Taylor, 1967; Weisenberg *et al.*, 1968). Tubulin is isolated either by reassembly of microtubules when the medium is properly adjusted (Shelanski *et al.*, 1973; Borisy *et al.*, 1974) or by precipitation with vinblastine (Olmsted *et al.*, 1970). Vinblastine precipitates other proteins as well (Wilson *et al.*, 1970). Tubulin binds colchicine, but many chemical agents which disrupt microtubules cause inactivation of the colchicine-binding activity; vinca alkaloids (vinblastine and vincristine) stabilize colchicine-binding activity without altering the binding (Wilson, 1970). The colchicine-binding activity is also stabilized by GTP (Weisenberg *et al.*, 1968).

A brief but useful summary of the chemistry of tubulin and the use of colchicine and vinblastine to study the role of microtubules in neuronal function has been presented by Shelanski (1973). The proceedings of a symposium on the biology of cytoplasmic microtubules has recently been published (Soifer, 1975), and the chemistry and function of microtubules have been reviewed (Stephens and Edd, 1976).

Under denaturing conditions (SDS, mercaptoethanol) tubulin separates into two polypeptides (tubulin α and tubulin β) having molecular weights of 55,000–60,000 daltons but differing both in their amino acid compositions (Bryan and Wilson, 1971) and peptide maps (Feit *et al.*,

1971*a;* Fine, 1971). Brain tubulin has been detected in both particulate and cytoplasmic compartments (Feit and Barondes, 1970; Feit *et al.,* 1971*b*). Tubulin represents 10–40% of the soluble protein of nerve endings, depending on species and age (Dutton and Barondes, 1969; Feit *et al.,* 1971*b*). The large quantity present and its rapid turnover (Feit, 1971) indicate an important role in nerve function.

In studies of tubulin in synaptosomes and derived components (Blitz and Fine, 1974), a major protein band with molecular weight of 55,000 daltons was seen in SDS gels of synaptosomes, synaptic membranes, and synaptosomal cytosol. This protein was not present in either synaptosomal mitochondria or synaptic vesicles. Synaptosomal tubulin is similar but perhaps not identical to tubulin isolated from the cytosol fraction of brain which is derived primarily from cell bodies. Observed differences between membrane-bound and soluble tubulins are small, and their significance has not yet been established (Bhattacharyya and Wolff, 1975). Feit (1976) extracted a tubulinlike protein from nerve endings which was precipitated by vinblastine but did not possess colchicine-binding activity. In several respects, such as gel migration and peptide maps, the properties of the tubulinlike protein of nerve endings corresponded to those of soluble brain tubulin, but differences were still detectable. Soluble brain tubulin assembled into microtubules when the conditions were properly adjusted, but the nerve ending protein did not. Whether these differences are inherent in the structure or caused by impurities remains to be determined. Several reports (Banker *et al.,* 1972; Levitan *et al.,* 1972; Morgan *et al.,* 1973*b;* Gurd *et al.,* 1974; Mahadik *et al.,* 1976) have shown that synaptic membranes contain a number of closely spaced polypeptide bands in both SDS tube gels and SDS slab gels in the region of 45,000–60,000 daltons. A major band with a molecular weight of 55,000 ($\pm$2000) daltons was seen which was absent from rat brain nuclei, mitochondria, microsomes, and synaptic vesicles. Proteins of this size (53,000 daltons) found in synaptosomal membranes from both human and swine brain (Kornguth and Sunderland, 1975) had similar peptide maps and contained no carbohydrate or sialic acid. These proteins represented 1–2% of the total synaptosomal protein and did not arise from contamination with the tubulin in brain cytosol. The purified protein lost its capacity to bind colchicine. Tubulin in microtubules and synaptic junctions has been demonstrated by immunohistochemical methods (Matus *et al.,* 1975*b*), and in postsynaptic densities ("postsynaptic junctional lattice") by SDS gels, peptide mapping, and immunohistology (Walters and Matus, 1975*b*).

In a recent report, Kadota *et al.* (1976) isolated from the synaptosomes of pig brain a flocculent material, presumably representing matrix, which produced a "crystalloid" with vinblastine. This crystalloid resembled vinblastine-induced microtubule crystals (Soifer *et al.*, 1975; Wilson, 1975), suggesting a probable relation between the flocculent material, which adheres to vesicles, and tubulin.

Neurofilaments are composed principally of single-protein subunits, but these differ in size depending on the source. From axoplasm of squid giant axon (Huneeus and Davison, 1970) the size of the subunits is 80,000 daltons whereas from isolated axons of bovine white matter (Shelanski *et al.*, 1971) it is 60,000 daltons. These neurofilament proteins were different from tubulin; neither had the capacity to bind colchicine (Shelanski *et al.*, 1972). The size of the protein subunits in neurofilaments from calf brain was reported by Yen *et al.* (1976*a*) to be 54,000 daltons. Immunohistological studies (Yen *et al.*, 1976*b*) suggest that this protein is a major component of postsynaptic densities.

An actinlike fibrous protein is present in microfilaments of neuroblastoma cells (Chang and Goldman, 1973) as indicated by the binding of heavy meromyosin to the microfilament fibers, in a manner analogous to the binding of meromyosin to F-actin (Huxley, 1963). Actinlike filaments have also been detected in synaptosomes (Inestrosa *et al.*, 1976).

A fibrous protein with properties similar to those of actomyosin of muscle has been found in neural tissue and called neurostenin or "actomyosinlike protein of brain" (Berl, 1975*a,b*). The actinlike (neurin) and myosinlike (stenin) subunits of this protein have molecular weights of 47,000 and 240,000 daltons, respectively, which are very close to those of actin and myosin of muscle. The myosinlike protein is associated with synaptic vesicles whereas the actinlike protein is associated with synaptic membranes, giving rise to the hypothesis that their interaction is a step in the mechanism of exocytosis (Berl *et al.*, 1973). Berl *et al.* (1976) have now provided ultrastructural evidence based on binding of heavy meromyosin, that the actinlike protein is present in synaptosome membranes but not in vesicles.

Blitz and Fine (1974) have shown that major bands seen in SDS gels of polypeptides from synaptosomes and synaptic membranes correspond to actinlike, tropomyosinlike, and myosinlike proteins. The similarities were confirmed by peptide mapping. These proteins were not present in synaptic vesicles, but the actinlike protein was present in synaptosomal cytosol.

Another fibrous protein in nerve tissue is "brain dynein" (Gaskin *et al.*, 1974) which resembles dynein, a protein first detected in cilia of tetrahymena (Gibbons, 1966), by behaving as a divalent ion-activated ATPase (but of a much lower order of activity). Brain dynein has two subunits with molecular weights of 370,000 and 355,000, very similar to those of "sperm dynein" (370,000 and 350,000), but its ATPase activity is only 1/80th as high. Microtubules obtained by assembly of brain proteins maintain a constant ratio of brain dynein to tubulin on reassembly (Gaskin *et al.*, 1974). An ATPase with such a high molecular weight has not been reported in synaptosomes.

3.3.3. Proteins of Unknown Function

The characterization of protein components of subcellular fractions by electrophoresis in polyacrylamide gels in the presence of SDS, SDS plus urea, concentrated formic acid, and other polar solvents has become common practice even as improvements in methods are introduced. Most of the proteins so detected belong in this category of "unknown function." They are identified by molecular weights determined from the plot of logarithm of molecular weight versus relative rate of migration as described by Weber and Osborn (1969). A few polypeptides migrate anomalously in SDS gels (Bretscher, 1971; Furthmayer and Timpl, 1971; Panyim and Chalkley, 1971) and estimates of their size by this method are in error. An alternative method has been described (Rodbard and Chrambach, 1971, 1974) which is applicable to polypeptides separated by electrophoresis in SDS gels (Neville, 1971) by applying Ferguson plots (Ferguson, 1964). A similar method was used by Banker and Cotman (1972) to show that the same relation exists among molecular weight, retardation, and free mobility for SDS complexes of the major polypeptides of synaptic membranes as for the SDS complexes of soluble proteins. This method permits validation of molecular weight estimates.

A number of studies attempting to characterize synaptic particles by polypeptide composition suffer from limitations arising from incomplete separation of organelles of different types and poor resolution of the polypeptides themselves, either of low-molecular-weight polypeptides on 5.6% acrylamide gels (Banker *et al.*, 1972) or of high-molecular-weight polypeptides on 12.5% acrylamide gels (Morgan *et al.*, 1973*b*). Despite these difficulties, qualitative differences were always seen in comparing synaptosomes or synaptic membranes with mitochondria or myelin.

However, major polypeptide bands from synaptic plasma membranes correspond to those from microsomes (see later). Banker *et al.* (1972) found almost 30 bands in SDS–polyacrylamide tube gels of synaptic plasma membranes prepared by three different procedures. Molecular weights ranged from 20,000 to 211,000, with three bands (C6, C7, C8) of 99,000, 52,400, and 41,500 daltons accounting for 40–50% of the staining. Only traces of these bands were seen in mitochondria and myelin, whereas the major mitochondrial and myelin polypeptides were present only in minor amounts in synaptic plasma membranes. Two major polypeptides, with molecular weights of 93,000 and 52,000, were found in synaptic plasma membranes by Gurd *et al.* (1974). They also reported that the profiles of proteins (polypeptides) and glycoproteins in synaptic membranes and microsomes were very similar and differed substantially from mitochondrial profiles. Similar studies of the polypeptides of synaptic plasma membranes were also reported by Levitan *et al.* (1972), Wanamaker and Kornguth (1973), and Karlsson *et al.* (1973).

The polypeptides of rat brain synaptic membranes, synaptic junctions, and synaptic vesicles were compared by Morgan *et al.* (1973*b*). In synaptic membranes over 30 bands were seen ranging in molecular weight from 12,000 to 210,000 daltons, with the nine most prominent bands at 160,000, 93,000, 52,000, 39,000, 30,300, 18,000, 16,000, 14,000, and 12,000 daltons. The three polypeptides of 93,000, 53,000, and 39,000 daltons correspond to polypeptide chains identified in purified Na,K-ATPase of bovine brain (Uesugi *et al.*, 1971) in agreement with the high Na,K-ATPase activity found in synaptic membranes (Morgan *et al.*, 1971; Gurd *et al.*, 1974; Tamir *et al.*, 1976*a*).* Although the polypeptides of synaptic vesicles were all present in synaptic membranes, significant quantitative differences were observed in a number of bands, and such differences were also observed in comparing vesicles and synaptic junctions. Five glycoproteins (120,000, 66,000, 43,000, 34,000, and 23,000) were detected in synaptic membranes, but only three (recorded as 120,000, 68,000, and 45,000) were present in synaptic vesicles (Morgan *et al.*, 1973*b*). It is of interest to recall that Pearse (1975) found only a single protein of 180,000 daltons in the complex vesicle fraction of pig brain.

The sequential extraction of proteins with progressively increasing concentrations of Triton X-100 and SDS has been useful in determining the nature of their association (integral, peripheral) with membrane particles (Bosman *et al.*, 1970; Waehneldt *et al.*, 1971; Cotman *et al.*, 1971*c*; Breckenridge and Morgan, 1972). This method may reveal differences between subcellular particles that will be useful for their characterization.

Substantial improvement in the electrophoretic resolution of polypeptides in subcellular organelles of brain has been described by Mahadik *et al.* (1976) using one-dimensional slab gels containing SDS and a discontinuous buffer. Optimization of conditions was obtained by delipidation of the

---

*A large number of different polypeptides in the range 50,000–60,000 daltons are found by gel electrophoresis of synaptic membrane extracts. Their molecular weights cannot be established with sufficient precision to expect agreement in reports from different laboratories. At least three prominent bands have been identified representing subunits of acetylcholinesterase (Rosenberry, 1975), Na,K-ATPase, and tubulin.

membranes, adjustment of the ratio of SDS to protein, use of EDTA and mercaptoethanol, storage under nitrogen, and maintaining pH at 6.8. Electrophoresis conditions and staining technique were also adjusted. These modifications provided reproducible electrophoretograms having sharp, well-resolved bands that permitted more accurate comparisons of different fractions. On 10% polyacrylamide slab gels over 50 polypeptide bands were resolved, whereas on 9–25% gradient slabs, over 70 polypeptide bands were seen ranging in molecular weights from less than 10,000 to greater than 200,000. With this method, well-marked differences were detectable between synaptic membranes and microsomes for the first time, and the nuclear and mitochondrial fractions were substantially different. For example, mitochondria displayed 12 bands with molecular weights below 19,000, whereas nuclei had the usual four major histone bands in addition to two minor bands in this low-molecular-weight region. Synaptic membranes and microsomes had relatively little protein in this region, but significant differences between these fractions were found in the location and intensity of six microsomal bands (15,000, 24,500, 43,000, 46,500, 69,000, and 71,000) and seven synaptic membrane bands (17,700, 18,500, 23,000, 29,000, 42,000, 47,000, and 50,000).

The composition of isolated postsynaptic densities appears to be almost entirely (>90%) proteinaceous (Banker et al., 1974) since these particles were degraded by proteolytic enzymes but not by glycosidases, ribonuclease, or deoxyribonuclease. They displayed two major and six lesser polypeptide bands on SDS gels, a much simpler profile than that of other subcellular particles. One major band, representing 45% of the total protein in postsynaptic densities, had a molecular weight of 53,000 daltons (corresponding to band C7 in the synaptic membranes of Banker et al., 1972). The other major band, representing 17% of the protein, had a molecular weight of 97,000 daltons. The lesser components, each representing 3–9% of the protein, ranged in size from 100,000 to 180,000 daltons. The proteins of postsynaptic densities contained much larger amounts of polar amino acids than proteins in synaptic membranes (Cotman et al., 1968b). Their high content of basic amino acids is consistent with the suggestion (Bloom and Aghajanian, 1968; Pfenninger, 1971) that these residues are primarily involved in the staining of postsynaptic densities with ethanolic phosphotungstic acid and bismuth iodide–uranyl–lead.

Two acidic proteins that have been found to be associated with synaptosomes are S-100 (Rusca et al., 1972; Donato and Michetti, 1974; Hyden, 1974) and GP-350 (Van Nieuw Amerongen and Roukema, 1974). The association between S-100 and synaptic membranes (Hyden, 1974) is dependent on Ca^{2+} (Moore, 1973) and appears to be very weak, since the S-

100 can be dissociated (solubilized) by treatment with 5% pentanol (Rusca *et al.*, 1972). It has been suggested that receptors for S-100 protein are present in synaptosomes (Donato *et al.*, 1975). The association of GP-350 with synaptic membranes is based on immunochemical and immunohisto-logical evidence (Van Nieuw Amerongen *et al.*, 1974).

3.4. Lipid Composition

A characteristic feature, first noted by Eichberg *et al.* (1964) and confirmed by Lapetina *et al.* (1967), was that synaptic membranes were enriched in gangliosides, a family of neuraminic acid-containing glyco-sphingolipids present in much higher concentrations in gray matter than in white matter, whereas synaptic vesicles and synaptic mitochondria contained little. Breckenridge *et al.* (1972) reported ganglioside concentrations in synaptic membranes of 70–125 μg/mg protein. It has also been found that the sphingomyelins of synaptic membranes differ from those of other membranes, particularly myelin, in having predominantly shorter-chain (C_{16}, C_{18}) fatty acids rather than C_{24} fatty acids (Cotman *et al.*, 1969; Kishimoto *et al.*, 1969; Breckenridge *et al.*, 1971, 1972). Synaptic membranes are also reported to have a much higher content than myelin or white matter of polyunsaturated acids (arachidonic, docosahexenoic) in their ethanolamine and serine–phosphoglycerides (Breckenridge *et al.*, 1971, 1972). It has been suggested (Nielson *et al.*, 1970) that polyunsaturated phosphatides may have an important role in excitability of membranes.

3.5. Antigenic Components

Antisera prepared against cells, cell membranes, and other organelles are capable of defining selected antigenic components in such structures, for example the blood group antigens in erythrocytes (Cook and Eylar, 1965; Hakomori and Strycharz, 1968) and transplantation antigens in guinea pig and mouse tissues (Shimada and Nathenson, 1969; Yamane and Nathenson, 1970; Kahan and Reisfeld, 1967). Antisera against adult rat brain, neonatal rat brain, synaptic membranes, and synaptic vesicles have shown the presence of a number of antigens such as C1, D1, D2, and D3 (Bock *et al.*, 1974; Jorgensen and Bock, 1974) but these have not yet been isolated or chemically characterized. Their localizations (C1 in vesicles; D1, D2, and D3 in neuronal membranes) have been established by crossed immunoelectrophoresis against synaptic structures solubilized with Triton X-100. The specificity of antisera prepared against intact synaptosomes was shown (Herschman *et al.*, 1972) by their serological (complement fixation) reactions with synaptosomes and synaptic membranes but not with other particulate materials (myelin, nuclei, mitochondria, synaptic vesicles, or membranes from organs other than brain). Since antisera against synaptic membranes, when injected into the brain, can produce a number of biological effects such as interference with learning (Karpiak *et al.*, 1974; Karpiak and Rapport, 1975), induction of seizure activity (De Robertis *et al.*, 1966; Karpiak *et al.*, 1974; Karpiak and Rapport, 1975), and alterations in morphology (De Robertis *et al.*, 1968), and since such antisera have specific staining properties for nerve terminals (Livett *et al.*, 1974), it will be of great importance to isolate the individual antigenic components of synaptic membranes to determine whether one or several different antigen–antibody systems are involved. There is little doubt that the antisera used in these studies contain antibodies in varying amounts to an undefined number of different antigens, and this complexity and attendant ambiguity have hindered more extensive exploitation of the technique. The use of antisera against purified brain proteins for immunohistochemical studies is covered extensively by Eng and Bigbee in Chapter 2.

4. FUNCTIONAL ORGANIZATION

4.1. Axonal Transport

The dynamic state of synaptic constituents is maintained by four processes of supply and four of disposal. In order of importance the supply is dependent on axonal transport from perikaryon to nerve terminal (presynaptic), intradendritic transport (postsynaptic), glial support, and transneuronal transfer (Droz, 1973; Kreutzberg *et al.*, 1973; Grafstein, 1975). Disposal is carried out by means of local enzymatic proteolysis, retrograde transport, transfer to glial cells, and transfer transneuronally. At the present time, the predominant mechanism of supply of proteins, lipids, nucleic acids, mitochondria, and synaptic vesicles to the axon terminals appears to be axonal transport from the perikaryon. Bondy (1975) has compared the several techniques used to study axonal transport. Some studies (Singer and Salpeter, 1966*a,b*; Singer and Green, 1968) suggest that supporting glial cells may supply axons with metabolites which are then transported to axon terminals. Direct transfer of material from glia to neurons has been observed only in tissue culture (Geiger, 1963) and in isolated squid giant axon (Lasek *et al.*, 1974). Axonal transport proceeds at different rates for different constituents. In studies of axonal transport of various particles,

Kirkpatrick *et al.* (1972) acquired evidence that axonal transport is a complex phenomenon in which movement of individual particulate components such as mitochondria might involve specific mechanisms. However, Ochs (1975) has proposed a unitarian concept based on such particles being repeatedly bound to and released from transport filaments. These transport filaments would move along two sets of microtubules, one directing orthograde and the other retrograde movements.

Evidence has been presented, based on autoradiography and gel electrophoresis, that synaptic membranes are maintained by fast axonal transport (Krygier-Brevart *et al.,* 1974). Using a corticothalamic tract in rabbits extending from striate cortex to the lateral geniculate nucleus, labeled leucine was found to be incorporated into synaptic membrane polypeptides, the majority of which were in the range 50,000–120,000 daltons. Since this tract showed little local protein biosynthesis, interference from labeled proteins in microsomes was very low. Proteins in synaptic vesicles also contained little label. Droz *et al.* (1975), using heavy metal impregnation of rat spinal and chick ciliary ganglia in conjunction with low- and high-voltage electron microscopy, found smooth endoplasmic reticulum in a continuous system extending along the axon to the axon terminal. The presence of such a continuous system suggested that renewal of both axonal membranes and synaptic vesicles proceeds through connections with this smooth endoplasmic reticulum.

The removal of proteins from axon terminals by proteolysis is supported by the presence of a large amount of different proteases (Marks and Lajtha, 1971) in such terminals. To maintain steady state conditions, proteins that are carried to nerve endings by rapid axonal transport must also be catabolized rapidly. Synaptic membrane proteins have relatively long half-lives, up to several weeks (Marko and Cuenod, 1973). Transport of RNA to nerve endings is of particular interest because of early reports suggesting that protein synthesis occurs there. However, there is little evidence that ribosomal RNA (Barondes, 1974) and heterogeneous mRNA (Jones, 1975) are present in the axon terminal (other than that associated with mitochondria). The presence of transfer RNA has been demonstrated (Lasek, 1972), suggesting that adding amino acid residues to preexisting proteins may be a regulatory mechanism (Soffer *et al.,* 1969).

4.2. Release, Storage, and Uptake

The most significant steps in the utilization of chemical transmitters, namely, storage, release, and removal either by reuptake or enzymatic inactivation, have been dealt with in a number of reviews (Axelrod, 1973;

Dahlstrom, 1973; Fonnum, 1973). In an extensive discussion of release mechanisms, Jones (1975) has summarized the evidence for and limitations of quantal release, the vesicle hypothesis, and exocytosis in the functioning of cholinergic central synapses.

4.2.1. Release

Drawing heavily on evidence for the release mechanisms present in adrenal medulla, the neuromuscular junction, sympathetic ganglia, and neurosecretory tissue, the view most widely held is that transmitters in central axon terminals are stored in vesicles in definite quantities and released by exocytosis (Jones, 1975). There is, however, little direct evidence from central synapses to support this hypothesis, and a number of observations are difficult to reconcile with it, such as the existence of three pools of acetylcholine (stable bound, labile bound, and free), the preferential release of newly synthesized neurotransmitter, distinctive differences in chemical composition between vesicular membranes and synaptic plasma membranes, and inhomogeneity of the vesicle population in axon terminals. Experimental manipulation of the neuromuscular junction or peripheral ganglion by nerve stimulation or administration of black widow spider venom (Frontali *et al.*, 1976) or treatment with elevated concentrations of K^+ has shown that transmitter release is associated with a decrease in the number of vesicles. Reutilization of vesicle membrane appears to take place, after fusion with the plasma membrane and exocytosis, by transport within the membrane to appropriate sites, retrieval via formation of coated vesicles, coalescence of such vesicles into cisternae, and budding of cisternae with formation of new vesicles. This proposed mechanism (Heuser and Reese, 1973) emphasizes conservation of membrane components in the junction. However, the functional demands in the neuromuscular junction differ sufficiently from those in peripheral ganglia and in central synapses to eliminate any compulsion to accept identical release mechanisms for all three systems, nor is it especially likely that such mechanisms in cholinergic, noradrenergic, and serotonergic synapses will all show the same features. Macromolecular components of the process have not yet been identified, and it will be of considerable interest to see whether the unusual protein in coated vesicles (Pearse, 1975) will permit some new access to this process, provided the coat protein does not represent an artifact (Matus, 1976*a*).

The many factors triggering or inhibiting release require much further study. For example, evidence has been presented (Paton *et al.*, 1971; Vizi, 1972) to support the view that stimulation of Na,K-ATPase in axon terminals inhibits transmitter release, and that the inhibition of release by prostaglandins (Gilbert *et al.,* 1975) is the result of such stimulation. Another example is the inhibition of release by vinca alkaloids, cytochalasin B, and colchicine (Nicklas *et al.,* 1973).

4.2.2. *Storage*

Maintenance of neurotransmitter stores in the axon terminal is dependent both on biosynthesis of transmitter in the terminal (where the required enzymes are all present) and on reuptake into the terminal of released neurotransmitter (a rapid mechanism for inactivation) (Axelrod, 1973). Although some neurotransmitter is synthesized in the cell body and transported to axon terminals in particulate form, the quantity handled in this way does not contribute significantly (Dahlstrom and Haggendal, 1966).

The heterogeneity of storage compartments for biogenic amines has been suggested by several lines of evidence. One is the differential response to drugs as detected in the distribution of amine between soluble and particulate fractions (Glowinski and Axelrod, 1966). A second is the failure of autoradiographic studies to demonstrate that most of the vesicles in axons and axon terminals are associated with labeled biogenic amines (Bloom, 1970*b*; Descarries and Droz, 1970). A third is that newly synthesized or newly injected biogenic amine is more rapidly utilized than that already present in the tissue (Collier, 1969; Glowinski *et al.,* 1972; Enna and Shore, 1974). There is now direct evidence indicating a physical basis for such differences in storage compartments for one neurotransmitter. A high-affinity, soluble binding protein for serotonin has been discovered (Tamir and Huang, 1974; Tamir and Rapport, 1976; Tamir *et al.,* 1976*b*) which is associated with serotonergic tracts, is localized in synaptosome cytoplasm, and binds newly synthesized amine. Thus two possible storage compartments for serotonin, one soluble and the other particulate, are present in the CNS and in the peripheral nervous system as well (Jonakait *et al.,* 1977). Whether similar soluble binding proteins exist for other transmitters or whether this compartment represents a special feature of serotonergic systems will have to be ascertained. There are reasons to believe that storage and/or release of serotonin in the CNS may have unique features, since few serotonergic axon terminals show typical synaptic densities (Descarries *et al.,* 1975), and the serotonin levels in brain are modulated rather quickly by dietary manipulation (Wurtman and Fernstrom, 1972). In contrast, only a single storage pool for GABA was indicated (Neal and Iversen, 1969) by experiments on the subcellular distribution of endogenous and exogenous transmitters.

4.2.3. Uptake

Although the overall processing (storage, release, and uptake) of neurotransmitters appears to be a highly specific phenomenon so that Dale's principle that each neuron has but one transmitter is still correct, the uptake process tends to show a lesser degree of specificity than do storage or release. Reuptake, which is the principal mechanism of inactivation of catecholamines and serotonin but not of acetylcholine, is of considerable interest as an important site of action of tricyclic antidepressant drugs. These drugs display differential activities, e.g., imipramine and chlorimipramine are far more effective than desipramine or protriptyline in blocking serotonin uptake, whereas desipramine and protriptyline are effective blockers of norepinephrine uptake (Weil-Malherbe, 1976).

The uptake process has five characteristic properties: it is saturable, temperature- sensitive, Na^+-dependent, inhibited by dinitrophenol and ouabain, and permits accumulation of transmitter against a concentration gradient (Kuhar, 1973). The process is considered to be mediated through a specific carrier mechanism, but the Na^+ dependence and inhibition by ouabain suggest that Na,K-ATPase, which is very active in presynaptic membranes, is also involved. Vinblastine inhibits the uptake of norepinephrine and dopamine by brain synaptosomes *in vitro* (Nicklas *et al.,* 1973), and both colchicine and vinblastine inhibit the uptake of serotonin into rat brain synaptosomes but not into small vesicle fractions (Nomura and Segawa, 1975). The inference from these experiments is that tubulinlike molecules in the synaptosomal membrane are involved in the uptake process.

4.3. Topography

4.3.1. Introduction

Understanding the relation between physiological function and molecular organization of the membranes of various subcellular particles is now one of the principal objectives of many neurochemists and cell biologists. Evidence has been accumulating that membrane fluidity and chemical groups exposed on the outer membrane surface are involved in growth and proliferation of cells and their processes (Singer, 1974). The organization of the molecules at the surface of the tip of the growing axon must play an important role in mechanical guidance, chemotaxis, and the location of complementary receptive sites on the postsynaptic cell during developmental and regenerative processes (Cotman and Banker, 1974; Sidman, 1974).

Organization of subsynaptic structures has been examined in great detail by electron microscopy, but the elucidation of cytoarchitecture in terms of specific macromolecular arrangements has barely begun. Explorations of molecular organization take advantage of new techniques for identifying functional molecules (e.g., receptors and components of transport systems), for labeling specific groups on exposed surfaces, for specific staining of organelles rich in protein (e.g., postsynaptic densities), and for selective dissection of macromolecules with specialized groups (e.g., sialoglycoproteins, glycoproteins, and gangliosides) or specialized properties (e.g., enzymes and antigens).

Postsynaptic densities *in situ* were shown to have a uniquely high proportion of protein (Bloom and Aghajanian, 1966, 1968), since they were resistant to the actions of the carbohydrases and nucleases but were destroyed by proteases. These deductions were confirmed by analysis of isolated postsynaptic densities (Banker *et al.,* 1974; Cohen *et al.,* 1976). Since, as discussed earlier, presynaptic and postsynaptic membranes contain a substantial quantity of tubulinlike protein (Banker *et al.,* 1974; Matus *et al.,* 1975*b*), Matus (1976*b*) has suggested that this protein may be involved in organizing the distribution of membrane proteins. This suggestion is consistent with the hypothesis (Berlin, 1975) that tubulin acts as a molecular framework serving to bind membrane molecules together into a "supramolecular array" at the cell surface.

Gray (1975*b*) has recently suggested the term "stereoframework" to describe certain intracellular and extracellular regions known to be rich in protein complexes and which show, when fixed and processed for electron microscopy, a reticular precipitate representing a three-dimensional framework of material forming the walls of polygonal lacunae. Examples of such stereoframeworks are presynaptic dense projections, cleft substance, postsynaptic densities, cytonets, coats of coated vesicles, reticulosomes, and the "microfilamentous network" of growth cones. Distortions may be introduced when the stereoframework precipitates during processing.

Di Carlo (1975) has discussed the use of high-resolution electron microscopy in studies of the macromolecular organization of membranes and organelles in nervous tissue. The results encourage the application of this method to nerve tissue in different functional, pathological, or pharmacologically altered states.

The "fluid mosaic model" of membrane structure (Singer, 1972, 1974; Singer and Nicolson, 1972) appears to be generally applicable to nerve membranes. It has been shown by Tasaki *et al.* (1971, 1973*a,b*) that electrical stimulation of nerve is accompanied by a transient change in the intensity of light derived from various fluorescent membrane probes, and Hoss and Abood (1974) presented evidence for fluidity in the hydrophobic regions of synaptic membranes using a similar technique.

A general approach to the study of molecular organization of membranes is to label membrane molecules either covalently or noncovalently. Covalently attached labels are introduced with either chemical reagents or enzymes, whereas noncovalent labels are introduced with binding probes for the receptor, such as neurotoxins, lectins, colchicine, neurotransmitters, transmitter antagonists and agonists, to name a few. In a review, Carraway (1975) summarized elegantly the techniques for covalent labeling of membranes and applications to erythrocytes, platelets, and cultured cells, both normal and transformed. This approach allows identification of membrane receptors or other components involved in functional processes such as transport or protein phosphorylation. Although freely dissociated cells such as the human erythrocyte permit unambiguous study and interpretation of the organization of the proteins in their membranes (Steck, 1974), isolated synaptosomes are much more difficult targets because of their fragility and great heterogeneity, and the appreciable contamination of preparations with broken membranes and other elements derived from glia and neurons.

4.3.2. Covalent Labeling

Covalent labeling, when it takes advantage of endogenous enzyme systems, may be correlated with functional processes and thereby provide some indication of functional organization. This is particularly effective in the phosphorylation of membrane proteins by endogenous protein kinases in which ^{32}P is introduced from a labeled nucleotide donor. The enzymes (some of which are dependent on cAMP or cGMP) and the proteins involved in endogenous phosphorylation of synaptosomes have been discussed earlier. A number of reports involve cAMP-dependent protein phosphorylation in functional processes such as erythrocyte permeability (Rudoph and Greengard, 1974) and Na^+ transport both in erythrocytes (Gardner et al., 1973) and in toad bladder (Walton et al., 1975). Phosphorylated proteins obtained in such studies can be identified and characterized. Evidence has been presented showing that two "microtubule associated proteins" (MAP$_1$, 350,000 daltons; MAP$_2$, 300,000 daltons) are phosphorylated in vivo, but only one, MAP$_2$, is phosphorylated in vitro by intrinsic cAMP-dependent protein kinase (Sloboda et al., 1975). These proteins are thought to be similar to dynein and to serve as attachment arms to microtubules. Goodman et al. (1970) found that tubulin preparations from bovine cerebral cortex contain a cAMP-dependent protein kinase that phosphorylates tubulin *in vitro*. Similar endogenous kinases were found in pig brain tubulin (Soifer, 1973) and rat brain tubulin (Eipper, 1974*a*), but the enzyme in rat brain was not cAMP-dependent. The β subunit of tubulin is preferentially phosphorylated (Lagnado *et al.*, 1972). Tubulins phosphorylated *in vivo* differ from those phosphorylated *in vitro* (Eipper, 1974*a,b*) in their states of aggregation, rates of gel filtration, and in the labeled peptides found after proteolysis. The relation between *in vitro* phosphorylation and polymerization of tubulin subunits has been discussed (Rappaport *et al.*, 1975).

A method of covalently labeling exposed regions of proteins in the external cell surface is by enzyme-mediated iodination using lactoperoxidase (Phillips and Morrison, 1970). Its application to murine neuroblastoma cells in differentiated and undifferentiated states (Truding *et al.*, 1974) revealed the presence of a protein (78,000 daltons) on the surface of undifferentiated cells. This method was also used (Poduslo and Braun, 1975) to show (1) that several high-molecular-weight proteins were exposed in intact myelin sheaths, (2) that proteolipid protein was only partially exposed, and (3) that the basic protein in myelin must be located on the inner surface of the membrane since it was not labeled at all. Enzyme-mediated iodination of synaptic plasma membranes (Wang *et al.*, 1975) showed that the iodinatable groups of polypeptides with molecular weights of 205,000, 185,000, 92,000, and 39,000 daltons were located within the membrane, since such groups were labeled only after synaptosomes were lysed. A topographical distribution largely within the lipid bilayer is suggested for these proteins that are inaccessible in intact synaptosomes as well as for others that cannot be labeled even in isolated membrane preparations. A limitation in the use of lactoperoxidase for such labeling experiments has been pointed out (Gow and Wardlaw, 1975).

A second method for covalent labeling of groups in the external cell surface was introduced by Steck (1972). Hydroxyl groups of terminal galactose and galactosamine residues on the carbohydrate chains of glycoproteins and glycolipids are first oxidized with galactose oxidase; the aldehyde groups so formed are then reduced with tritium-labeled sodium borohydride to hydroxyl groups, thereby reestablishing the original structure with incorporation of a tritium atom. This technique has been applied under appropriate conditions for external surface labeling of intact synaptosomes (Mahadik *et al.*, 1975, 1977; Hungund *et al.*, 1975).

Purified synaptosomes were labeled and disrupted by osmotic shock; the membranes were then fractionated on a step gradient of diatrizoate (Tamir *et al.*, 1976*a*) to give four progressively denser membrane fractions (A–D) and a mitochondrial pellet (E). Specific incorporations (ratio of label found with enzyme to that without enzyme) were A, 4.5; B, 2.4; C–E, ≤ 1.6. (Labeling of isolated membrane fractions showed five- to sixfold greater incorporation and less discrimination.) In fractions A and B, which are the purest synaptic plasma membranes, one-third of the label was in protein and two-thirds was in lipid (chloroform–methanol extract). Delipidated membranes showed six labeled polypeptide bands in polyacrylamide tube gels (Figure 2) with molecular weights of 96,000, 72,000, 53,000, 33,000, 25,000, and less than 17,000 daltons. Gradient slab gels showed that the size of the smallest band was 7800–3200 daltons and that the largest incorporation of label was in two regions: the smallest band and that near 72,000–70,000 daltons. The presence of oligosaccharide chains in a number of these labeled polypeptides could be confirmed with the periodic acid–Schiff stain, consistent with similar identification by Morgan et al. (1973b) of three bands (66,000, 34,000, and 23,000 daltons) as glycoproteins. Most

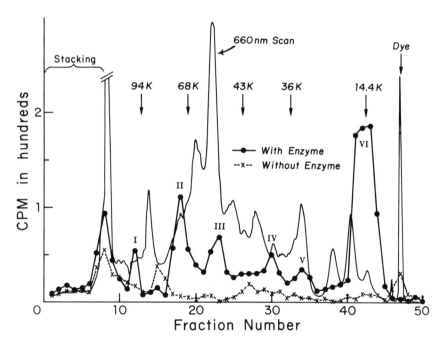

FIGURE 2. Polypeptides of synaptic membrane fraction A after surface labeling of intact synaptosomes. Delipidated membrane protein (about 100 µg) from synaptosomes treated with galactose oxidase-labeled borohydride was subjected to electrophoresis in 10% acrylamide tube gels at pH 8.8. Gels were stained with Coomassie blue, destained, and scanned at 660 nm for proteins. Gels were sliced and radioactivity was counted.

of the polypeptides in the ranges 160,000–96,000 and 70,000–40,000 daltons that were accessible to galactose oxidase in isolated membrane preparations were not labeled in intact synaptosomes.

The specific labeling of glycolipids was almost entirely restricted to a single ganglioside species, G_{M1}.

By comparing the results obtained with intact synaptosomes and isolated synaptic membrane fractions, two conclusions could be drawn. One was that only a minor fraction of the membrane constituents are accessible for functional interactions at the external surface of the intact axon terminal (the most important molecules are the six polypeptide groups and G_{M1} ganglioside). The other was that, assuming the generally accepted asymmetric orientation of saccharide chains toward the outer surface, the molecular organization of the external membrane of axon terminals must be very close-knit. Only after disruption of synaptosomes does this tight organization fall apart with consequent exposure of the greater part of the saccharide chains of glycoproteins and gangliosides.

4.3.3. Binding Probes

Since plasma membranes of cells contain surface receptors for many substances such as insulin (Cuatrecasas, 1972, 1973*a*), lectins (Lis and Sharon, 1973; Cuatrecasas, 1973*b*; Nicolson, 1974), and cholera toxin (Cuatrecasas, 1973*c*), these substances have been used to study synaptic membranes for the localization of similar receptors. Using the ferritin–concanavalin A technique (Stobo *et al.*, 1972), Matus *et al.* (1973) showed that concanavalin A was extensively bound to the external face of the postsynaptic membrane, less so in the synaptic cleft, and not bound to the inner face, to synaptic vesicles, or to mitochondria. The intramembrane mobility of these receptors for concanavalin A was abolished by glutaraldehyde fixation. Cotman and Taylor (1974) found these sites to be tightly structured since they were not disrupted by Triton X-100. The affinity for concanavalin A suggests that glycoprotein receptors contain α-glucosyl or α-mannosyl residues. Similar results were obtained by Bittiger and Schnebli (1974), who also found that ricin, another lectin, was bound to the synaptic cleft to a much lesser extent than concanavalin A. Ricin binding is indicative of galactosyl residues.

Cholera toxin appears to be a specific plasma membrane marker (Chang *et al.*, 1975), binding to receptor sites containing ganglioside (Cuatrecasas, 1973*d*). Recently Manuelidis and Manuelidis (1976) reported that G_{M1} ganglioside receptors for cholera toxin were present in the surface of cells as detected histologically using a conjugate of cholera toxin with peroxidase. One may therefore expect cholera toxin to bind to the external surface of some axon terminals, where G_{M1} ganglioside molecules are exposed (Hungund *et al.*, 1975). It should be of great interest to establish the concordance between this method of detecting ganglioside receptors and that based on the use of labeled antiganglioside antibodies (De Baecque *et al.*, 1976).

5. PROSPECT

The remarkable progress that neurochemists have made over the past 10 years in biochemical dissection and cytochemical characterization of synaptic elements should serve as a great source of encouragement in attacking the many complex problems that this progress has brought within experimental range. As indicated in this chapter, we have gained decisive entry into the phase of separation and identification of the macromolecular components of the synaptic region. The information now being acquired is prerequisite to determination of structural organization and elucidation of the relation between such organization and functional properties. Our present conception of this relationship in mitochondria serves as an excellent model.

Fundamental progress in the study of macromolecules has made it possible to attack conceptually more complex problems in membrane function. For example, the concept of conformational alterations in macromolecules, as the result of the binding of ligands, readily permits projection of mechanisms for the most central of neurochemical processes, namely, the induction by neurotransmitters of transient alterations in the permeability of membranes to ions. It is now possible to formulate molecular models of the excitatory postsynaptic membrane involving interacting ionophores (Dubois and Schoffeniels, 1975) for Na^+ and K^+ that permit computer simulation of the quantitative aspects of both excitatory postsynaptic potentials and current. Such models can provide the experimental tests that will determine whether ion channels are coupled to receptors or whether they are directly opened by transmitter–receptor interaction. The experiments require the receptors to be isolated and reconstituted into experimental systems, and a rich source of acetylcholine receptors is available in the electric organs of torpedo and eel. Thus this exciting reconstitution experiment is close to realization for a cholinergic system. However, cholinergic transmission shows sufficient differences from other systems, particularly in the mechanisms of neurotransmitter release into and removal from the synaptic cleft, to restrict acceptance of the generality of the acetylcholine mechanism until more information can be acquired concerning the agonist action of other neurotransmitters: norepinephrine, serotonin, GABA, and the like. The problem of isolating receptors for these systems is therefore a pressing one and at present appears to be most formidable.

In this current phase of dissection of macromolecular components of the synaptic region, four of the more powerful of the available tools would seem to be separation by affinity chromatography, specific labeling techniques for both receptors and components of transport systems, immunological analysis using both crossed electrophoresis and histological techniques, and resolution of polypeptides by slab gel electrophoresis. There is a great need for methods for completely removing detergents required to solubilize integral proteins of the membrane, so that the properties of isolated proteins can be determined and the reconstitution experiments carried out. A large number of proteins are probably present in synaptic regions and these must still be identified and assigned some function.

A major challenge to neurochemists arises from a consideration of the diversified nature of the brain and awareness of the heterogeneity (with respect to the many different types of cells in which they originate) of all subcellular components now under study. Morphologists are constantly adding to this challenge with improved fixation procedures that permit identification of additional synaptic features, such as matrix material, synaptic ribbons, and vesicular differences. This area of neuroscience is thus continuing to expand and to offer much to attract those who rally to the banner of what W. B. Yeats called "the fascination of what's difficult."

6. REFERENCES

Abdel-Latif, A. A., 1966, A simple method for isolation of nerve-ending particles from rat brain. *Biochim. Biophys. Acta* **121**:403–406.

Akert, K., Moore, H., Pfenninger, K., and Sandri, C., 1969, Contributions of new impregnation methods and freeze-etching to the problems of synaptic fine structure, *Prog. Brain Res.* **31**:223–240.

Appel, S. H., Day, E. D., and Mickey, D. D., 1972, Cellular and subcellular fractionation, in: *Basic Neurochemistry* (R. W. Albers, G. J. Siegel, R. Katzman, and B. W. Agranoff, eds.), pp. 425–448, Little, Brown, Boston, Mass.

Arora, R. C., Vugrincic, C., Ungar, F., and Alivisatos, S. G. A., 1974, The presence of monoamine oxidase in synaptic membranes of bovine brain, *Pharmacologist* **16(2)**:249.

Autilio, L. A., Appel, S. H., Pettis, P., and Gambetti, P. L., 1968, Biochemical studies of synapses *in vitro* I. Protein synthesis, *Biochemistry* **7**:2615–2622.

Axelrod, J., 1973, The fate of noradrenaline in the sympathetic neuron, in: *The Harvey Lectures,* Series 67, pp. 175–197, Academic Press, New York.

Balazs, R., Hajos, R., Johnson, A. L., Reinjnierse, G. L. A., Tapia, R., and Wilkin, G. P., 1975, Large fragments of cerebellar glomeruli, *Brain Res.* **86**:17–30.

Baldessarini, R. J., and Vogt, M., 1971, Uptake and release of norepinephrine by rat brain tissue fractions prepared by ultrafiltration, *J. Neurochem.* **18**:951–962.

Banker, G. A., and Cotman, C. W., 1972, Measurement of free electrophoretic mobility and retardation coefficient of protein–sodium dodecyl sulphate complexes by gel electrophoresis: A method to validate molecular weight estimates, *J. Biol. Chem.* **247**:5856–5861.

Banker, G., Crain, B., and Cotman, C. W., 1972, Molecular weights of the polypeptide chains of synaptic plasma membranes, *Brain Res.* **42**:508–513.

Banker, G., Churchill, L., and Cotman, C. W., 1974, Proteins of the postsynaptic density, *J. Cell Biol.* **63**:456–465.

Barondes, S. H., 1968, Further studies of the transport of proteins to nerve endings, *J. Neurochem.* **15**:343–350.

Barondes, S. H., 1974, Synaptic macromolecules: Identification and metabolism, *Annu. Rev. Biochem.* **43**:147–168.

Barondes, S. H., and Dutton, G. R., 1969, Acetoxycycloheximide effect on synthesis and metabolism of glucosamine-containing macromolecules in brain and in nerve endings, *J. Neurobiol.* **1**:99–110.

Berl, S., 1975*a,* Actomyosin-like protein in brain, in: *Advances in Neurochemistry* (B. W. Agranoff and M. H. Aprison, eds.), Vol. 1, pp. 157–187, Plenum Press, New York.

Berl, S., 1975*b,* The actomyosin-like system in nervous tissue, in: *The Nervous System* (D. B. Tower, ed.), Vol. 1: *The Basic Neurosciences,* pp. 565–573, Raven Press, New York.

Berl, S., and Nicklas, W. J., 1975, Contractile proteins in relation to transmitter release, in: *Metabolic Compartmentation and Neurotransmission: Relation to Brain Structure and Function* (S. Berl, D. D. Clarke, and D. Schneider, eds.), NATO Adv. Study Inst. Series A, Vol. 6, pp. 247–272, Plenum Press, New York.

Berl, S., Puszkin, S., and Nicklas, W. J., 1973, Actomyosin-like protein in brain: Actomyosin-like protein may function in the release of transmitter material at synaptic endings, *Science* **179**:441–446.

Berl, S., Schwartz, J., Nicklas, W. J., Mahendran, C., Whetsell, W. O., and Elizan, T. S., 1975, Molecular and supramolecular interactions in the presynaptic regions, *Trans. Am. Soc. Neurochem.* **7**:60.

Berlin, R. D., 1975, Microtubules and the fluidity of the cell surface, *Ann. N.Y. Acad. Sci.* **253**:445–454.

Bhattacharyya, B., and Wolff, J., 1975, Membrane-bound tubulin in brain and thyroid tissue, *J. Biol. Chem.* **250**:7639–7646.

Bittiger, H., 1975, Fractionation of subcellular organelles from rat brain by affinity binding on concanavalin A-Sepharose, Abstracts, Fifth International Meeting, International Society of Neurochemists, p. 242.

Bittiger, H., and Schnebli, H. P., 1974, Binding of concanavalin A and ricin to synaptic junctions of rat brain, *Nature* **249**:370–371.

Blitz, A. L., and Fine, R. E., 1974, Muscle-like contractile proteins and tubulin in synaptosomes, *Proc. Natl. Acad. Sci. U.S.A.* **71**:4472–4476.

Bloom, F. E., 1970*a,* Correlating structure and function of synaptic ultrastructure, in: *The Neurosciences: Second Study Program* (F. O. Schmitt, ed.), pp. 729–747, Rockefeller Univ. Press, New York.

Bloom, F. E., 1970*b,* The fine structural localization of biogenic monoamines in nervous tissue, in: *International Review of Neurobiology* (C. C. Pfeiffer and J. R. Smythies, eds.), Vol. 13, pp. 27–66, Academic Press, New York.

Bloom, F. E., and Aghajanian, G. K., 1966, Cytochemistry of synapses: A selective staining method for electron microscopy, *Science* **154**:1575–1577.

Bloom, F. E., and Aghajanian, G. K., 1968, Fine structural and cytochemical analysis of the staining of synaptic junctions with phosphotungstic acid, *J. Ultrastruct. Res.* **22**:361–375.

Bock, E., Jorgensen, O. S., and Morris, S. J., 1974, Antigen–antibody crossed electrophoresis of rat brain synaptosomes and synaptic vesicles: Correlation to water-soluble antigens from rat brain, *J. Neurochem.* **22**:1013–1017.

Bondy, S. C., 1975, Axoplasmic transport, in: *Research Methods in Neurochemistry* (N. Marks and R. Rodnight, eds.), Vol. 3, pp. 43–66, Plenum Press, New York.

Bonting, S. L., Caravaggio, L. L., and Hawkins, N. M., 1962, Studies on sodium-potassium activated adenosinetriphosphatase. IV. Correlation with cation transport sensitive to cardiac glycosides, *Arch. Biochem. Biophys.* **98**:413–419.

Borisy, G. G., Olmsted, J. B., Marcum, J. M., and Allen, C., 1974, Microtubule assembly *in vitro, Fed. Proc.* **33**:167–174.

Bosman, H. B., Hagopian, A., and Eylar, E. H., 1968, Cellular membranes: The isolation and characterization of the plasma and smooth membranes of HeLa cells, *Arch. Biochem. Biophys.* **128**:51–69.

Bosman, H. B., Case, K. R., and Shea, M. B., 1970, Proteins and glycoproteins of rat cerebral cortex synaptosomal fractions: Extraction with sodium dodecyl sulphate and analytical gel electrophoresis, *FEBS Lett.* **11**:261–264.

Brandt, A. E., Distler, J. J., and Jourdian, G. W., 1975, Biosynthesis of chondroitin sulfate proteoglycan: Subcellular distribution of glycosyltransferases in embryonic chick brain, *J. Biol. Chem.* **250**:3996–4006.

Breckenridge, W. C., and Morgan, I. G., 1972, Common glycoproteins of synaptic vesicles and the synaptosomal plasma membranes, *FEBS Lett.* **22(3)**:253–256.

Breckenridge, W. C., Gombos, G., and Morgan, I. G., 1971, The docosahexenoic acids of the phospholipids of synaptic membranes, vesicles, and mitochondria, *Brain Res.* **33**:581–583.

Breckenridge, W. C., Gombos, G., and Morgan, I. G., 1972, The lipid composition of adult rat brain synaptosomal plasma membranes, *Biochim. Biophys. Acta* **266**:695–707.

Bretscher, M. S., 1971, Major human erythrocyte glycoprotein spans the cell membrane, *Nature New Biol.* **231**:229–232.

Bretz, U., Baggliolini, M., Hauser, R., and Hodel, C., 1974, Resolution of three distinct populations of nerve endings from rat brain homogenates by zonal isopycnic centrifugation, *J. Cell Biol.* **61**:466–480.

Brunner, G., and Bucher, Th., 1970, Determination of the quantitative relationship of outer and inner membrane proteins in rat liver mitochondria by means of enzymology and electron microscopy, *FEBS Lett.* **6**:105–108.

Bryan, J., and Wilson, L., 1971, Are cytoplasmic microtubules heteropolymers?, *Proc. Natl. Acad. Sci. U.S.A.* **68**:1762–1766.

Cahn, F. H., and Fox, M. S., 1968, Fractionation of transformable bacteria from competent cultures of *Bacillus subtilis* on renografin gradients, *J. Bacteriol.* **95**:867–875.

Carlsson, A., and Lindqvist, M., 1963, Effect of chlorpromazine or haloperidol on formation of 3-methyoxytyramine and normetanephrine in mouse brain, *Acta Pharmacol. Toxicol.* **20**:140–144.

Carraway, K. L., 1975, Covalent labeling of membranes, *Biochim. Biophys. Acta* **415**:379–410.

Chang, C., and Goldman, R. D., 1973, The localization of actin-like fibers in cultured neuroblastoma cells as revealed by heavy meromyosin binding, *J. Cell Biol.* **57**:867–874.

Chang, H., 1974, Purification and characterization of acetylcholine receptor-I from *Electrophorus electricus, Proc. Natl. Acad. Sci. U.S.A.* **71**:2113–2117.

Chang, K., Bennett, V., and Cuatrecasas, P., 1975, Membrane receptors as general markers for plasma membrane isolation procedures: The use of ^{125}I-labelled wheat germ agglutinin, insulin, and cholera toxin, *J. Biol. Chem.* **250**:488–500.

Cheung, W. Y., and Salganicoff, L., 1967, Cyclic 3',5'-nucleotide phosphodiesterase: Localization and latent activity in rat brain, *Nature* **214**:90–91.

Cohen, J. B., and Changeux, J. P., 1975, The cholinergic receptor protein in its membrane environment, *Annu. Rev. Pharmacol.* **15**:83–103.

Cohen, R. S., Blomberg, F., and Siekevitz, P., 1976, Studies of postsynaptic densities isolated from dog cerebral cortex, *J. Cell Biol.* **70**:93a.

Collier, B., 1969, The preferential release of newly synthesized transmitter by a synpathetic ganglion, *J. Physiol. (Lond.)* **205**:341–352.

Cook, G. M., and Eylar, E. H., 1965, Separation of the M and N blood-group antigens of the human erythrocyte, *Biochim. Biophys. Acta* **101**:57–66.

Costa, E., and Meek, J. L., 1974, Regulation of biosynthesis of catecholamines and serotonin in the CNS, *Annu. Rev. Pharmacol.* **14**:491–511.

Cotman, C. W., 1972, Principles for the optimization of centrifugation conditions for fractionation of brain tissue, in: *Research Methods in Neurochemistry* (N. Marks and R. Rodnight, eds.), Vol. 1, pp. 45–93, Plenum Press, New York.

Cotman, C. W., and Banker, G. A., 1974, The making of a synapse, in: *Reviews of Neuroscience* (S. Ehrenpreis and I. J. Kopin, eds.), Vol. 1, pp. 1–62, Raven Press, New York.

Cotman, C. W., and Mathews, D. A., 1971, Synaptic plasma membranes from rat brain synaptosomes: Isolation and partial characterization, *Biochim. Biophys. Acta* **249**:380–394.

Cotman, C. W., and Taylor, D., 1972, Isolation and structural studies on synaptic complexes from rat brain, *J. Cell Biol.* **55**:696–711.

Cotman, C. W., and Taylor, D., 1974, Localization and characterization of Con A receptors in the synaptic cleft, *J. Cell Biol.* **62**:236–242.

Cotman, C., Mahler, H. R., and Anderson, N. G., 1968a, Isolation of a membrane fraction enriched in nerve-ending membranes from rat brain by zonal centrifugation, *Biochim. Biophys. Acta* **163**:272–275.

Cotman, C. W., Mahler, H. R., and Hugli, T. E., 1968b, Isolation and characterization of insoluble proteins of the synaptic plasma membrane, *Arch. Biochem. Biophys.* **126**:821–837.

Cotman, C., Blank, M. L., Moehl, A., and Snyder, F., 1969, Lipid composition of synaptic plasma membranes isolated from rat brain by zonal centrifugation, *Biochemistry* **8**:4606–4612.

Cotman, C. W., Herschman, H., and Taylor, D., 1971a, Subcellular fractionation of cultured glial cells, *J. Neurobiol.* **2**:169–180.

Cotman, C. W., Levy, W., Banker, G., and Taylor, D., 1971c, An ultrastructural and chemical analysis of the effect of Triton X-100 on synaptic plasma membranes, *Biochim. Biophys. Acta* **249**:406–418.

Cotman, C. W., McCaman, R. E., and Dewhurst, S. A., 1971b, Synaptosomal distribution of enzymes involved in the metabolism of lipids, *Biochim. Biophys. Acta* **249**:395–405.

Cotman, C. W., Banker, G., Churchill, L., and Taylor, D., 1974, Isolation of PSDs from rat brain, *J. Cell Biol.* **63**:441–455.

Cuatrecasas, P., 1972, Properties of the insulin receptor from liver and fat cell membranes, *J. Biol. Chem.* **247**:1980–1991.

Cuatrecasas, P., 1973a, Insulin receptor of liver and fat cell membranes, *Fed. Proc.* **32**:1838–1846.

Cuatrecasas, P., 1973*b,* Interaction of wheat germ agglutinin and concanavalin A with isolated fat cells, *Biochemistry* **12**:1312–1323.

Cuatrecasas, P., 1973*c,* Interaction of *Vibrio cholerae* enterotoxin with cell membranes, *Biochemistry* **12**:3547–3558.

Cuatrecasas, P., 1973*d,* Gangliosides and membrane receptors for cholera toxin, *Biochemistry* **12**:3558–3566.

Cuatrecasas, P., 1974, Membrane receptors, *Annu. Rev. Biochem.* **43**:169–214.

Dahlstrom, A., 1973, Aminergic transmission: Introduction and short review, *Brain Res.* **62**:441–460.

Dahlstrom, A., and Haggendal, J., 1966, Studies on the transport and life-span of amine storage granules in a peripheral adrenergic nervous system, *Acta Physiol. Scand.* **67**:278–288.

Daniel, A., and Guth, L., 1975, Histochemical demonstration of sodium ion plus potassium ion-activated ATPase activity of synaptosomes and synaptosomal membranes, *Exp. Neurol.* **47(1)**:181–188.

Darin De Lorenzo, D. M., Dettbarn, W. D., and Bozin, M., 1969, Fine structural localization of acetylcholinesterase in single axons, *J. Ultrastruct. Res.* **28**:27–40.

Davis, G. A., and Bloom, F. E., 1970, Proteins of synaptic junctional complexes, *J. Cell Biol.* **47**:46a.

Davis, G. A., and Bloom, F. E., 1973*a,* Isolation of synaptic junctional complexes from rat brain, *Brain Res.* **62**:135–153.

Davis, G. A., and Bloom, F. E., 1973*b,* Subcellular particles separated through a histochemical reaction, *Anal. Biochem.* **51**:429–435.

Day, E. D., McMillan, P. N., Mickey, D. D., and Appel, S. H., 1971, Zonal centrifuge profiles of rat brain homogenates: Instability in sucrose, stability in isoosmotic Ficoll–sucrose, *Anal. Biochem.* **39**:29–45.

De Baecque, C., Johnson, A. B., Naiki, M., Schwarting, G., and Marcus, D. M., 1976. Ganglioside localization in cerebellar cortex: An immunoperoxidase study with antibody to G_{M1} ganglioside, *Brain Res.* **114**:117–122.

De Champlain, J., Muller, R. A., and Axelrod, J., 1969, Cellular localization of monoamine oxidase in rat tissues, *J. Pharmacol. Exp. Ther.* **166**:339–345.

Den, H., Kaufman, B., McGuire, E. J., and Roseman, S., 1975, The sialic acids: XVIII. Subcellular distribution of seven glycosyltransferases in embryonic chicken brain, *J. Biol. Chem.* **250**:739–746.

De Robertis, E. D. P., 1964*a,* Electron microscope and chemical study of brain biogenic amines, *Prog. Brain Res.* **8**:118–136.

De Robertis, E. D. P., 1964*b, Histophysiology of Synapses and Neurosecretion,* Pergamon Press, New York.

De Robertis, E. D. P., 1975*a,* Synaptic receptor proteins. Isolation and reconstruction in artificial membranes, *Rev. Physiol. Biochem. Pharmacol.* **73**:9–38.

De Robertis, E. D. P., 1975*b, Synaptic Receptors: Isolation and Molecular Biology,* Dekker, New York.

De Robertis, E. D. P., and Bennett, H. S., 1955, Some features of the submicroscopic morphology of synapses in frog and earthworm, *J. Biophys. Biochem. Cytol.* **1**:47–58.

De Robertis, E. D. P., De Iraldi, A. P., Arnaiz, G. R., and Salganicoff, L., 1962, Cholinergic and noncholinergic nerve endings in rat brain—I. Isolation and subcellular distribution of acetylcholine and acetylcholinesterase, *J. Neurochem.* **9**:23–35.

De Robertis, E. D. P., Arnaiz, G. R., Salganicoff, L., De Iraldi, A. P., and Zieher, L. M., 1963, Isolation of synaptic vesicles and structural organization of the acetylcholine system within brain nerve endings, *J. Neurochem.* **10**:225–235.

De Robertis, E. D. P., Lapetina, E., Pecci Saavedra, J., and Soto, E. F., 1966, *In vivo* and *in vitro* action of antisera against isolated nerve endings of brain cortex, *Life Sci.* **5**:979–989.

De Robertis, E. D. P., Azcurra, J. M., and Fiszer, S., 1967*a*, Ultrastructure and cholinergic binding capacity of junctional complexes isolated from rat brain, *Brain Res.* **5**:45–56.

De Robertis, E. D. P., DeLores Arnaiz, G. R., Alberici, M., Butcher, R. W., and Sutherland, E. W., 1967*b*, Subcellular distribution of adenyl cyclase and cyclic phosphodiesterase in rat brain cortex, *J. Biol. Chem.* **242**:3487–3493.

De Robertis, E. D. P., Lapetina, E. G., and Wald, F., 1968, The effect of antiserum against nerve ending membranes from cat cerebral cortex on the ultrastructure of isolated nerve endings and mollusc neurons, *Exp. Neurol.* **21**:322–335.

Derry, D. M., and Wolfe, L. S., 1968, Gangliosides in isolated neurons and glial cells, *Science* **158**:1450–1452.

Descarries, L., and Droz, B., 1970, Intraneuronal distribution of exogenous norepinephrine in the central nervous system of the rat, *J. Cell Biol.* **44**:385–399.

Descarries, L., Beaudet, A., and Watkins, K. C., 1975, Serotonin nerve terminals in adult rat neocortex, *Brain Res.* **100**:563–588.

Di Carlo, V., 1975, Macromolecular organization of membranes and organelles in nervous tissue, in: Central Nervous System Studies on Metabolic Regulation and Function, International Symposium, Saint Vincent, Italy, pp. 185–198.

Di Cesare, J. L., and Dain, J. A., 1972, Localization, solubilization, and properties of *N*-acetylgalactosaminyl ganglioside transferase and galactosyl ganglioside transferase in rat brain synaptic membrane, *J. Neurochem.* **19**:403–410.

Donato, R., and Michetti, F., 1974, S-100 protein in cerebral cortex synaptosomes, *Experientia* **30**:511–512.

Donato, R., Michetti, F., and Miani, N., 1975, Soluble and membrane-bound S-100 protein in cerebral cortex synaptosomes: Properties of the S-100 receptor, *Brain Res.* **98**:561–573.

Doyle, L. C., and Cotman, C. W., 1972, Analysis of myelin–synaptosomal interactions in sucrose and Ficoll–sucrose gradients, *Anal. Biochem.* **49**:29–36.

Droz, B., 1973, Renewal of synaptic proteins, *Brain Res.* **62**: 383–394.

Droz, B., Rambourg, A., and Koenig, H. L., 1975, The smooth endoplasmic reticulum structure and role in the renewal of axonal membrane and synaptic vesicles by fast axonal transport, *Brain Res.* **93**:1–14.

Dubois, D. M., and Schoffeniels, E., 1975, Molecular model of postsynaptic potential, *Proc. Natl. Acad. Sci. U.S.A.* **72**:1749–1752.

Dutton, G., and Barondes, S. H., 1969, Glycoprotein metabolism in developing brain, *Science* **166**:1637–1638.

Dutton, G. R., Haywood, P., and Barondes, S. H., 1973, [^{14}C]Glucosamine incorporation into specific products in the nerve ending fraction *in vitro* and *in vivo*, *Brain Res.* **57**:397–408.

Eichberg, J., Whittaker, V. P., and Dawson, R. M. C., 1964, Distribution of lipids in subcellular particles of guinea-pig brain, *Biochem. J.* **92**:91–100.

Eipper, B. A., 1974*a*, Rat brain tubulin and protein kinase activity, *J. Biol. Chem.* **249**:1398–1406.

Eipper, B. A., 1974*b*, Properties of rat brain tubulin, *J. Biol. Chem.* **249**:1407–1416.

Eldefrawi, M. E., and Eldefrawi, A. T., 1973, Purification and molecular properties of the acetylcholine receptor from torpedo electroplax. *Arch. Biochem. Biophys.* **159**:362–373.

Emmelot, P., and Box, C. J., 1966, Studies on plasma membranes. II. K$^+$-dependent *p*-nitrophenyl phosphatase activity of plasma membranes isolated from rat liver, *Biochim. Biophys. Acta* **121**:375–385.

Enna, S. J., and Shore, P. A., 1974, Extragranular amine binding site in adrenergic neurons of heart, *J. Neural Transm.* **35**:125–135.

Enna, S. J., and Snyder, S. H., 1975, Properties of gamma-aminobutyric acid receptor binding in rat brain synaptic membrane fractions, *Brain Res.* **100**:81–97.

Fahn, S., Rodman, J. S., and Cote, L. J., 1969, Association of tyroxine hydroxylase with synaptic vesicles in bovine caudate nucleus, *J. Neurochem.* **16**:1293–1300.

Feit, H., 1971, Metabolism of microtubule proteins in mouse brain, Ph.D. Thesis, Department of Molecular Biology, Albert Einstein College of Medicine, Yeshiva University, New York.

Feit, H., 1976, Quoted in Synaptic Proteins, Ninth Annual Winter Conference on Brain Research, Brain Information Service Publications Office, University of California, pp. 115–127.

Feit, H., and Barondes, S. H., 1970, Colchicine-binding activity in particulate fractions of mouse brain, *J. Neurochem.* **17**:1355–1364.

Feit, H., Slusarek, L., and Shelanski, M. L., 1971*a*, Heterogeneity of tubulin subunits, *Proc. Natl. Acad. Sci. U.S.A.* **68**:2038–2031.

Feit, H., Dutton, G., Barondes, S. H., and Shelanski, M. L., 1971*b*, Microtubule protein identification in and transport to nerve endings, *J. Cell Biol.* **51**:138–147.

Ferguson, K. A., 1964, Starch-gel electrophoresis—Application to the classification of pituitary proteins and polypeptides, *Metab. Clin. Exp.* **13**:985–1002.

Fine, R., 1971, Heterogeneity of tubulin, *Nature* **233**:283–284.

Fiszer, S., and De Robertis, E. D. P., 1967, Action of Triton X-100 of ultrastructure and membrane-bound enzymes of isolated nerve endings from rat brain, *Brain Res.* **5**:31–44.

Florendo, N. T., Barrnett, R. J., and Greengard, P., 1971, Cyclic 3′,5′-nucleotide phosphodiesterase: Cytochemical localization in cerebral cortex, *Science* **173**:745–747.

Fonnum, F., 1967, The "compartmentation" of choline acetyltransferase within the synaptosomes, *Biochem. J.* **103**:262–270.

Fonnum, F., 1968*a*, The distribution of glutamate decarboxylase and aspartate transaminase in subcellular fractions of rat and guinea-pig brain, *Biochem. J.* **106**:401–412.

Fonnum, F., 1968*b*, Choline acetyltransferase binding to and release from membranes, *Biochem. J.* **109**:389–398.

Fonnum, F., 1973, Recent developments in biochemical investigations of cholinergic transmission, *Brain Res.* **62**:497–507.

Frontali, N., Ceccarelli, B., Gorio, A., Mauro, A., Siekevitz, P., Tzeng, M., and Hurlbut, W. P., 1976, Purification from black widow spider venom of a protein factor causing the depletion of synaptic vesicles at neuromuscular junctions, *J. Cell Biol.* **68**:462–479.

Furthmayer, H., and Timpl, R., 1971, Characterization of collagen peptides by sodium dodecylsulfate–polyacrylamide gel electrophoresis, *Anal Biochem.* **41**:510–516.

Gardner, J. D., Klaevman, H. L., Bilezikian, J. P., and Aurbach, G. D., 1973, Effect of β-adrenergic catecholamine on sodium transport in turkey erythrocytes, *J. Biol. Chem.* **248**:5590–5597.

Gaskin, F., Kramer, S. B., Cantor, C. R., Adelstein, R., and Shelanski, M. L., 1974, A dynein-like protein associated with neurotubules, *FEBS Lett.* **40**:281–286.

Geiger, R. S., 1963, The behavior of adult mammalian brain cells in culture, *Int. Rev. Neurobiol.* **5**:1–52.

Gfeller, E., Kuhar, M. J., and Snyder, S. H., 1971, Neurotransmitter-specific synaptosomes in rat corpus striatum: Morphological variation, *Proc. Natl. Acad. Sci. U.S.A.* **68**:155–159.

Gibbons, I. R., 1966, Studies on the adenosine triphosphatase activity of 14S and 30S dynein from cilia of tetrahymena, *J. Biol. Chem.* **241**:5590–5596.

Gilbert, J. C., Wyllie, M. G., and Davison, D. V., 1975, Nerve terminal ATPase as possible trigger for neurotransmitter release, *Nature* **255**:237–238.

Glowinski, J., and Axelrod, J., 1966, Effect of drugs on the disposition of norepinephrine in the rat brain, *Pharm. Rev.* **18**:775–785.

Glowinski, J., Besson, M. J., Cheramy, A., and Thierry, A. M., 1972, Disposition and role of newly synthesizes amines in central catecholaminergic neurons, *Adv. Biochem. Psychopharmacol.* **6**:93–109.

Goldstein, M., Anagnoste, B., and Shirron, C. J., 1973, The effect of trivastal, haloperidol and dibutyryl cyclic AMP on [^{14}C]dopamine synthesis in rat striatum, *J. Pharm. Pharmacol.* **25**:348–351.

Goodman, D. P. B., Rasmussen, H., Di Bella, F., and Guthrow, C. E., Jr., 1970, Cyclic adenosine 3′,5′-monophosphate-stimulated phosphorylation of isolated neurotubule subunits, *Proc. Natl. Acad. Sci. U.S.A.* **67**:652–659.

Gow, J., and Wardlaw, A. C., 1975, Iodination of a mixture of soluble proteins by the [^{125}I]lactoperoxidase technique, *Biochem. Biophys. Res. Commun.* **67**:43–49.

Grafstein, B., 1975, The eyes have it: Axonal transport and regeneration in the optic nerve, in: *The Nervous System* (D. B. Tower, ed.), Vol. 1, pp. 147–151, Raven Press, New York.

Gray, E. G., 1959*a,* Axosomatic and axodendritic synapses of the cerebral cortex: An electron microscopic study, *J. Anat. (Lond.)* **93**:420–433.

Gray, E. G., 1959*b,* Electron microscopy of synaptic contacts on dendritic spines of the cerebral cortex, *Nature* **183**:1592–1593.

Gray, E. G., 1969, Electron microscopy of excitatory and inhibitory synapses: A brief review, *Prog. Brain Res.* **31**:141–155.

Gray, E. G., 1972, Are the coats of coated vesicles artifacts? *J. Neurocytol.* **1**:363–382.

Gray, E. G., 1975*a,* Presynaptic microtubules and their association with synaptic vesicles, *Proc. Roy. Soc. Lond. B* **190**:369–372.

Gray, E. G., 1975*b,* Synaptic fine structure and nuclear, cytoplasmic, and extracellular networks: The stereoframework concept, *J. Neurocytol.* **4**:315–339.

Gray, E. G., and Guillery, R. W., 1966, Synaptic morphology in the normal and degenerating nervous system, *Int. Rev. Cytol.* **19**:111–182.

Gray, E. G., and Whittaker, V. P., 1962, The isolation of nerve endings from brain: An electron microscopic study of cell fragments derived by homogenization and centrifugation, *J. Anat. (Lond.)* **96**:79–87.

Green, A. I., Snyder, S. H., and Iversen, L. L., 1969, Separation of catecholamine-storing synaptosomes in different regions of rat brain, *J. Pharmacol. Exp. Ther.* **168**:264–271.

Greengard, P., 1976, Possible role for cyclic nucleotides and phosphorylated membrane proteins in postsynaptic actions of neurotransmitters, *Nature* **260**:101–108.

Gregson, N. A., and Williams, P. L., 1969, Comparative study of brain and liver mitochondria from new-born and adult rats, *J. Neurochem.* **16**:617–626.

Gurd, J. W., Jones, L. R., Mahler, H. R., and Moore, W. J., 1974, Isolation and partial characterization of rat brain synaptic plasma membranes, *J. Neurochem.* **22**:281–290.

Hajos, F., and Kerpel-Fronius, S., 1973, Comparative electron cytochemical studies of presynaptic and other neuronal mitochondria, *Brain Res.* **62**:425–429.

Hajos, F., Tapia, R., Wilkin, G., Johnson, A. L., and Balazs, R., 1974, Subcellular fractionation of rat cerebellum: An electron microscopic and biochemical investigation. I. Preservation of large fragments of the cerebellar glomeruli, *Brain Res.* **70**:261–279.

Hakomori, S., and Strycharz, G. D., 1968, Investigation on cellular blood-group substances. I. Isolation and chemical composition of blood-group ABH and Le^{b} isoantigens of sphingoglycolipid nature, *Biochemistry* **7**:1279–1286.

Hall, Z. W., 1972, Release of neurotransmitters and their interaction with receptors, *Annu. Rev. Biochem.* **41**:925–952.

Hamberger, A., and Svennerholm, L., 1971, Composition of gangliosides and phospholipids of neuronal and glial cell-enriched fractions, *J. Neurochem.* **18**:1821–1829.

Hamberger, A., Hansson, H. A., Sellstrom, A., and Yanajihara, T., 1975. Isolation of highly purified glomerular complexes from rabbit cerebellum, *Experientia* **31**:221.

Hamberger, A., Hansson, H. A., Lazarewicz, J. W., Lundh, T., and Sellstrom, A., 1976, The cerebellar glomerulus: Isolation and metabolic properties of a purified fraction, *J. Neurochem.* **27**:267–272.

Hanning, K., 1967, Preparative electrophoresis, in: *Electrophoresis* (M. Biet, ed.), pp. 423–471, Academic Press, New York.

Harris, J. E., Morgenroth, V. H., Roth, R. H., and Baldessarini, R. J., 1974, Regulation of catecholamine synthesis in the rat brain *in vitro* by cyclic AMP, *Nature* **252**:156–158.

Harvey, J. A., and McIlwain, H., 1969, Electrical phenomena and isolated tissues from the brain, in: *Handbook of Neurochemistry* (A. Lajtha, ed.), Vol. 2, pp. 115–136, Plenum Press, New York.

Heidrich, H. G., Stahn, R., and Hanng, K., 1970, The surface charge of rat liver mitochondria and their membranes: Clarification of some controversies concerning mitochondrial structure, *J. Cell Biol.* **46**:137–150.

Heilbronn, E., and Mattson, C., 1974, The nicotinic cholinergic receptor protein: Improved purification method, preliminary amino acid composition and observed auto-immuno response, *J. Neurochem.* **22**:315–316.

Herschman, H. R., Cotman, C., and Matthews, D. A., 1972, Serological specificities of brain subcellular organelles. I. Antisera to synaptosomal fractions, *J. Immunol.* **108**:1362–1369.

Heuser, J. E., and Reese, T. S., 1973, Evidence for recycling of synaptic vesicle membrane during transmitter release at the frog neuromuscular junction, *J. Cell Biol.* **57**:314–344.

Horne, R. W., and Whittaker, V. P., 1962, The use of the negative staining method for the electron-microscopic study of subcellular particles from animal tissues, *Z. Zellforsch.* **58**:1–16.

Hosie, R. J. A., 1965, The localization of adenosine triphosphatase in morphologically characterized subcellular fractions of guinea-pig brain, *Biochem. J.* **96**:404–412.

Hoss, W., and Abood, L. G., 1974, Fluidity in hydrophobic protein regions of synaptic membrane, *Eur. J. Biochem.* **50**:177–181.

Huneeus, F. C., and Davison, P. F., 1970, Fibrillar proteins from squid axons, I. Neurofilament protein, *J. Mol. Biol.* **52**:415–428.

Hungund, B. L., Mahadik, S. P., and Rapport, M. M., 1975, Surface labeling of intact synaptosomes: Gangliosides, *Neurosci. Abstr.* **1**:616.

Huxley, H. E., 1963, Electron microscope studies on the structures of natural and synthetic protein filaments from striated muscle, *J. Mol. Biol.* **7**:281–308.

Hyden, H., 1974, A calcium-dependent mechanism for synapse and nerve cell membrane modulation, *Proc. Natl. Acad. Sci. U.S.A.* **71**:2965–2968.

Inestrosa, N. C., Fernandez, H. L., and Garrido, J., 1976, Actin-like filaments in synaptosomes detected by heavy meromyosin binding, *Neurosci. Lett.* **2**:217–221.

Israel, M., Gautron, J., and Leshats, B., 1970, Fractionnement de l'organe électrique de la Torpille: Localization subcellulaire de l'actylcholine, *J. Neurochem.* **17**:1441–1450.

Iversen, L. L., 1975, How do antipsychotic drugs work?, *Neurosci. Res. Prog. Bull.* **13**:29–51.

Iversen, L. L., and Snyder, S. H., 1968, Synaptosomes: Different populations storing catecholamines and gamma-aminobutyric acid in homogenates of rat brain, *Nature* **220**:796–798.

Johnson, E. M., Maeno, H., and Greengard, P., 1971, Phosphorylation of endogenous protein of rat brain by cyclic adenosine 3′,5′-monophosphate-dependent protein kinase, *J. Biol. Chem.* **246**:7731–7739.

Johnson, G. A., Boukma, S. J., Lahti, R. A., and Mathews, T., 1973, Cyclic AMP and phosphodiesterase in synaptic vesicles from mouse brain, *J. Neurochem.* **20**:1387–1392.

Johnson, M. K., and Whittaker, V. P., 1963, Lactate dehydrogenase as a cytoplasmic marker in brain, *Biochem. J.* **88**:404–409.

Jonakait, G. M., Tamir, H., Rapport, M. M., and Gershon, M. D., 1977, Detection of a soluble serotonin-binding protein in the myenteric plexus and other peripheral sites of serotonin storage, *J. Neurochem.* **28**:277–284.

Jones, D. G., 1975, *Synapses and Synaptosomes: Morphological Aspects,* Chapman & Hill, London.

Jones, E. H., and Matus, A. I., 1974, Isolation of SPM from brain by combined flotation-sedimentation density gradient centrifugation, *Biochim. Biophys. Acta* **336**:276–287.

Jorgensen, O. S., and Bock, E., 1974, Brain-specific synaptosomal membrane proteins demonstrated by crossed immunoelectrophoresis, *J. Neurochem.* **23**:879–880.

Kadota, K., and Kadota, T., 1973, Isolation of coated vesicles, plain synaptic vesicles, and flocculent material from a crude synaptosome fraction of guinea-pig whole brain, *J. Cell Biol.* **58**:135–151.

Kadota, K., and Kanaseki, T., 1969, Isolation of a synaptic vesicle fraction from guinea-pig brain with the use of DEAE–Sephadex column chromatography and some of its properties, *J. Biochem. (Tokyo)* **65**:839–842.

Kadota, K., Mori, S., and Imaizumi, K., 1967, The properties of ATPase of synaptic vesicle fraction, *J. Biochem. (Tokyo)* **61**:424–432.

Kadota, T., Kadota, K., and Gray, E. G., 1976, Coated vesicle shells, particle-chain material and tubulin in brain synaptosomes: An electron microscopic and biochemical study, *J. Cell Biol.* **69**:608–621.

Kahan, B. D., and Reisfeld, R. A., 1967, Electrophoretic purification of a water-soluble guinea-pig transplantation antigen, *Proc. Natl. Acad. Sci. U.S.A.* **58**:1430–1437.

Kanaseki, T., and Kadota, K., 1969, The "vesicle in a basket." A morphological study of the coated vesicle isolated from the nerve endings of guinea-pig brain, with special reference to the mechanism of membrane movement, *J. Cell Biol.* **42**:202–220.

Karlin, A., 1975, The acetylcholine receptor: Isolation and characterization, in: *The Nervous System* (D. B. Tower, ed.), Vol. 1, pp. 323–331, Raven Press, New York.

Karlsson, J. O., Hamberger, A., and Henn, F. A., 1973, Polypeptide composition of membranes derived from neural and glial cells, *Biochim. Biophys. Acta* **298**:219–229.

Karpiak, S. E., and Rapport, M. M., 1975, Behavioral changes in 2-month-old rats following prenatal exposure to antibodies against synaptic membranes, *Brain Res.* **92**:405–413.

Karpiak, S. E., Rapport, M. M., and Bowen, F. P., 1974, Immunologically induced behavioral and electrophysiological changes in the rat, *Neuropsychologia* **12**:313–322.

Kashnig, D. M., and Kasper, C. B., 1969, Isolation, morphology, and composition of the nuclear membrane from rat liver, *J. Biol. Chem.* **244**:3786–3792.

Kataoka, K., and De Robertis, E., 1967, Histamine in isolated small nerve endings and synaptic vesicles of rat brain cortex, *J. Pharmacol. Exp. Ther.* **156**:114–125.

Kebabian, J. W., Petzold, G. L., and Greengard, P., 1972, Dopamine-sensitive adenyl cyclase in caudate nucleus of rat brain, and its similarity to the "dopamine receptor," *Proc. Natl. Acad. Sci. U.S.A.* **69**:2145–2149.

Kirkpatrick, J. B., Bray, J. J., and Palmer, S. M., 1972, Visualization of axoplasmic flow *in vitro* by Nomarsky microscopy. Comparison to rapid flow of radioactive proteins, *Brain Res.* **43**:1–10.

Kishimoto, Y., Agranoff, B. W., Radin, N. S., and Burton, R. M., 1969, Comparison of fatty acids of lipids of subcellular brain fractions, *J. Neurochem.* **16**:397–404.

Kokko, A., Mauthner, H. G., and Barrnett, R. J., 1965, Fine structural localization of acetyl cholinesterase using acetyl-β-methylthiocholine and acetylselenocholine as substrates, *J. Histochem. Cytochem.* **17**:625–640.

Kornguth, S. E., and Sunderland, E., 1975, Isolation and partial characterization of a tubulin-like protein from human and swine synaptosomal membranes, *Biochim. Biophys. Acta* **393**:100–114.

Kornguth, S. E., Anderson, J. W., Scott, G., and Kubinski, H., 1967, Fractionation of subcellular elements from rat central nervous tissue in a cesium chloride gradient: Biochemical and ultrastructural studies, *Exp. Cell Res.* **45**:656–670.

Kornguth, S. E., Anderson, J. W., and Scott, G., 1969, Isolation of synaptic complexes in a cesium chloride density gradient: Electron microscopic and immunohistochemical studies, *J. Neurochem.* **16**:1017–1024.

Kreutzberg, G. W., Schubert, P., Toth, L., and Rieske, E., 1973, Intradendritic transport to postsynaptic sites, *Brain Res.* **62**:399–404.

Krueger, B. K., Forn, J., and Greengard, P., 1975, Dopamine-sensitive adenylate cyclase and protein phosphorylation in the rat caudate nucleus, in: *Pre- and Postsynaptic Receptors* (E. Usdin and W. E. Bunney, eds.), pp. 123–145, Dekker, New York.

Krygier-Brevart, V., Weiss, D. G., Mehl, E., Schubert, P., and Kreutzberg, G. W., 1974, Maintenance of synaptic membranes by fast axonal flow, *Brain Res.* **77**:97–110.

Kuhar, M. J., 1973, Neurotransmitter uptake: A tool in identifying neurotransmitter-specific pathways, *Life Sci.* **13**:1623–1634.

Kuhar, M. J., Green, A. I., Snyder, S. H., and Gfeller, E., 1970, Separation of synaptosomes storing catecholamines and gamma-aminobutyric acid in rat corpus striatum, *Brain Res.* **21**:405–417.

Kurihara, T., and Tsukada, Y., 1967, The regional and subcellular distribution of 2′,3′-cyclic nucleotide 3′-phosphohydrolase in the central nervous system, *J. Neurochem.* **14**:1167–1174.

Kurokawa, M., Sakamoto, T., and Kato, M., 1965, A rapid isolation of nerve-ending particles from brain, *Biochim. Biophys. Acta* **94**:307–309.

Lagercrantz, H., and Pertoft, H., 1972, Separation of catecholamine-storing synaptosomes in colloidal silica density gradients, *J. Neurochem.* **19**:811–823.

Lagnado, J. R., Lyons, C. A., Weller, M., and Phillipson, B., 1972, The possible significance of adenosine 3′,5′-cyclic monophosphate-stimulated protein kinase activity associated with purified microtubular protein preparations of mammalian brain, *Biochem. J.* **128**:95P.

Lai, J. C. K., and Clark, J. B., 1976, Preparation and properties of mitochondria derived from synaptosomes, *Biochem. J.* **154**:423–432.

Lai, J. C. K., Walsh, J. M., Dennis, S. C., and Clark, J. B., 1975, Compartmentation of citric acid cycle and related enzymes in distinct populations of rat brain mitochondria, in: *Metabolic Compartmentation and Neurotransmission: Relation to Brain Structure and Function* (S. Berl, D. D. Clarke, and D. Schneider, eds.), NATO Adv. Study Inst. Series A, Vol. 6, pp. 487–496, Plenum Press, New York.

Lapetina, E. G., Sato, E. F., and De Robertis, E., 1967, Gangliosides and acetylcholinesterase in isolated membranes of rat brain cortex, *Biochim. Biophys. Acta* **135**:33–43.

Lasek, R. J., 1972, Characterization of axoplasmic RNA from squid and polycheate giant axons, *Trans. Am. Soc. Neurochem.* **3**:98.

Lasek, R. J., Gainer, H., and Przybylski, R. J., 1974, Transfer of newly synthesized proteins from Schwann cells to the squid giant axon, *Proc. Natl. Acad. Sci. U.S.A.* **71**:1188–1192.

Lemkey-Johnston, N., and Dekermenjian, H., 1970, The identification of fractions enriched in nonmyelinated axons from rat whole brain, *Exp. Brain Res.* **11**:392–410.

Levitan, J. B., Mushynski, W. E., and Ramirez, G., 1972, Highly purified synaptosome membranes from rat brain, *J. Biol. Chem.* **247**:5376–5381.

Lis, H., and Sharon, N., 1973, The biochemistry of plant lectins (phytohemagglutinins), *Annu. Rev. Biochem.* **41**:541–574.

Livett, B. G., Rostas, J. A. P., Jeffrey, P. L., and Austin, L., 1974, Antigenicity of isolated synaptosomal membranes, *Exp. Neurol.* **43**:330–338.

Lloyd, T., and Kaufman, S., 1975, Evidence for the lack of direct phosphorylation of bovine caudate tyrosine hydroxylase following activation by exposure to enzymatic phosphorylating conditions, *Biochem. Biophys. Res. Commun.* **66**:907–913.

Louisot, P., and Broquet, P., 1975, Subcellular localization of glycosyl transferases in synaptosomes and mitochondria of brain, in: Central Nervous System: Studies on Metabolic Regulation and Function, International Symposium, Saint Vincent, Italy, September 16–17, 1972, pp. 164–166.

Lovenberg, W., Bruckwick, E. A., and Hanbauer, I., 1975, ATP, cylic AMP, and magnesium increase the affinity of rat striatal tyrosine hydroxylase for its cofactor, *Proc. Natl. Acad. Sci. U.S.A.* **72**:2955–2958.

Lowy, J., McGregor, J., Rosenstone, J., and Schmidt, J., 1976, Solubilization of an α-bungarotoxin-binding component from rat brain, *Biochemistry* **15**:1522–1527.

Maelicke, A., and Reich, E., 1976, On the interaction between cobra α-neurotoxin and the acetylcholine receptor, *Cold Spring Harbor Symp. Quant. Biol.* **40**:231–237.

Maeno, H., and Greengard, P., 1972, Protein phosphatases from rat brain cerebral cortex: Subcellular distribution and characterization, *J. Biol. Chem.* **247**:3269–3277.

Maeno, H., Johnson, E. M., and Greengard, P., 1971, Subcellular distribution of adenosine 3',5'-monophosphate-dependent protein kinase in rat brain, *J. Biol. Chem.* **246**:134–142.

Mahadik, S. P., Hungund, B. L., and Rapport, M. M., 1975, Surface labeling of intact synaptosomes, *Trans. Am. Soc. Neurochem.* **6**:118.

Mahadik, S. P., Korenovsky, A., and Rapport, M. M., 1976, Slab gel analysis of the polypeptide components of rat brain subcellular organelles, *Anal. Biochem.* **76**:615–633.

Mahadik, S. P., Hungund, B. L., and Rapport, M. M., 1977, Topographical studies of glycoproteins and gangliosides in synaptosomes, *Neurosci. Abstr.* **3**:221.

Mahler, H. R., Gurd, J. W., and Wang, Y., 1975, Molecular topography of the synapse, in: *The Nervous System* (D. B. Tower, ed.), Vol. 1, pp. 455–466, Raven Press, New York.

Manuelidis, L., and Manuelidis, E. E., 1976, Cholera toxin-peroxidase: Changes in surface labeling of glioblastoma cells with increased time in tissue culture, *Science* **193**:588–590.

Marchbanks, R. M., 1967, Compartmentation of acetylcholine in synaptosomes, *Biochem. Pharmacol.* **16**:921–923.

Marchbanks, R. M., 1968, Exchangeability of radioactive acetylcholine with the bound acetylcholine of synaptosomes and synaptic vesicles, *Biochem. J.* **106**:87–95.

Marchbanks, R. M., 1974, Isolation and study of synaptic vesicles, in: *Research Methods in Neurochemistry* (N. Marks and R. Rodnight, eds.), Vol. 2, pp. 79–98, Plenum Press, New York.

Marchbanks, R. M., and Israel, M., 1971, Aspects of acetylcholine metabolism in the electric organ of *Torpedo marmorata, J. Neurochem.* **18**:439–448.

Marchbanks, R. M., and Israel, M., 1972, The heterogeneity of bound acetylcholine and synaptic vesicles, *Biochem. J.* **129**:1049–1061.

Marko, P., and Cuenod, M., 1973, Contribution of the nerve cell body to renewal of axonal and synaptic glycoproteins in the pigeon visual system, *Brain Res.* **62**:419–423.

Marks, N., and Lajtha, A., 1971, Protein and polypeptide breakdown, in: *Handbook of Neurochemistry* (A. Lajtha, ed.), Vol. 5, p. 76, Plenum Press, New York.

Matthysse, S., 1973, Antipsychotic drug actions: A clue to the neuropathology of schizophrenia?, *Fed. Proc.* **32**:200–205.

Matus, A. I., 1976a, The cytonet protein, *Nature* **262**:176.

Matus, A. I., 1976b, Molecular architecture of nerve connections, *New Sci.* **8**:57–59.

Matus, A. I., and Walters, B. B., 1975, Ultrastructure of the synaptic junctional lattice isolated from mammalian brain, *J. Neurocytol.* **4**:369–375.

Matus, A. I., and Walters, B. B., 1976, Type 1 and 2 synaptic junctions: Differences in distribution of concanavalin A binding sites and stability of the junctional adhesion, *Brain Res.* **108**:249–256.

Matus, A. I., De Petris, S., and Raff, M. C., 1973, Mobility of concanavalin A receptors in myelin and synaptic membranes, *Nature New Biol.* **244**:278–280.

Matus, A. I., Walters, B. B., and Jones, D. H., 1975*a*, Junctional ultrastructure in isolated synaptic membranes, *J. Neurocytol.* **4**:357–367.

Matus, A. I., Bradford, B. W., and Mughal, S., 1975*b*, Immunohistochemical demonstration of tubulin associated with microtubules and synaptic junctions in mammalian brain, *J. Neurocytol.* **4**:733–744.

McBride, W. J., Mahler, H. R., Moore, W. J., and White, F. P., 1970, Isolation and characterization of membranes from rat cerebral cortex, *J. Neurobiol.* **2**:73–92.

McGovern, S., Maguire, M. E., Gurd, R. S., Mahler, H. R., and Moore, W. J., 1973, Separation of adrenergic and cholinergic synaptosomes from immature rat brain, *FEBS Lett.* **31**:193–198.

Mergenroth, V. H., Hegstrand, L. R., Roth, R. H., and Greengard, P., 1975, Evidence for involvement of protein kinase in the activation by adenosine 3',5'-monophosphate of brain tyrosine 3-monooxygenase, *J. Biol. Chem.* **250**:1946–1948.

Metuzals, J., and Mushynski, W. E., 1974, Electron microscope and experimental investigation of the neurofilaments vs network in Deiter's neurons: Relationship with the cell surface and nuclear pores, *J. Cell Biol.* **61**:701–722.

Michaelis, E. K., Michaelis, M. L., and Boyarsky, L. L., 1974, High affinity glutamic acid binding to brain synaptic membranes, *Biochim. Biophys. Acta* **367**:338–348.

Michaelson, I. A., and Whittaker, V. P., 1963, The subcellular localization of 5-hydroxytryptamine in guinea-pig brain, *Biochem. Pharmacol.* **12**:203–211.

Moore, B. W., 1973, Brain-specific proteins, in: *Proteins of the Nervous System* (D. J. Schneider, ed.), pp. 1–12, Raven Press, New York.

Morgan, I. G., Wolfe, L. S., Mandel, P., and Gombos, G., 1971, Isolation of plasma membranes from rat brain, *Biochim. Biophys. Acta* **241**:737–751.

Morgan, I. G., Breckenridge, W. C., Vincendon, G., and Gombos, G., 1973*a*, Proteins of nerve-ending membranes, E. Preparation of synaptic vesicles, in: *Proteins of the Nervous System* (D. Schneider, ed.), pp. 179–181, Raven Press, New York.

Morgan, I. G., Zanetta, J. P., Breckenridge, W. C., Vincendon, G., and Gombos, G., 1973*b*, The chemical structure of synaptic membranes, *Brain Res.* **62**:405–411.

Morris, S. J., 1973, Removal of residual amounts of acetylcholinesterase and membrane contamination from synaptic vesicles isolated from the electric organ of *Torpedo, J. Neurochem.* **21**:713–715.

Nagy, A., Baker, R. R., Morris, S. J., and Whittaker, V. P., 1976, The preparation and characterization of synaptic vesicles of high purity, *Brain Res.* **109**:285–309.

Neal, M. J., and Iversen, L. L., 1969, Subcellular distribution of endogenous and ^{3}H-GABA in rat cortex, *J. Neurochem.* **16**:1245–1252.

Neidle, A., Van den Berg, C. J., and Grynbaum, A., 1969, The heterogeneity of rat brain mitochondria isolated on continuous sucrose gradients, *J. Neurochem.* **16**:225–234.

Neville, D. M., 1971, Molecular weight determination of protein-dodecyl sulphate complexes by gel electrophoresis in a discontinuous buffer system, *J. Biol. Chem.* **246**:6328–6334.

Nicklas, W. J., Puszkin, S., and Berl, S., 1973, Effect of vinblastine and colchicine on uptake and release of putative transmitters by synaptosomes and on brain actomyosin-like protein, *J. Neurochem.* **20**:109–121.

Nicolson, G. L., 1974, The interactions of lectins and animal cell surfaces, *Int. Rev. Cytol.* **39**:89–190.

Nielson, N. C., Fleischer, S., and McConnell, D. J., 1970, Lipid composition of bovine retinal outer-segment fragments, *Biochim. Biophys. Acta* **211**:10–19.

Nomura, Y., and Segawa, T., 1975, Influence of colchicine and vinblastine on the uptake of 5-hydroxytryptamine and norepinephrine by rat brain synaptosomes and small vesicle fractions, *J. Neurochem.* **24**:1257–1259.

Norton, W. T., and Poduslo, S. E., 1971, Neuronal perikarya and astroglia of rat brain: Chemical composition during myelination, *J. Lipid Res.* **12**:84–90.

Novikoff, A., 1967, AChE in axons, dendritic membrane and ER., in: *The Neuron* (H. Hyden, ed.), pp. 255–318, Elsevier, Amsterdam.

Ochs, S., 1975, Axoplasmic transport, in: *The Nervous System* (D. B. Tower, ed.), Vol. 1, pp. 137–147, Raven Press, New York.

Olmsted, J. B., Carlson, K., Klebe, R., Ruddle, F., and Rosenbaum, J., 1970, Isolation of microtubule protein from cultured mouse neuroblastoma cells, *Proc. Natl. Acad. Sci. U.S.A.* **65**:129–136.

Orrego, F., and Valdes, F., 1973, Glycine receptors in the cerebral cortex are probably transport receptors, *Acta Physiol. Lat. Am.* **23**:623–625.

Palay, S. L., 1956, Synapses in the central nervous system, *J. Biophys. Biochem. Cytol. Suppl.* **2**:193–202.

Palay, S. L., and Palade, G. E., 1954, Electron microscope observations of interneuronal and neuromuscular synapses, *Anat. Rec.* **118**:335–336.

Panyim, S., and Chalkley, R., 1971, The molecular weight of vertebrate histones exploiting a modified sodium dodecyl sulfate electrophoretic method, *J. Biol. Chem.* **246**:7557–7560.

Paton, W. D. M., Vizi, E. S., Zar, M., and Aboo, M., 1971, The mechanism of acetylcholine release from parasympathetic nerves, *J. Physiol. (Lond.)* **215**:819–848.

Pearse, B., 1975, Coated vesicles from pig brain, *J. Mol. Biol.* **97**:93–8.

Perper, R. J., Zee, T. W., and Mickelson, M. M., 1968, Purification of lymphocytes and platelets by gradient centrifugation, *J. Lab. Clin. Med.* **72**:842–848.

Peters, A., Palay, S. L., and Webster, H., DeF., 1970, *The Fine Structure of the Nervous System,* pp. 25, 58, 107, 112, 116, Harper & Row, New York.

Pfenninger, K. H., 1971, The cytochemistry of synaptic densities. I. An analysis of bismuth iodide impregnation method, *J. Ultrastruct. Res.* **34**:103–122.

Pfenninger, K. H., 1973, Synaptic morphology and cytochemistry, *Prog. Histochem. Cytochem.* **5**:1–86.

Phillips, D. R., and Morrison, M., 1970, The arrangement of proteins in the human erythrocyte membrane, *Biochem. Biophys. Res. Commun.* **40**:284–289.

Poduslo, J. F., and Braun, P. E., 1975, Topographic arrangement of membrane proteins in the intact myelin sheath: Lactoperoxidase incorporation of iodine into myelin surface proteins, *J. Biol. Chem.* **250**:1099–1105.

Pollard, H. B., Miller, A., and Cox, G. C., 1973, Synaptic vesicles: Structure of chromaffin granule membranes, *J. Supramol. Struct.* **1**:295–306.

Raftery, M. A., Schmidt, J., Vandlen, R., and Moody, T., 1974, Large-scale isolation and characterization of an acetyl choline receptor, in: *Neurochemistry of Cholinergic Receptors* (E. De Robertis and J. Schacht, eds.), pp. 5–18, Raven Press, New York.

Rappaport, L., Leterrier, J. F., and Nunez, J., 1975, Protein-kinase activity, *in vitro* phosphorylation and polymerization of purified tubulin, *Ann. N.Y. Acad. Sci.* **253**:611–629.

Reijnierse, G. L. A., Veldstra, H., and Van Den Berg, C. J., 1976, Radioassay of acetyl-CoA synthetase, propionyl-CoA synthetase and butyryl-CoA synthetase in brain, *Anal. Biochem.* **72**:614–622.

Reith, M., Morgan, I. G., Gombos, G., Breckenridge, W. C., and Vincendon, G., 1972, Synthesis of synaptic glycoproteins I. The distribution of UDP-galactose:N-acetylglucosamine galactosyl transferase and thiamine pyrophosphatase in adult rat brain subcellular fractions, *Neurobiology* **2**:169–175.

Richter, J. A., and Marchbanks, R. M., 1971, Isolation of [³H]acetylcholine pools by subcellular fractionation of cerebral cortex slices incubated with [³H]choline, *J. Neurochem.* **18**:705–712.

Rodbard, D., and Chramback, A., 1971, Estimation of molecular radius, free mobility, and valence using polyacrylamide gel electrophoresis, *Anal. Biochem.* **40**:95–134.

Rodbard, D., and Chrambach, A., 1974, in: *Electrophoresis and Isoelectric Focusing in Polyacrylamide Gel* (R. D. Allen and H. R. Maurer, eds.), pp. 28–61, de Gruyter Press, New York.

Rodriguez de Lores Arnaiz, G., Alberici, M., and De Robertis, E., 1967, Ultrastructural and enzymatic studies of cholinergic and non-cholinergic synaptic membranes isolated from brain cortex, *J. Neurochem.* **14**:215–225.

Rosenberry, T. L., 1975, Acetylcholinesterases, in: *Advances in Enzymology* (A. Meister, ed.), Vol. 43, pp. 89–218, Wiley, New York.

Rubin, C. S., and Rosen, O. M., 1975, Protein phosphorylation, *Annu. Rev. Biochem.* **44**:831–887.

Rudolph, S. A., and Greengard, P., 1974, Regulation of protein phosphorylation and membrane permeability by β-adrenergic agents and cyclic adenosine 3′,5′-monophosphate in the avian erythrocyte, *J. Biol. Chem.* **249**:5684–5687.

Rusca, G., Calissano, P., and Alema, S., 1972, Identification of a membrane-bound fraction of the S-100 protein, *Brain Res.* **49**:223–227.

Ryan, K. J., Kalant, M., and Thomas, E. L., 1971, Free-flow electrophoresis separation and electrical surface properties of subcellular particles from guinea-pig brain, *J. Cell Biol.* **49**:235–246.

Salganicoff, L., and De Robertis, E., 1963, Subcellular distribution of glutamic decarboxylase and gamma-aminobutyric alpha-ketoglutaric transaminase, *Life Sci.* **2**:85–91.

Salvaterra, P. M., and Mahler, H. R., 1976, Nicotinic acetylcholine receptor from rat brain: Solubilization, partial purification and characterization, *J. Biol. Chem.* **251**:6327–6334.

Salvaterra, P. M., Mahler, H. R., and Moore, W. J., 1975, Subcellular and regional distribution of ¹²⁵I-labeled α-bungarotoxin binding in rat brain and its relationship to acetylcholine esterase and choline acetyltransferase, *J. Biol. Chem.* **250**:6469–6475.

Schaffer, A., Seregi, A., and Komlos, M., 1974, Ascorbic acid-like effect of the soluble fraction of rat brain on ATPase and its relation to catecholamines and chelating agents, *Biochem. Pharmacol.* **23**:2257–2271.

Schengrund, C. L., and Rosenberg, A., 1970, Intracellular localization and properties of bovine brain sialidase, *J. Biol. Chem.* **250**:6196–6200.

Sellinger, O. Z., and Borens, R. N., 1969, Zonal density gradient electrophoresis of intracellular membranes of brain cortex, *Biochim. Biophys. Acta* **173**:176–184.

Shelanski, M. L., 1973, Microtubules, in: *Proteins of the Nervous System* (D. J. Schneider, ed.), pp. 227–241, Raven Press, New York.

Shelanski, M. L., and Taylor, E. W., 1967, Isolation of protein subunit from microtubules, *J. Cell Biol.* **34**:549–554.

Shelanski, M. L., Albert, S., DeVries, G. H., and Norton, W. T., 1971, Isolation of filaments from brain, *Science* **174**:1242–1245.

Shelanski, M. L., Feit, H., Berry, R. W., and Daniels, M. P., 1972, Some biochemical aspects of neurotubule and neurofilament proteins, *Adv. Exp. Med. Biol.* **32**:55–67.

Shelanski, M. L., Gaskin, F., and Cantor, C. R., 1973, Microtubule assembly in the absence of added nucleotides, *Proc. Natl. Acad. Sci. U.S.A.* **70**:765–768.

Shimada, A., and Nathenson, S. G., 1969, Murine histocompatibility-2 (H-2) alloantigens. Purification and some chemical properties of soluble products from H-2^b and H-2^d genotype released by papain digestion of membrane fractions, *Biochemistry* **8**:4048–4062.

Shute, C. C. D., and Lewis, P. R., 1966, Electron microscopy of cholinergic terminals and acetylcholinesterase containing neurons in the hippocampal formation of the rat, *Z. Zellforsch.* **69**:334–343.

Sidman, R. L., 1974, Cell–cell recognition in the developing central nervous system, in: *The Neurosciences Third Study Program* (F. O. Schmitt and F. G. Worden, eds.), pp. 743–758, MIT Press, Cambridge, Mass.

Singer, M., and Green, M. R., 1968, Autoradiographic studies of uridine incorporation in peripheral nerve of the newt *Friturus, J. Morphol.* **124**:321–344.

Singer, M., and Salpeter, M. M., 1966a, Transport of tritium-labelled 1-histidine through the Schwann and myelin sheath into the axon of peripheral nerves, *Nature* **210**:1212–1227.

Singer, M., and Salpeter, M. M., 1966b, The transport of ^{3}H-1-histidine through the Schwann and myelin sheath into the axon including re-evaluation of myelin function, *J. Morphol.* **120**:281–316.

Singer, S. J., 1972, A fluid lipid-globular protein mosaic model of membrane structure, *Ann. N.Y. Acad. Sci.* **195**:16–23.

Singer, S. J., 1974, The molecular organization of membranes, *Annu. Rev. Biochem.* **43**:805–833.

Singer, S. J., and Nicolson, G. L., 1972, The fluid mosaic model of the structure of cell membranes: Cell membranes are viewed as two-dimensional solutions of oriented globular proteins and lipids, *Science* **175**:720–731.

Skou, J. C., 1957, The influence of some cations on an adenosine triphosphatase from peripheral nerves, *Biochim. Biophys. Acta* **23**:394–401.

Sloboda, R. D., Rudolph, S. A., Rosenbaum, J. L., and Greengard, P., 1975, Cyclic AMP-dependent endogenous phosphorylation of a microtubule-associated protein, *Proc. Natl. Acad. Sci. U.S.A.* **72**:177–181.

Smith, D. S., 1971, On the significance of cross bridges between microtubules and synaptic vesicles, *Phil. Trans. Roy. Soc. Lond. Ser. B* **261**:395–405.

Smoley, J. M., Kuylenstierna, B., and Ernster, L., 1970, Topological and functional organization of the mitochondrion, *Proc. Natl. Acad. Sci. U.S.A.* **66**:125–131.

Snyder, S. H., Young, A. B., Bennett, J. P., and Mulder, A. H., 1973, Synaptic biochemistry of amino acids, *Fed. Proc.* **32**:2039–2047.

Snyder, S. H., Banerjee, S. P., Yamamura, H. I., and Greenberg, D., 1974, Drugs, neurotransmitters, and schizophrenia: Phenothiazines, amphetamines, and enzymes synthesizing psychotomimetic drugs and schizophrenia research, *Science* **184**:1243–1253.

Snyder, S. H., Chang, K. J., Kuhar, M. J., and Yamamura, H. I., 1975, Biochemical identification of the mammalian muscarinic cholinergic receptor, *Fed. Proc.* **34**:1915–1921.

Soffer, R. L., Horinishi, H., and Leibowitz, M. J., 1969, The aminoacyl tRNA-protein transferases, *Cold Spring Harbor Symp. Quant. Biol.* **34**:529–533.

Soifer, D., 1973, Cyclic-AMP regulation of the intrinsic protein kinase activity of microtubule protein from porcine brain, *J. Gen. Physiol.* **61**:265.

Soifer, D., 1975, The biology of cytoplasmic microtubules, *Ann. N.Y. Acad. Sci.* **253**:5–848.

Soifer, D., Laszlow, A., Mack, K., Scotto, J., and Siconolfi, L., 1975, The association of a cyclic AMP-dependent protein kinase activity with microtubule protein, *Ann. N.Y. Acad. Sci.* **253**:598–610.

Sottocasa, G. L., Kuylenstierna, B., Ernster, L., and Bergstrand, A., 1967, Separation and some enzymatic properties of the inner and outer membranes of rat liver mitochondria, in: *Methods in Enzymology* (R. W. Estabrook and M. E. Pullman, eds.), Vol. 10, pp. 448–463, Academic Press, New York.

Spanner, S., 1972, Methods of separating subcellular components of brain tissue, in: *Glycolipids, Glycoproteins, and Mucopolysaccharides of the Nervous System* (V. Zambotti, G. Tettamanti, and M. Arrigoni, eds.), pp. 195–207, Plenum Press, New York.

Steck, T. L., 1972, The organization of proteins in human erythrocyte membranes, in: *Membrane Research* (C. F. Fox, ed.), pp. 71–93, Academic Press, New York.

Steck, T. L., 1974, The organization of proteins in the human red blood cell membrane. A review, *J. Cell Biol.* **62**:1–19.

Steck, T. L., and Wallach, D. F. H., 1970, Isolation of plasma membranes, in: *Methods in Cancer Research* (H. Busch, ed.), Vol. V, pp. 93–153, Academic Press, New York.

Stephens, R. E., and Edd, K. T., 1976, Microtubules: Structure, chemistry, and function, *Physiol. Rev.* **56**:709–777.

Stobo, J. D., Rosenthal, A. S., and Paul, W. E., 1972, Functional heterogeneity of murine lymphoid cells. I. Responsiveness to and surface binding of concanavalin A and phytohemagglutinin, *J. Immunol.* **108**:1–17.

Suzuki, K., 1970, Formation and turnover of myeline ganglioside, *J. Neurochem.* **17**:209–213.

Tamir, H., and Gilvarg, C., 1966, Density gradient centifugation for the separation of sporulating forms of bacteria, *J. Biol. Chem.* **241**:1085–1090.

Tamir, H., and Huang, Y. L., 1974, Binding of serotonin to soluble protein from synaptosomes, *Life Sci.* **14**:83–93.

Tamir, H., and Rapport, M. M., 1976, Is the serotonin binding protein (SBP) a soluble storage for serotonin? *Res. Commun. Chem. Pathol. Pharmacol.* **13**:225–235.

Tamir, H., Kaufman, H., and Rapport, M. M., 1972, Subcellular distribution of pyruvate kinase (EC 2.7.1.40) in cerebral cortex, *J. Neurochem.* **19**:1759–1768.

Tamir, H., Rapport, M. M., and Roizin, L., 1974, Preparation of synaptosomes and vesicles with sodium diatrizoate, *J. Neurochem.* **23**:943–949.

Tamir, H., Mahadik, S., Klein, A., Roizin, L., Liu, J. C., and Rapport, M. M., 1975, Separation and characterization of two types of rat brain mitochondria, *Neurosci. Abstr.* **1**:617.

Tamir, H., Mahadik, S. P., and Rapport, M. M., 1976a, Fractionation of synaptic membranes with sodium diatrizoate, *Anal. Biochem.* **76**:634–647.

Tamir, H., Klein, A., and Rapport, M. M., 1976b, Serotonin binding protein: Enhancement of binding by Fe^{2+} and inhibition of binding by drugs, *J. Neurochem.* **26**:871–878.

Tanaka, R., 1974, ATPases of plain synaptic vesicle fraction and coated vesicle fraction of rat brain, *Fed. Proc.* **33**:1550.

Tasaki, I., Watanabe, A., and Hallet, M., 1971, Properties of squid axon membrane as revealed by a hydrophobic probe, 2-*p*-toluidinyl-naphthalene-6-sulfonate, *Proc. Natl. Acad. Sci. U.S.A.* **68**:938–941.

Tasaki, I., Hallet, M., and Carbone, E., 1973a, Further studies of nerve membranes labeled with fluorescent probes, *J. Membrane Biol.* **11**:353–376.

Tasaki, I., Carbone, E., Sisco, K., and Singer, I., 1973b, Spectral analysis of extrinsic fluorescence of the nerve membrane labeled with aminonaphthalene derivatives, *Biochim. Biophys. Acta* **323**:220–233.

Teravainen, H., 1969, Histochemical localization of acetylcholinesterase in isolated brain synaptosomes, *Histochemie* **18**:191–194.

Tettamanti, G., Morgan, I. G., Gombos, G., Vincendon, G., and Mandel, P., 1972, Subsynaptosomal localization of brain particulate neuraminidase, *Brain Res.* **47**:515–518.

Tettamanti, G., Poeti, A., Lombardo, A., Donati, F., and Zambotti, V., 1973, Parallelism of subcellular location of major particulate neuraminidase and gangliosides in rabbit brain cortex, *Biochim. Biophys. Acta* **306**:466–477.

Tkachenko, A. N., 1972, Isolation of synaptosomal membrane from animal brains, *Bickhimiya* **37**:201–206.

Torack, R. M., and Barrnett, R. J., 1964, The fine structural localization of nucleoside phosphatase activity in the blood-brain barrier, *J. Neuropathol. Exp. Neurol.* **23**:46–59.

Truding, R., Shelanski, M. L., Daniels, M. P., and Morell, P., 1974, Comparison of surface membranes isolated from cultured murine neuroblastoma cells in the differentiated or undifferentiated state, *J. Biol. Chem.* **249**:3973–3982.

Tucek, S., 1966, On subcellular localization and binding of choline acetyltransferase in the cholinergic nerve endings of the brain, *J. Neurochem.* **13**:1317–1327.

Ueda, T., Maeno, H., and Greengard, P., 1973, Regulation of endogenous phosphorylation of specific proteins in synaptic membrane fractions from rat brain by adenosine $3',5'$-monophosphate, *J. Biol. Chem.* **248**:8295–8305.

Ueda, T., Rudolph, S. A., and Greengard, P., 1975, Solubilization of a phosphoprotein and its activated cyclic AMP-dependent kinase and phosphoprotein phosphatase from synaptic membrane fractions and some kinetic evidence for their existence as a complex. *Arch. Biochem. Biophys.* **170**:492–503.

Uesugi, S., Dulak, N. C., Dixon, J. F., Hexum, T. D., Dahl, J. L., Perdue, J. F., and Hokin, L. E., 1971, Studies on the characterization of the sodium-potassium transport adenosine triphosphatase VI. Large scale partial purification and properties of a Lubrol-solubilized bovine brain enzyme, *J. Biol. Chem.* **246**:531–543.

Van der Kloot, W., and Kita, H., 1974, Mechanisms for neurotransmitter release, *Bioscience* **24**:13–17.

Van Nieuw Amerongen, A., and Roukema, P. A., 1974, GP-350, a sialoglycoprotein from calf brain: Its subcellular localization and occurrence in various brain areas, *J. Neurochem.* **23**:85–89.

Van Nieuw Amerongen, A., Roukema, P. A., and Van Rossum, A. L., 1974, Immunofluorescence study on the cellular localization of GP-350, a sialoglycoprotein from brain, *Brain Res.* **81**:1–19.

Verity, M. A., Gade, G. F., and Brown, W. J., 1973, Characterization and localization of acid hydrolase activity in the synaptosomal fraction from rat cerebral cortex, *J. Neurochem.* **20**:1635–1648.

Vizi, E., 1972, Stimulation by inhibition of $(Na^+-K^+-Mg^{2+})$-activated ATPase of acetylcholine release in cortical slices from rat brain, *J. Physiol. (Lond.)* **226**:95–117.

Vos, J., Kuriyama, K., and Roberts, E., 1968, Electrophoretic mobilities of brain subcellular particles and binding of γ-aminobutyric acid, acetylcholine, norepinephrine, and 5-hydroxytryptamine, *Brain Res.* **9**:224–230.

Waehneldt, T. V., Morgan, I. G., and Gombos, G., 1971, Common glycoproteins of synaptic vesicles and the synaptosomal plasma membranes, *Brain Res.* **34**:403–406.

Walberg, F., 1968, Morphological correlates of postsynaptic inhibitory processes, in: *Structure and Function of Inhibitory Neuronal Mechanisms* (C. Van Euler, S. Skoglund, and U. Soderberg, eds.), pp. 7–14, Pergamon Press, Oxford.

Walters, B. B., and Matus, A. I., 1975*a*, Ultrastructural organization in isolated synaptic densities, *J. Anat. (Lond.)* **119**:415.

Walters, B. B., and Matus, A. I., 1975*b*, Tubulin in postsynaptic junctional lattice, *Nature* **257**:496–498.

Walton, K. G., De Lorenzo, R. J., Curran, P. F., and Greengard, P., 1975, Regulation of protein phosphorylation and sodium transport in toad bladder, *J. Gen. Physiol.* **65**:153–177.

Wanamaker, B. B., and Kornguth, S. E., 1973, Electrophoretic patterns of proteins from isolated synapses of human and swine brain, *Biochim. Biophys. Acta* **303**:333–337.

Wang, Y., Crawford, G., and Mahler, H. R., 1975, Topography of the synaptic plasma membrane, *Neurosci. Abstr.* **1**:618.

Weber, K., and Osborn, M., 1969, The reliability of molecular weight determination by dodecyl sulfate–polyacrylamide gel electrophoresis, *J. Biol. Chem.* **244**:4406–4412.

Weil-Malherbe, H., 1976, The biochemistry of affective disorders, in: *Biological Foundations of Psychiatry* (R. G. Grenell and S. Gabay, eds.), Vol. 2, pp. 683–728, Raven Press, New York.

Weinstein, H., Roberts, E., and Kakefuda, T., 1963, Studies of subcellular distribution of α-aminobutyric acid and glutamic decarboxylase in mouse brain, *Biochem. Pharmacol.* **12**:503–509.

Weisenberg, R. C., Borisy, G. G., and Taylor, E. W., 1968, The colchicine-binding protein of mammalian brain and its relation to microtubules, *Biochemistry* **7**:4466–4479.

Welsh, F. A., 1972, Polypeptide chains of synaptic membranes: Identification of a sodium ion–potassium ion-dependent ATPase chain, *Fed. Proc.* **31**:431.

Westrum, L. E., and Boderson, S. E., 1976, Ultrastructural localization of acetylcholinesterase at synapses, *Trans. Am. Soc. Neurochem.* **7**:136.

Whittaker, V. P., 1968, The morphology of fractions of rat forebrain synaptosomes separated on continuous sucrose density gradients, *Biochem. J.* **106**:412–417.

Whittaker, V. P., and Barker, L. A., 1972, The subcellular fractionation of brain tissue with special reference to the preparation of synaptosomes and their component organelles, in: *Methods of Neurochemistry* (R. Fried, ed.), Vol. 2, pp. 1–52, Dekker, New York.

Whittaker, V. P., and Gray, E. G., 1962, The synapse: Biology and morphology, *Br. Med. Bull.* **18**:223–228.

Whittaker, V. P., Michaelson, I. A., and Kirkland, R. J. A., 1964, The separation of synaptic vesicles from nerve-ending particles ("synaptosomes"), *Biochem. J.* **90**:293–303.

Whittaker, V. P., Essman, W. B., and Dowe, G. H. C., 1972, The isolation of pure cholinergic synaptic vesicles from the electric organs of Elasmobranch fish of the family Torpedinidae, *Biochem. J.* **128**:833–846.

Williams, M., and Rodnight, R., 1977, Protein phosphorylation in nervous tissue: Possible involvement in nervous tissue function and relationship to cyclic nucleotide metabolism, *Prog. Neurobiol.* **8**:183–250.

Wilson, J. E., Wilkin, G. P., and Balazs, R., 1976, Metabolic properties of a purified preparation of large fragments of cerebellar glomeruli: Glucose metabolism and amino acid uptake, *J. Neurochem.* **26**:957–965.

Wilson, L., 1970, Properties of colchicine binding protein from chick embryo brain. Interactions with vinca alkaloids and podophylotoxin, *Biochemistry* **9**:4999–5007.

Wilson, L., 1975, Microtubules as drug receptors: Pharmacological properties of microtubule protein, *Ann. N.Y. Acad. Sci.* **253**:215–231.

Wilson, L., Bryan, J., Ruby, A., and Mazia, D., 1970, Precipitation of proteins by vinblastine and calcium ions, *Proc. Natl. Acad. Sci. U.S.A.* **66**:807–814.

Wilson, W. S., and Cooper, J. R., 1972, The preparation of cholinergic synaptosomes from bovine superior cervical ganglia, *J. Neurochem.* **19**:2779–2790.

Wilson, W. S., Schulz, R. A., and Cooper, J. R., 1973, The isolation of cholinergic synaptic vesicles from bovine superior cervical ganglion and estimation of their acetylcholine content, *J. Neurochem.* **20**:659–667.

Wuerker, R. B., 1970, Neurofilaments and glial filaments, *Tissue Cell* **2**:1–9.

Wurtman, R. J., and Fernstrom, J. D., 1972, L-Tryptophan, L-tryosine, and the control of brain monoamine biosynthesis, in: *Perspectives in Neuropharmacology* (S. H. Snyder, ed.), pp. 145–193, Oxford Univ. Press, London.

Yamane, K., and Nathenson, S. G., 1970, Murine histocompatibility-2 (H-2) alloantigens. Purification and some chemical properties of a second class of fragments (class II) solubilized by papain from cell membranes of H-2^b and H-2^d mice, *Biochemistry* **9**:1336–1341.

Yen, S., Dahl, D., Schachner, M., and Shelanski, M. L., 1976a, Biochemistry of the filaments of brain, *Proc. Natl. Acad. Sci. U.S.A.* **73**:529–533.

Yen, S., Kelly, P., Liem, R., Cotman, C., and Shelanski, M. L., 1976b, The neurofilament protein is a major component of the postsynaptic density, *Neurosci. Abstr.* **2**:620.

Zatz, M., and Barondes, S. H., 1971, Particulate and solubilized fucosyl transferases from mouse brain, *J. Neurochem.* **18**:1625–1637.

Zieher, L. M., and De Robertis, E., 1963, Subcellular localization of 5-hydroxytryptamine in rat brain, *Biochem. Pharmacol.* **12**:596–598.

THE MULTIPLE ROLES OF GLUTAMATE AND ASPARTATE IN NEURAL TISSUES

RICHARD P. SHANK

Department of Physiology
Temple University School of Medicine
Philadelphia, Pennsylvania

AND

LEWIS T. GRAHAM, JR.

Department of Biochemistry and Molecular Biology
Louisiana State University Medical Center
Shreveport, Louisiana

1. INTRODUCTION

L-Glutamate and L-aspartate, like many other substances, serve a number of functions in biological tissues. In virtually all types of biological cells these amino acids serve as constituents of protein, intermediates in energy and nitrogen metabolism, and as precursors of other biochemical compounds. In many cells, particularly neurons, these amino acids are utilized for even more functions. Both glutamate and aspartate are probably major excitatory neurotransmitters, and both make a significant contribution to the osmotic and ionic state of nerve cells. They are also immediate precursors of other compounds which have unique physiological roles in nerve tissues. For example, glutamate is the metabolic precursor of γ-aminobutyrate (GABA) which serves as a major inhibitory neurotransmitter (in addition to other possible functions), and aspartate is an immediate precursor of N-acetylaspartate, whose neural functions include a role in the maintenance of intracellular ionic balance. Because most of the functions mediated by glutamate and aspartate are common to both, we have chosen to include in this chapter the functions of both amino acids.

Although the total pool of glutamate and aspartate in nerve tissues is utilized for several purposes, the specific function each individual molecule will serve depends on its cellular location and the metabolic and physiological state of the tissue. For instance, if the molecule is within a cell and in the proximity of a ribosome, it may become attached to a specific tRNA molecule and subsequently be incorporated into an incipient protein molecule. If located in the cytosol, the molecule could serve as a precursor to any one of several substances, or it could be taken up into a mitochondrion and therein be converted to its respective keto acid for utilization in energy metabolism. If present in a nerve terminal, the molecule may, depending on the type of neuron, be transported into a synaptic vesicle and be released subsequently into the synaptic cleft, thereby acting as a neurotransmitter agent; or, in the case of glutamate, the molecule may be decarboxylated to form γ-aminobutyrate, thus serving as the immediate precursor of another transmitter agent. Also, in the case of glutamate, the molecule may be utilized to prevent an accumulation of toxic amounts of ammonia by being coupled to the latter through the action of glutamine synthetase. Regardless of the cellular location, each molecule of glutamate and aspartate contributes to the osmotic and ionic state of the tissue fluids, and due to their relatively high contents in neural tissues these two amino acids serve an important role in this regard.

In order for glutamate and aspartate to be utilized for these different roles, it is essential that neural tissues possess mechanisms which ensure that these amino acids are maintained in adequate amounts, and that their concentrations within various intracellular and extracellular compartments are controlled within narrow limits. In recent years, our knowledge of the enzymes and transport systems which are responsible for regulating the contents of these amino acids in the various tissue compartments has been advanced considerably. However, we are far from having a comprehensive understanding of the cellular processes which function collectively to maintain and regulate the levels of these two important amino acids.

2. THE PUTATIVE NEUROTRANSMITTER FUNCTION

Although the present evidence does not provide conclusive proof that glutamate and aspartate are synaptic transmitters, the evidence supporting such a function in both vertebrates and invertebrates is very compelling. The results of recent studies leave little doubt that glutamate is an excitatory neuromuscular transmitter in arthropods, and studies strongly supporting a transmitter role for both glutamate and aspartate in the central nervous system (CNS) of vertebrates are being reported at an ever increasing rate.

2.1. The Status of the Transmitter Role in Invertebrates

The original studies in the late 1950s and early 1960s which led to the concept that glutamate may be the excitatory neuromuscular neurotransmitter in crustacea and other arthropods have been discussed extensively in previous reviews (Florey, 1967; Kravitz et al., 1970; Takeuchi and Takeuchi, 1972; Gerschenfeld, 1973). These early studies showed (1) that L-glutamate at relatively low concentrations (~0.1 mM) could cause muscle contraction in the limbs of several species of arthropods, (2) that L-glutamate is present in the excitatory motor nerves in high amounts, and (3) that the excitatory action of glutamate is restricted to the neuromuscular junctions.

The results of several recent studies have established that the reversal potential of the excitatory responses elicited by glutamate is identical to that of the neurally evoked excitatory junction potentials (Taraskevich, 1971; Takeuchi and Onodera, 1973; Anwyl and Usherwood, 1974; Onodera and Takeuchi, 1975; Dudel, 1975). Thus the "identity of action" criterion has been satisfied. The possibility that glutamate acts indirectly by evoking the release of endogenous transmitter from nerve terminals has been ruled out by a denervation study which showed that the muscle fibers of crayfish were responsive to glutamate several months after the nerve terminals had degenerated (Frank, 1974).

Many analogues of glutamate have been studied in recent years in an attempt to discover substances which selectively block neurally evoked excitatory junction potentials and the action of glutamate. As a result of these pharmacological studies a number of glutamate antagonists have been found (Lowagie and Gerschenfeld, 1974; Wheal and Kerkut, 1975; Shank and Freeman, 1976; Cull-Candy *et al.*, 1976). However, none of the antagonists so far reported is highly potent, and for at least some of the compounds the blocking action is not consistent from species to species. Kainic acid at concentrations greater than 1 mM blocks excitatory junction potentials and the action of applied L-glutamate in the walking limbs of the lobster, *Homarus americanus* (Shank and Freeman, 1976), but at concentrations less than 1 mM this substance potentiates the action of glutamate in crayfish (Shinozaki and Shibuya, 1974). Also, the diethyl ester of L-glutamate exhibits an antagonistic effect in some crustacea (Lowagie and Gerschenfeld, 1974; Wheal and Kerkut, 1975), but not in others (Nistri and Constanti, 1975; Shank and Freeman, 1976).

One additional criterion required to establish glutamate unequivocally as the excitatory neuromuscular transmitter in the limbs of arthropods is that of transmitter release. A number of studies have been undertaken in an attempt to satisfy this criterion, but these studies have not provided convincing evidence that glutamate is released from nerve terminals in physiologically active amounts during periods of sustained stimulation of excitatory motor axons (Kravitz *et al.*, 1970). Unfortunately, it is exceedingly difficult to determine the amount of glutamate released from nerve terminals because of a high rate of release of this amino acid from the large mass of muscle (Daoud and Miller, 1976).

Although there is virtually no doubt that glutamate is the transmitter which mediates neuromuscular excitation in the limbs of arthropods, the results of several recent studies indicate that aspartate also serves a role in this excitatory synaptic process, at least in some crustacea. Kravitz *et al.* (1970) reported that aspartate exhibited a weak excitatory action when applied to muscle fibers in the limbs of crayfish and lobsters, and that the excitatory responses elicited by glutamate sometimes could be potentiated by aspartate. Recent studies on the actions of these amino acids on muscle fibers in the walking limbs of lobsters indicate that aspartate has very little excitatory activity by itself, but that it markedly potentiates the action of glutamate without affecting the maximum response elicited by the latter (Shank *et al.*, 1975; Shank and Freeman, 1975) (see Figure 1). These observations suggest that aspartate acts in a manner analogous to a positive modulator on an allosteric enzyme. Since aspartate is highly concentrated in the excitatory motor axons (Kravitz *et al.*, 1970; McBride *et al.*, 1974), this action of aspartate probably has physiological significance. Aspartate has also been reported to potentiate the action of glutamate in a species of crab (Kerkut and Wheal, 1974).

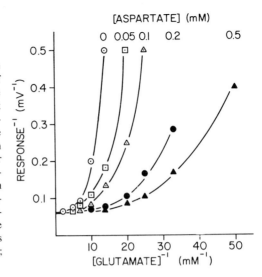

FIGURE 1. Effect of aspartate on the glutamate-induced depolarization of lobster muscle fibers. This is a double reciprocal (Lineweaver–Burke) plot of data reported by Shank and Freeman (1975). Glutamate and aspartate were dissolved in lobster saline which was superfused directly onto lobster muscle fibers. The decrease in membrane potential (depolarization response) was recorded using an intracellular electrode. The upward divergence of the curves indicates that the activation of receptors by glutamate is a cooperative process (Triggle, 1971; Colquhoun, 1973).

A number of studies on other species of invertebrates have provided evidence that glutamate and aspartate serve an inhibitory as well as excitatory neurotransmitter function in animals representative of other phyla of invertebrates (Miledi, 1972; Gerschenfeld, 1973; Carew *et al.,* 1974; Yarowsky and Carpenter, 1976). However, their status as neurotransmitters in these other phyla is less certain than their status in arthropods.

2.2. The Status of the Transmitter Role in Vertebrates

2.2.1. Neurophysiological Studies

When applied by iontophoresis onto the external surface of neurons in the CNS, both glutamate and aspartate exert an excitatory effect on the vast majority of these cells (Curtis *et al.,* 1960; Krnjević and Phillis, 1963; Curtis and Crawford, 1969; Krnjević, 1974; Curtis and Johnston, 1974). When it first became evident that glutamate and aspartate excite virtually all neurons in the spinal cord of cats, the suggestion was made that these amino acids might serve some generalized "nonspecific" excitatory function (Curtis *et al.,* 1960). However, since the middle 1960s there has been a gradual realization that these two amino acids are probably the principal excitatory neurotransmitters in the CNS of vertebrates.

Based on studies in which the amino acids were applied by bulk flow (superfusion) to neurons in the cat cerebral cortex, the concentration

TABLE 1. Relative Sensitivity of Spinal Interneurons and Renshaw
Cells to L-Glutamate and L-Aspartate[a]

	Number of cells tested		
Relative potency	Renshaw cells	Interneurons	Total
Asp > Glu	22	4	26
Glu > Asp	1	24	25
Glu = Asp	5	4	9

[a] Data from Duggan (1974).

needed to increase the frequency of action potentials was estimated to be about 0.1 mM (Krnjević and Phillis, 1963). The average content (μmol/g wet tissue) of these amino acids in the CNS of vertebrates is between 20 and 100 times this concentration. Hence there is potentially a sufficient amount of glutamate and aspartate present so that each could be the transmitter released from a relatively high percentage of the total population of neurons in the CNS.

Glutamate and aspartate excite central neurons in a transmitterlike manner in that when they are iontophoresed onto these cells, the latency between the onset of the driving current and the peak of the excitatory response is brief, and when the iontophoretic current is terminated, the response subsides very quickly. The exact nature of the excitatory action is not yet established, but it is known that there is a depolarization of the cell membrane which is associated with an increase in membrane conductance (Krnjević and Schwartz, 1967; Curtis and Crawford, 1969; Zieglgansberger and Puil, 1973; Altmann et al., 1976). The increase in membrane conductance is almost certainly due to an increase in the membrane permeability to Na$^+$, K$^+$, and possibly Ca^{2+}, but not to Cl$^-$ (Curtis et al., 1972; Hösli et al., 1973, 1976). In this respect the action of glutamate and aspartate appears to be the same as that induced by the neurally released transmitter at most central excitatory synapses. However, it has yet to be shown for vertebrate neurons that the reversal potential of the membrane response to glutamate and aspartate is identical to that of the neurally evoked excitatory postsynaptic responses.

Most neurons are more responsive to glutamate than to aspartate; however, some cells in the lateral geniculate (Morgan et al., 1972), spinal cord (Duggan, 1974) (see Table 1), and red nucleus (Altmann et al., 1976) are more sensitive to aspartate. These observations coupled with the indication from iontophoretic studies that there is no apparent interference between the actions of glutamate and aspartate suggest that these amino acids act upon separate receptors (Johnston *et al.*, 1974). However, because of technical limitations associated with iontophoretic studies on central neurons, these observations must be interpreted cautiously (Gent *et al.*, 1974). Comprehensive reviews of the excitatory actions of glutamate and aspartate in the CNS of vertebrates have been written by Curtis and Johnston (1974) and Krnjević (1974).

2.2.2. Neurochemical Studies

2.2.2.1. Tissue Content and Distribution Studies. The concept that a neurotransmitter should be present in the neurons which utilize it for this function is applicable to glutamate and aspartate. However, both amino acids are also present in all the major areas of the vertebrate CNS and in peripheral nerves as well. Depending on the species of animal and the particular area of the nervous system analyzed the content of glutamate ranges between 2 and 15 μmol/g wet tissue, and the corresponding values for the content of aspartate are generally one-fifth to one-half that of glutamate (Tables 2 and 3).

TABLE 2. Content of Glutamate and Aspartate in Whole Brain of Various Species of Vertebrates[a]

Species	Glutamate (μmol/g wet tissue)	Aspartate	Reference
Man[b]	5.95	0.96	Perry *et al.*, 1971
Pig	10.50	2.60	Badger and Tumbleson, 1975
Dog	9.05	3.28	Himwich and Agrawal, 1969
Cat	7.87	1.70	Himwich and Agrawal, 1969
Rabbit	8.53	2.05	Himwich and Agrawal, 1969
Guinea pig	9.51	2.36	Himwich and Agrawal, 1969
Rat	11.60	2.63	Levi *et al.*, 1967
Mouse	11.50	3.38	Agrawal *et al.*, 1968
Chicken	12.20	2.76	Levi *et al.*, 1967
Toad	5.75	1.04	Shank and Baxter, 1973
Frog	5.36	0.86	Levi *et al.*, 1967
Tortoise	4.62	0.47	Okumura *et al.*, 1959
Catfish	5.05	0.29	Okumura *et al.*, 1959
Caiman	5.16	0.47	Coulson and Hernandez, 1971

[a] The data represent the tissue content of free (noncovalently linked) glutamate and aspartate. In most cases protein hydrolysis was minimized by freezing or extracting the tissue within seconds or a few minutes after death.
[b] Data for man represent cerebral cortex only.

TABLE 3. Content of Glutamate and Aspartate in Eight Areas of the Rat CNS[a]

CNS area	Glutamate	Aspartate
	(μmol/g wet tissue $\pm$ SEM)	
Telencephalon	11.24 $\pm$ 0.19	2.39 $\pm$ 0.06
Diencephalon	8.62 $\pm$ 0.11	2.40 $\pm$ 0.05
Mesencephalon	7.06 $\pm$ 0.20	2.53 $\pm$ 0.06
Cerebellum	9.68 $\pm$ 0.16	1.99 $\pm$ 0.06
Pons	6.24 $\pm$ 0.15	2.53 $\pm$ 0.09
Medulla	6.19 $\pm$ 0.29	2.07 $\pm$ 0.07
Spinal cord		
Gray	6.36 $\pm$ 0.22	3.45 $\pm$ 0.08
White	3.45 $\pm$ 0.08	1.25 $\pm$ 0.08

[a] Data from Shank and Aprison (1970).

Although these amino acids are presumably present in all neurons and glia cells as well, it seems reasonable to expect them to be more concentrated in neurons which utilize them as transmitters than in other cells. For further discussion of this assumption see Aprison and Werman (1965, 1968). This concept has been the basis for a number of distribution studies. The results of these studies indicate that glutamate and aspartate are more concentrated in some neurons than in others, and at least in some areas of the nervous system the two amino acids are not concentrated in the same neurons. For example, glutamate is more concentrated in spinal dorsal roots than in ventral roots, whereas the content of aspartate within these two tissues is nearly the same (Graham *et al.,* 1967; Duggan and Johnston, 1970; Johnson and Aprison, 1970) (see Table 4). Within the spinal cord of

TABLE 4. Distribution of Glutamate and Aspartate in the Cat Spinal Cord and Roots (L_6-S_2)[a]

Tissue area	Glutamate	Aspartate
	(μmol/g wet tissue $\pm$ SEM)	
Dorsal root	4.61 $\pm$ 0.01	1.02 $\pm$ 0.05
Ventral root	3.14 $\pm$ 0.13	1.27 $\pm$ 0.08
Dorsal gray	6.48 $\pm$ 0.15	2.05 $\pm$ 0.16
Ventral gray	5.25 $\pm$ 0.18	3.06 $\pm$ 0.17
Dorsal white	4.80 $\pm$ 0.07	1.11 $\pm$ 0.05
Ventral white	3.89 $\pm$ 0.12	1.29 $\pm$ 0.04

[a] Each value is the mean of eight animals. Data from Graham *et al.* (1967).

cats, glutamate is more concentrated in the dorsal horn than in the ventral horn, whereas the reverse is true for aspartate (Table 4). This distribution data in conjunction with the "transmitterlike" excitatory activity of these amino acids on spinal neurons led to the suggestion that glutamate is the transmitter released by primary afferent neurons, and that aspartate is the transmitter released by excitatory interneurons in the spinal cord (Graham *et al.,* 1967). Further evidence that aspartate and not glutamate is concentrated in spinal excitatory interneurons was provided by a study showing that the content of aspartate, but not that of glutamate, correlated with the number of spinal interneurons remaining after a selective destruction of these neurons by ischemia (Davidoff *et al.,* 1967).

Because substance P is much more highly concentrated in spinal dorsal roots than in ventral roots, Otsuka *et al.* (1975) have suggested that this peptide rather than glutamate is the transmitter released by primary afferent neurons. This peptide exhibits an excitatory action on spinal neurons, and on a molar basis it is about 200 times more potent than glutamate (Otsuka *et al.,* 1975; Otsuka, 1977). However, the activity of substance P is less transmitterlike than that of glutamate because it evokes a gradual and prolonged excitatory action. Furthermore, the content of glutamate in the spinal cord of cats is approximately 20,000 times that of the peptide. Thus the total excitatory activity of glutamate in the spinal cord is about 100 times that of substance P (Table 5). Within the spinal cord of cats, substance P is concentrated mostly within the upper portion of the dorsal horn (Takahashi and Otsuka, 1975). This suggests that substance P could be the transmitter released by certain primary afferent neurons which terminate predominantly in laminae I, II, and III of the dorsal horn. This is quite possible since the dorsal root contains several anatomically and physiologically different types of sensory neurons, some of which synapse primarily

TABLE 5. Comparison of the Tissue Contents and Excitatory Activity of Glutamate and Substance P in the Spinal Cord Gray Matter of the Cat

Compound	Content[a]	Relative potency[b]	Relative excitatory activity[c]
Glutamate	6000	1	100
Substance P	0.3	200	1

[a] Approximate average values (nmol/g wet tissue) of data reported by Graham *et al.* (1967) and Takahashi and Otsuka (1975) for glutamate and substance P, respectively.
[b] Potency values reported by Otsuka *et al.* (1975).
[c] Calculated from the tissue content and relative potency values.

on neurons in the upper dorsal horn. Therefore, both glutamate and substance P may function as a transmitter released from primary afferent neurons, but for substance P this function may be restricted to sensory neurons which terminate almost exclusively in the upper portion of the dorsal gray matter. In support of this concept Hökfelt *et al.* (1976) have demonstrated with an immunohistochemical technique that substance P is localized to small dorsal root fibers which terminate predominantly in lamina I of the dorsal horn. It is also possible that some neurons release both glutamate and substance P, and that the latter serves a modulatory role rather than being an actual transmitter. A modulatory role is more consistent with the gradual and prolonged excitatory effect exerted by substance P.

Within the cerebellum glutamate, but not aspartate, appears to be selectively concentrated in granule cells (Young *et al.*, 1974; McBride *et al.*, 1976). This conclusion is based on studies which show that the content of glutamate, but not other amino acids, in cerebellar tissues is markedly decreased if the granule cells are selectively destroyed during maturation (Table 6). In the absence of granule cells, the metabolic state of the cerebellum may be quite different from the normal state, and the content of glutamate in remaining cells could be reduced by this pathologic condition. Therefore, it cannot be concluded definitely that glutamate is more highly concentrated in the granule cells, although the selective depletion of glutamate must be regarded as strong evidence that glutamate is concentrated in granule cells. The granule cells are the only excitatory neurons endogenous to the cerebellum, and if glutamate is the transmitter released by all the

TABLE 6.   Effect of Granule Cell Loss in the Cerebellum on the Content of Putative Transmitter Amino Acids

Cerebellar tissue	Tissue content (μmol/g wet tissue)			
	Glutamate	Aspartate	GABA	Glycine
Hamster[a]				
Normal	12.0	1.34	—	0.58
Viral infected	6.84	1.67	—	0.92
Mouse[b]				
Normal C57BL/6J	12.0	2.52	1.56	1.06
Mutant (weaver)	8.77	2.82	3.35	1.55
Normal C57BL	12.0	2.59	1.61	1.08
Mutant (staggerer)	6.62	2.41	1.45	2.00

[a] Data from Young *et al.* (1974).
[b] Data from McBride *et al.* (1976).

granule cells, then a question can be raised regarding the physiological significance of the excitatory action exerted by aspartate on cerebellar neurons. Aspartate may be the transmitter released by some of the afferent neurons which terminate within the cerebellum, or it may serve some nonsynaptic excitatory function. Another possibility is that aspartate may have some capacity to activate receptors normally activated only by glutamate.

Within the hippocampus glutamate is selectively concentrated in layer CA3, which has led to the suggestion that glutamate is the transmitter released by granule cells originating in the dentate gyrus (Crawford and Connor, 1973). The results of distribution studies on the olfactory bulb and olfactory cortex before and after denervation, suggest that both glutamate and aspartate are somewhat concentrated in the mitral and tufted cells whose fibers comprise the lateral olfactory tract (Harvey *et al.*, 1975; L. T. Graham, Jr., unpublished observations). Other distribution studies on normal and denervated tissue suggest that glutamate may be selectively concentrated within certain neurons in several areas of the cerebral hemispheres (Johnson and Aprison, 1971; Reifferstein and Neal, 1974).

2.2.2.2. Subcellular Distribution Studies and the Question of the Transmitter Pool. If glutamate and aspartate are synaptic transmitters, then both must be present in the nerve terminals which release them, and the concentration must be adequate to meet the needs required for this function. If these amino acids are released by exocytosis, which is generally regarded as the universal mechanism for transmitter release, then they should be present in synaptic vesicles in physiologically active amounts. Subcellular fractionation studies have provided no indication that either amino acid is concentrated in nerve terminals (synaptosomes) or in synaptic vesicles (Mangan and Whitaker, 1966; Rassin, 1972). Unfortunately, the low Na^+ medium required for subcellular fractionation studies causes a rapid efflux of these amino acids from intracellular compartments (Shank and Aprison, 1977). Therefore the contents of glutamate and aspartate in isolated synaptosomes and synaptic vesicles are probably very much lower than the corresponding values *in vivo*. Thus, the argument that these amino acids cannot be transmitters because of their low contents in synaptosomes and isolated synaptic vesicles is not tenable.

Because the contents of glutamate and aspartate in neural tissues are generally high, it is possible that these amino acids may not have to be more concentrated in nerve terminals and synaptic vesicles than in other subcellular areas of neurons in order to function as transmitters. Based on the average content of glutamate and aspartate in CNS tissues, and on the results of distribution studies, the average intracellular concentration of glutamate in "glutamatergic" neurons is probably at least 10–20 mM, and that of aspartate in "aspartergic" neurons is probably at least 5–20 mM. Assuming that glutamate and aspartate are maintained in synaptic vesicles at these concentrations, and that the diameter of these vesicles is 500 Å, the calculated number of molecules in individual vesicles would be 300–600 for glutamate and 150–600 for aspartate. The number of molecules present in a single quantum of transmitter released from nerve terminals in the CNS is not known, but theoretically several hundred molecules are sufficient to activate a number of receptors in the subsynaptic membrane. Also, if it is assumed that the synaptic cleft is 200 Å wide, then the concentration of the transmitter subsequent to release should be diluted only tenfold or less as the molecules move across the cleft to the nearest point of the postsynaptic membrane. If the concentration within the vesicles is 10 mM, the concentration at receptors adjacent to the point of release should reach 1 mM, which is probably sufficient to saturate receptors in this area. This reasoning suggests that the concentration within vesicles must be at least nearly equal to the average intracellular concentration, but need not be much, if any, higher than that in the cytosol. If some neurons release both glutamate and aspartate, the total transmitter activity in these neurons would be represented by the total amount of the two amino acids in the vesicles. As a comparison to the values just calculated, Whitaker and his colleagues have calculated that synaptic vesicles from cholinergic neurons in the guinea pig brain contain 1000–2000 molecules of acetylcholine (Nagy *et al.*, 1976).

The transmitter pool of each amino acid supposedly must be composed of those molecules in nerve terminals which are either immediately or readily available for release. Presumably this includes those molecules within synaptic vesicles and those in the cytosol and possibly mitochondria of the nerve terminals. This probably represents a relatively small percentage of the total content of each amino acid in the CNS or even within the particular neurons using them as transmitters. There is considerable interest in the metabolic nature of the transmitter pool and how it differs metabolically from other tissue pools. It has been known for many years that glutamate and aspartate are metabolically compartmented (Berl and Clarke, 1969) and a relationship between this metabolic compartmentation and the presumed transmitter function of these amino acids is becoming increasingly evident (see Section 6).

2.2.2.3. Evoked Release from CNS Tissue Preparations. One of the fundamental criteria needed to establish a substance as an actual transmitter is an unequivocal demonstration that the substance is released in physiologically active amounts from nerve terminals during neural excitation. The importance of this criterion has prompted numerous studies on the release of these amino acids from various neural preparations. Although the results of nearly all of these studies are consistent with a transmitter function for glutamate and aspartate, few of them have provided compelling evidence that these amino acids are released from specific types of nerve terminals during physiological stimulation. Perhaps the most significant of all the release studies to date have been those which have shown that the release of glutamate and aspartate from the surface of the cerebral cortex is enhanced during periods of behavioral arousal, and that the release of GABA is enhanced during periods of reduced behavioral activity (Jasper *et al.*, 1965; Jasper and Koyama, 1969).

In recent years most release studies have been performed with tissue slices or synaptosomal preparations in which the tissue was stimulated by a depolarizing electrical field, or by high concentrations (30–80 mM) of K^+. Of the many release studies on tissue preparations *in vitro*, some of the most valuable have been those carried out by Bradford and his colleagues who have studied the release of endogenous glutamate and aspartate from synaptosomal beds derived from various regions of the CNS. In these studies the release was significantly increased by high K^+ and by depolarizing electrical current, and this evoked release was Ca^{2+}- dependent (DeBelleroche and Bradford, 1972; Osborne *et al.*, 1973; Osborne and Bradford, 1975). Unfortunately a dependency on extracellular Ca^{2+} does not provide unequivocal evidence that the release of these amino acids is due to neurosecretion from nerve terminals because a Ca^{2+}-dependent release from glia cells can also occur (Minchin and Iversen, 1974).

In order to provide more convincing evidence that these amino acids are released from terminals of specific types of neurons, a greater emphasis must be placed on studies in which discrete neuronal pathways are stimulated by truly physiological means. Recently Yamamoto and Matsui (1976) and Bradford and Richards (1976) have reported studies in which they isolated the lateral olfactory tract together with a slice of the olfactory cortex of guinea pigs. Stimulation of the olfactory tract induced a selective increase in the release of glutamate from the olfactory cortex. These observations provide further evidence that glutamate is the neurotransmitter released by afferent olfactory tract fibers, but do not support the possibility that aspartate may also be released from these excitatory neurons.

2.2.2.4. Initial and Steady State Uptake Studies. Except for the brief instant immediately following release, the concentration of a transmitter in the synaptic cleft and other extracellular spaces must be maintained at levels below that which affects neuronal activity. Such subactive extracellular concentrations of glutamate and aspartate are probably similar to the concentrations in CSF, which range between 10^{-6} and 10^{-5} M (Gjessing *et al.*, 1972).

There is no experimental evidence that glutamate or aspartate can be metabolized by any extracellular enzyme. Therefore it has been presumed that transport of these amino acids out of the extracellular fluid is the mechanism by which they are inactivated subsequent to release and by which they are maintained at very low extracellular levels. The results of various types of transport studies provide considerable support for this concept. An energy-requiring, Na^+-dependent transport of glutamate and aspartate by a common carrier system was studied by Tsukada *et al.* (1963) and by Lajtha and his colleagues (see Lajtha, 1968). Hammerschlag *et al.* (1971; see also Hammerschlag and Weinreich, 1972) studied the transport of glutamate and aspartate into tissue slices of the frog spinal cord under initial uptake conditions and found that these amino acids are taken up by a common Na^+-dependent "high-affinity" ($K_m \sim 2$–5×10^{-5} M) transport system, and by another carrier with a lower affinity ($K_m \sim 2 \times 10^{-4}M$). Snyder and his colleagues (1973) subsequently applied initial uptake procedures to study the transport of glutamate and aspartate by synaptosomal preparations. These latter investigators have placed great emphasis on the concept that the observed high-affinity uptake into nerve terminals represents the principal means of inactivation. In this regard it should be mentioned that the transmitter concentration within the synaptic cleft may reach levels of about 1 mM (~ 50 times the K_m of the high-affinity carrier) during periods of peak transmitter release. Therefore, *both* the high- and low-affinity carriers could be instrumental in transmitter inactivation. Since the low-affinity carrier possesses a high transport capacity (high V_{max}), these carriers may be very important during periods of sustained transmitter release.

Other studies have demonstrated that glia cells also possess a high-affinity uptake system for glutamate and aspartate (Henn *et al.*, 1974). These studies provide strong support for the concept that glia cells function in the inactivation of these amino acids, and in maintaining their extracellular concentrations at subactive levels.

A weakness of initial uptake studies is that they do not demonstrate that an actual net uptake into the cells occurs. This is a problem because an exchange of amino acid molecules across the membrane could account for the initial uptake data, and this exchange process would be useless for transmitter inactivation (Raiteri *et al.*, 1975).

A vigorous net uptake of glutamate by an isolated toad brain preparation has been reported. In these net uptake studies nearly 99% of the glutamate initially present in the medium was taken up by the tissue, and a net uptake continued until the extracellular concentration was reduced to a steady state value of less than 2×10^{-6} M (Figure 2). It is evident from these net uptake studies that CNS tissues are able to remove glutamate rapidly from the extracellular fluid, and that this uptake capacity is sufficient to maintain the extracellular concentration at a level far below that exhibiting excitatory activity.

FIGURE 2. Time course of change in the extracellular concentration of glutamate during incubation of isolated toad brains in a Ringer-like medium. Each toad brain (~0.05 g wet weight) was incubated in 2 ml of medium containing 0, 40, or 100 μM L-glutamate. Regardless of the initial concentration of glutamate in the medium, a steady state value between 1 and 2 μM was attained. The data are from Shank *et al.* (1973), Shank and Baxter (1975), and unpublished observations of R. P. Shank and M. H. Aprison. Each point is the mean ± SEM of three or four toad brains. Where no error bar is shown the SEM is less than the size of the symbol.

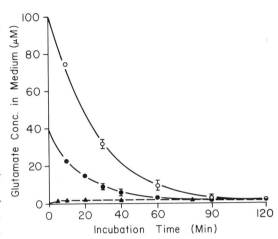

The studies which indicate that glutamate and aspartate are transported by the same carrier (Lajtha, 1968; Hammerschlag and Weinreich, 1972; Logan and Snyder, 1972; Balcar and Johnston, 1972; Roberts and Watkins, 1975) have interesting implications. If both amino acids are taken up by the same nerve terminals, then this would seem to support the concept that both are released from the same neurons. There is compelling evidence that both glutamate and aspartate are released by the excitatory motor neurons innervating muscle fibers in the limbs of crustacea (Kravitz *et al.,* 1970; Shank *et al.,* 1975; Shank and Freeman, 1975); however, the possibility that this occurs in the vertebrate CNS is less certain. Distribution studies support the concept that some neurons may utilize both amino acids for transmitter purposes, but available evidence indicates that certain others may use only one of the two (see Section 2.2.2.1).

2.2.2.5. *Studies on the Isolation and Characterization of the Synaptic Receptors.* Attempts to isolate and characterize the synaptic receptors activated by glutamate and aspartate are underway in several laboratories. Published reports to date have been limited to the regional distribution (Roberts, 1974*b*; Simon *et al.,* 1976) and partial purification of cellular components (proteins, glycoproteins, or lipoproteins) which have a high binding capacity for labeled glutamate, aspartate, or their analogues (Michaelis, 1975; De Robertis and Fiszer DePlazas, 1976*a,b*). A comparison of the apparent affinity between glutamate and its binding substance, and the effects of glutamate analogues indicates that these investigators are not all studying the same binding substance, although this is difficult to evaluate because of differences in their experimental techniques. Michaelis (1975) and Simon *et al* (1976) may have studied the same substance since both report values of approximately 10^{-6} *M* for the concentration at which the binding capacity is half-saturated, and in both studies D-glutamate had almost no capacity to compete with L-glutamate for the binding sites. If this binding capacity is due to synaptic receptors, these observations appear to be inconsistent with the physiological studies which show that D-glutamate is a relatively potent excitatory substance, and that the concentration of L-glutamate necessary for an apparent excitatory effect is approximately 10^{-4} *M*. Also, since the concentration of glutamate in cerebrospinal fluid (CSF) is between 10^{-6} and 10^{-5} *M*, it would seem unlikely that the synaptic receptors would be half-saturated at 10^{-6} *M*.

2.2.3. Pharmacological Studies

Many analogues of L-glutamate and L-aspartate possess potent neuroexcitatory properties (Curtis and Watkins, 1960). These substances are presumably agonists of glutamate and aspartate, and based on their excitatory activity, several of them appear to have a greater affinity for the transmitter receptors than do the putative transmitters (Johnston *et al.*, 1974).

The search for substances which can selectively block the action of glutamate and aspartate has revealed some analogues of glutamate with some ability to antagonize this amino acid selectively. Among these substances are certain esters and diesters of glutamate (Haldeman *et al.*, 1972). The nature of the antagonistic action of L-glutamate diethyl ester on L-glutamate-induced, and neurally evoked excitation in the thalamus (Haldeman and McLennen, 1972) and the striatum (Spencer, 1976) of the rat provides pharmacological evidence that glutamate is a transmitter in these areas of the CNS. However, the antagonistic activity of these compounds is weak and inconsistent (Curtis *et al.*, 1972; Altmann *et al.*, 1976). Potent, selective, and pure (no agonistic activity) antagonists of glutamate and aspartate are apparently yet to be found. It is interesting that most neuroactive analogues of glutamate and aspartate are agonistic in nature rather than antagonistic, and that agonists in general appear to have a greater affinity for the receptors than do the antagonists.

2.3. Possible Nonsynaptic Excitatory and Inhibitory Functions

The initial studies by Curtis and his colleagues (see Curtis and Watkins, 1960) suggested that glutamate and aspartate were universal neuroexcitatory agents, and at that time it seemed unlikely that synaptic neurotransmitters would act upon nearly all central neurons. This led to the concept that these amino acids were "nonspecific" excitatory agents, and that they might serve some generalized nonsynaptic excitatory function. No compelling evidence has yet been reported in support of such a function in the vertebrate CNS, and in recent years the "universality" of the excitatory action of glutamate and aspartate has been used as evidence that these amino acids are released from excitatory neurons prevalent in all major areas of the CNS (see review by Curtis and Johnston, 1974, for references). However, regarding a possible nonsynaptic function, it is of interest that glutamate is released from peripheral nerve and desheathed axons during neuroexcitation (Wheeler *et al.,* 1966; DeFeudis, 1971; Roberts, 1974*a*; Weinreich and Hammerschlag, 1975).

Recent studies have demonstrated that glutamate can alter the excitability of muscle cells in some arthropods by acting upon nonsynaptic regions of the membrane (Lea and Usherwood, 1972; Cull-Candy, 1976). Also, there is some evidence that glutamate and aspartate can enhance neurotransmitter release at the neuromuscular junction of some arthropods (Dowson and Usherwood, 1972). Such studies have led to the formulation of a concept which suggests that glutamate serves three types of neurophysiological functions: (1) the primary role as a synaptic transmitter, (2) a secondary role concerned with the regulation of nerve cell excitability via the activation of receptors present in nonsynaptic components of the membrane, and (3) a tertiary role concerned with the modulation of transmitter release (Freeman, 1976).

3. GLUTAMATE AND ASPARTATE AS CONSTITUENTS OF PROTEIN

Studies on the content of glutamate and aspartate in hydrolysates of protein from neural tissues indicate that these amino acids together with their amide derivatives, glutamine and asparagine, account for approximately 10–30% of the total amino acid residues, depending on the regional and cellular origin of the tissue (Minard and Richter, 1968; Wolfgram and Kotorii, 1968*a,b*; Mahler and Cotman, 1970; Wherrett and Tower, 1971). Studies by Tower and Wherrett (1971) on the content of glutamate and aspartate in proteins from various subcellular fractions demonstrated that these amino acids are much more prevalent in certain membrane-bound proteins than in the soluble proteins in the cytosol. The physiological significance of the high amount of these acidic amino acid moieties in these membrane proteins is not clear; however, the free carboxyl groups can account for the net negative charge exhibited by these proteins (Tower and

Wherrett, 1971). Some negatively charged membrane proteins are known to serve as carriers responsible for transporting specific substances across cell membranes (Tower and Wherrett, 1971).

At least two of the currently known "brain- specific" proteins contain a high degree of glutamyl and aspartyl moieties; these brain-specific proteins are the acidic proteins S-100 and 14-3-2, which were isolated and characterized by Moore and his colleagues (Moore, 1965, 1975). Although the physiological roles of these proteins are of considerable interest, the functions of these proteins have yet to be elucidated.

Wherrett and Tower (1971) reported that about half (45%) of the glutamyl and aspartyl moieties in cerebral proteins are in the amide rather than free carboxyl form. These investigators also reported that when cat cerebral tissue was prepared for incubation as tissue slices, approximately 16% of the glutaminyl moieties were deaminated *in situ*. This deamidation process occurred within a few minutes after the blood supply to the brain was terminated, and the amount of free ammonia formed was remarkably constant. The lability of these amide groups suggests that some glutaminyl moieties within certain proteins may be deamidated during normal metabolic activity *in vivo*. This process could serve an important physiological role by regulating the activity of certain transport proteins. If this deamidation does occur *in vivo,* then it is obvious that a corresponding amidation process must also occur in order to return the protein carboxyl groups to the amide form. Unfortunately, despite several attempts to demonstrate the existence of such a specific amidation process, no one has yet provided convincing evidence in support of this concept (Wherrett and Tower, 1971).

It is generally accepted that glutamate and glutamine, as well as aspartate and asparagine, are each incorporated into newly synthesized proteins by specific aminoacyl-tRNA synthetases and unique species of tRNA (Peterkofsky, 1973), although this aspect of protein synthesis by neural tissues has not been studied extensively. In some tissues it has been demonstrated that some transformation of the glutamyl or glutaminyl group occurs either after being bound to the tRNA or after being incorporated into a protein molecule (Peterkofsky, 1973). Evidence that the glutamyl and glutaminyl moieties can be transformed in CNS tissues subsequent to being linked to tRNA has been reported (Murthy and Roux, 1974); however, the significance of this process is not known. An important reaction involving the glutaminyl moiety is one by which certain proteins are cross-linked via the action of various transglutaminase enzymes. In this reaction the glutaminyl moiety is deamidated, then covalently linked to the ϵ-amino nitrogen of a lysyl group in another protein. Transglutaminase activity is known to be present in neural tissues (Wajda, 1970); however, the physiological significance of this enzymatic activity is not clear.

4. THE ROLE IN THE REGULATION AND MAINTENANCE OF INTRACELLULAR OSMOTIC AND IONIC BALANCE

In many animal tissues, a number of amino acids make a significant contribution to the total intracellular osmotic and ionic activities (Awapara, 1962; Potts and Parry, 1964; Florkin and Schoffeniels, 1965; Schoffeniels and Gilles, 1970; Drainville and Gagnon, 1972). In neural tissues, glutamate and aspartate are among the most prevalent osmotically active organic substances (Tallan, 1962). The content of these amino acids is especially high in nerve cells of many seawater invertebrates whose body fluids have high osmotic activities (Silber and Schmitt, 1940) (see Table 7).

In many species of vertebrates and invertebrates, the osmotic activity of the extracellular fluids changes in response to fluctuations in the osmolarity of the aquatic environment. In these osmoconforming animals, the neurons and certain other cells actively respond to the osmotic changes so that a relatively constant cell volume is maintained (Lang and Gainer, 1969; Pierce and Greenberg, 1973; Schmidt-Nielsen, 1975). Even in animals which normally maintain a relatively constant extracellular osmolarity, neurons can actively respond to changes in the osmotic activity of their extracellular environment (Fishman, 1974; Thurston *et al.*, 1975). As part of this active response, the tissue contents of several amino acids are altered. In nerve tissues, alterations in the levels of glutamate and aspartate are especially prominent (Shank and Baxter, 1973), whereas in muscle tissues, the contents of certain neutral amino acids (glycine, alanine, proline, and taurine) can also be altered considerably (Kittridge *et al.*, 1962; Gordon, 1965; Virkar and Webb, 1970).

Because glutamate and aspartate are negatively charged at physiological pH, they participate in the maintenance of the ionic balance of intracellular fluids as well as the osmotic balance. Since fewer organic substances can contribute to the maintenance of ionic balance rather than osmotic balance, the degree to which glutamate and aspartate participate in these two physiological processes may be most specifically related to the need for impermeant intracellular anions to balance K^+ (Burton, 1973). These amino acids may be ideal for this function since their concentrations can be readily controlled by both enzymes and transport systems, and their permeability through cell membranes is probably much less than that of Cl^- or keto acids.

In neural tissues glutamate and aspartate usually make a greater relative contribution to the ionic and osmotic activity in those animals which have high extracellular osmolarities (e.g., seawater crustacea), and

TABLE 7.   Content of Glutamate and Aspartate in Neural Tissues of Some Marine
Invertebrates

Species and tissue	Glutamate	Aspartate	Reference
	(μmol/g wet tissue)[a]		
Lobster (*Homarus americanus*)			
Walking limb			
Whole nerve	25	112	Lewis, 1952
Whole nerve	10	82	Marks *et al.*, 1970
Excitatory axon	42	132	McBride *et al.*, 1974
Inhibitory axon	32	150	McBride *et al.*, 1974
Sensory nerve	9	68	McBride *et al.*, 1974
CNS ganglia	12–15	18–36	Aprison *et al.*, 1973
CNS connectives	9–15	30–49	Aprison *et al.*, 1973
CNS giant axons	7–24	71–184	McBride *et al.*, 1975
Crab			
Cancer magister			
Peripheral nerves			
Whole nerve	22	116	Sorenson, 1973
Excitatory axons	53	196	Sorenson, 1973
Inhibitory axons	47	168	Sorenson, 1973
Carcinus maenas			
Peripheral nerve	35	138	Lewis, 1952
	36	199	Evans, 1973
	10	52	Marks *et al.*, 1970
CNS ganglia	18–19	33–40	Evans, 1973
CNS connective	19	52	Evans, 1973
Eriocheir sinensis			
Peripheral nerve	33	121	Schoffeniels, 1964
Maia squinado			
Peripheral Nerve	31	111	Schoffeniels, 1970
Cuttlefish			
Axon	39	82	Lewis, 1952
Squid			
Loligo pealii			
Giant axon	14	63	Deffner, 1961
Dosidicus gigas			
Giant axon	28	111	Deffner, 1961
Octopus (*Eledone cirrhosa*)			
Brain			
Optic lobe	11	8	Cory and Rose, 1969
Vertical lobe	10	8	Cory and Rose, 1969
Crayfish (*Orconectes immunis*)[b]			
Ventral nerve cord	4.3–5.0	6.5–7.2	Lin and Cohen, 1973
Aplysia californica			
Nerve cell somas	4–12	—	Borys *et al.*, 1973

[a] Data represent the free (uncombined) glutamate and aspartate. In some cases the data were reported as millimoles per liter of axoplasm or millimolar.
[b] This is the only freshwater species represented.

there is apparently no established reason for this. However, the relative contribution these amino acids make may depend partly on the contribution of protein to the intracellular pool of anions. If the total net negative charge on intracellular proteins is similar in all animals regardless of the osmotic strength of their body fluids, then the relative contribution of glutamate and aspartate to the total ionic activity would be expected to be greater in animals whose fluids have high osmolarities and ionic activities.

5.   THE ROLES OF GLUTAMATE AND ASPARTATE IN NITROGEN METABOLISM

Nitrogen metabolism in neural tissues is very dynamic. Most of this dynamic activity can be attributed to the enzymes which catalyze reactions involving glutamate and its related metabolites. The importance of glutamate in nitrogen metabolism was recognized many years ago (Weil-Malherbe, 1950), and in more recent years the importance of aspartate has also been recognized (Van den Berg, 1970; Buniatian, 1970). Yet at the present time, we are far from having a complete understanding of the biochemical processes by which these amino acids are utilized for the regulation of ammonia and various other nitrogen-containing compounds.

5.1.   The Regulation of Free Ammonia

Ammonium ions at concentrations on the order of 1.0 mM exert a toxic effect on nerve cells (Weil-Malherbe, 1950). The nature of this toxic effect is not established but it may be a multifactorial process. The toxic effect may be due to a direct depolarization of the cell membrane, inhibition of a Cl^- pump or certain other transport systems (Lux et al., 1970), inhibition of certain enzymes, or all of these. Since NH_4^+ is formed in neural tissues as a product in the metabolism of a number of compounds, e.g., the monoamine neurotransmitters, there must be a mechanism for removing this ion and maintaining its concentration at subtoxic levels. The principal mechanism appears to be the formation of glutamine through the action of glutamine synthetase (Berl and Clarke, 1969; Van Den Berg, 1970). Much of the glutamine formed is presumably released into the bloodstream, although some of it is probably converted back into glutamate and NH_4^+ in a tissue compartment (e.g., nerve terminals) different from that in which glutamine is synthesized (see Section 6). There can be little doubt that glutamine does serve as the principal end product of nitrogen metabolism in the CNS of vertebrates (Van den Berg et al., 1976).

Some NH_4^+ is removed by being coupled to α-ketoglutarate through the action of glutamate dehydrogenase. Hence glutamate serves as both a precursor and a product in the reactions responsible for removing NH_4^+ and regulating the intracellular concentrations of this substance.

5.2. Glutamate and α-Ketoglutarate as an Amino Donor–Acceptor System

The metabolism of aspartate, alanine, GABA, and serine is coupled to glutamate because the transaminase enzymes involved in either the synthesis or degradation of these amino acids specifically require glutamate as an amino donor or acceptor. The activity of aspartate transaminase is particularly high in the CNS of vertebrates, and this enzyme is present in both mitochondria and the cytosol (Van den Berg, 1970). The significance of this high activity is not fully known.

5.3. The Role of Aspartate in the Purine Nucleotide Cycle

The purine nucleotide cycle is known to be operative in the CNS of mammals (Buniatian, 1970; Schultz and Lowenstein, 1976), although the metabolic significance of the cycle in nerve tissues is not yet clear. Since aspartate serves as the amino donor for the regeneration of AMP, this amino acid is necessary for the operation of the cycle. The extent to which the cycle is operative *in vivo* is not known, but it has been suggested that this cycle can account for much of the free ammonia formed in the brain postmortem (Schultz and Lowenstein, 1976). The metabolic basis for the rapid formation of NH^+_4 in the CNS after death has been the object of a number of investigations, yet this curious phenomenon still remains somewhat of an enigma (Weil-Malherbe, 1975).

5.4. Synthesis of Urea in Nerve Tissues

The enzymes carbamylphosphate synthetase and ornithine citrulline transcarbamylase, which catalyze the first two steps in the synthesis of urea, are apparently not present in the CNS of vertebrates (Jones *et al.*, 1961). However, the enzymes which catalyze the formation of arginine and fumarate from citrulline and aspartate are active, as is the enzyme which catalyzes the synthesis of urea and ornithine from arginine (Ratner *et al.*, 1960; Sadasivudu and Hanumantharao, 1974). Therefore, providing there is a net uptake of citrulline from the blood into the CNS, there should be some urea formed in neural tissues. However, the extent to which this may occur is not yet established. It is possible that the enzymes of the urea cycle which are present in CNS tissues may serve a purpose other than just the synthesis of urea (Sadasivudu and Hanumantharao, 1974).

6. THE INVOLVEMENT OF GLUTAMATE AND ASPARTATE IN ENERGY METABOLISM

There have been many studies regarding the involvement of glutamate in cerebral metabolism since the early studies of Quastel and Wheatley (1932) which showed that L-glutamate could serve as a substrate for respiration in brain slices. It is now clear that neither glutamate nor aspartate readily crosses the blood–brain barrier and therefore cannot serve as significant sources of carbon for oxidative metabolism (Oldendorf, 1971). However, metabolic studies have shown that a high percentage of the carbon units metabolized via the tricarboxylic cycle are incorporated into glutamate and aspartate before being oxidized to CO_2 (Berl and Clarke, 1969; Van den Berg, 1970). Thus in a sense glutamate and aspartate serve as intermediates in energy metabolism in neural tissues. Although the reason for this is not fully understood, it probably reflects, at least in part, the operation of the malate–aspartate shuttle (Figure 3). This shuttle functions as a means of transporting hydrogen equivalents from the cytosol into mitochondria; its existence in brain tissue has recently been demonstrated (Brand and Chappel, 1974).

An outgrowth of the studies on glutamate metabolism has been the concept of metabolic compartmentation in the CNS tissues. This concept developed out of experiments which showed that after administration of [14C] glutamate, the specific radioactivity of glutamine in the CNS was considerably higher than that of glutamate even after very short time periods (Lajtha et al., 1959; Berl et al., 1961). The metabolic compartmentation of glutamate has been studied extensively, and the subject has been thoroughly reviewed in recent years (Berl and Clarke, 1969; Balázs and Cremer, 1972; Berl et al., 1976).

The current concept of the compartmentation of glutamate in the CNS stipulates that there are two principal compartments or pools of glutamate, and that each of these is composed of additional subcompartments (Van den Berg et al., 1976). In one compartment glutamate is derived extensively from glucose. This compartment apparently contains most of the total tissue pool of glutamate, and therefore has been designated as the "large" compartment. This is the compartment most closely associated with energy metabolism, and is thought to be located in neurons, where energy metabolism is so active. The second compartment is designated the "small" compartment and is the compartment in which glutamate is metabolized extensively to glutamine. This compartment is thought to be located in glia cells.

A recent development in the subject of metabolic compartmentation is that there is a net flow of glutamate (and GABA) from the large compartment to the small one, and that this is compensated by a net flow of glutamine in the reverse direction (Dzubow and Garfinkel, 1970; Van den Berg *et al.*, 1976). It has been proposed that the flux of glutamate and GABA represents the release of these amino acids from nerve terminals and subsequent uptake into glia cells (Quastel, 1974; Van den Berg *et al.*, 1976). The reverse flow of glutamine is attributed to a net synthesis of this amino acid either directly or indirectly from glutamate and GABA within the glia cells; this is followed by a release of this glutamine into the extracellular fluid, whereupon some of it is taken up by nerve terminals, and is utilized as a metabolic precursor for the restoration of the transmitter pools of glutamate and GABA (Figure 4). Although this cyclic process is still largely hypothetical there is considerable experimental evidence that supports it (Benjamin and Quastel, 1972, 1974; Van den Berg *et al.*, 1976; Bradford and Ward, 1976; Shank and Aprison, 1977).

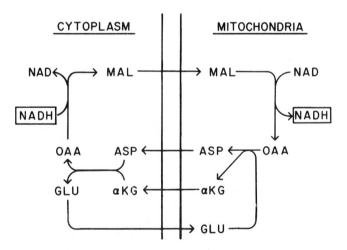

FIGURE 3. A diagrammatic depiction of the malate–aspartate shuttle. The net effect of the shuttle is to mediate the reduction of NAD inside the mitochondria by NADH in the cytosol. Although it is not evident from this diagram, the movement of aspartate out of the mitochondria is coupled to the movement of glutamate in the reverse direction. The efflux of α-ketoglutarate is also coupled to the influx of malate (Brand and Chappel, 1974).

FIGURE 4. A model depicting the flow of glutamate and GABA from nerve terminals to glia cells, and the reverse flow of glutamine from glia cells to nerve terminals. It should be emphasized that this model does not imply a specific stoichiometric relationship between the loss of glutamate and GABA from nerve terminals and the uptake of glutamine. This model is based on a similar one by Van den Berg *et al.* (1976). PSM means postsynaptic membrane.

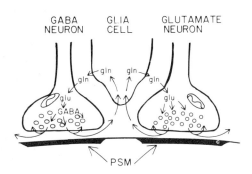

7. COMPOUNDS OF NEUROCHEMICAL INTEREST DERIVED FROM GLUTAMATE AND ASPARTATE

The high content of GABA and *N*-acetylaspartate in the vertebrate CNS is well known to be a distinctive characteristic of this tissue, and the synthesis of these compounds from glutamate and aspartate, respectively, is well established. Less well known are several other substances derived from glutamate and aspartate, most of which are small peptides.

7.1. γ-Aminobutyrate

GABA is formed as the α-decarboxylation product of glutamate by the action of the enzyme L-glutamate 1-carboxy-lyase (EC 4.1.1.15) which is more commonly referred to as glutamate decarboxylase. GABA is now generally accepted as being one of the principal inhibitory neurotransmitters in the vertebrate CNS. In addition there is evidence that GABA also serves other functions, such as an activator of protein synthesis. These and other aspects of GABA have been reviewed in a chapter by Baxter (1970) and in two books devoted entirely to GABA (Roberts *et al.*, 1960, 1976).

7.2. *N*-Acetylaspartate

N-Acetylaspartate (NAA) is synthesized from aspartate and acetyl coenzyme A (acetyl-CoA). Although metabolic studies indicate that this substance is formed at a relatively slow rate, it is one of the most abundant organic compounds in the CNS of mammals (Jacobson, 1959; D'Adamo and Yatsu, 1966; Fleming and Lowry, 1966).

Because NAA carries a net charge of -2, it serves as one of the major intracellular organic anions. McIntosh and Cooper (1965) have described an enzyme which is capable of reversibly converting NAA from its dicarboxylic acid form into a monocarboxylic acid form. This enzyme, which is present in CNS tissues, catalyzes the following internal cyclization process:

NAA   (?)   (?)

The existence of this enzyme suggests that NAA may serve a regulatory role in the maintenance of the intracellular ionic state of neurons.

NAA together with glutamate and aspartate probably comprises most of the total pool of metabolically active organic anions in nerve cells. Although it has yet to be conclusively demonstrated, glutamate and aspartate are probably more highly concentrated in excitatory neurons (at least those that utilize glutamate and aspartate as transmitters) than in inhibitory neurons. This suggests that NAA, which exhibits little or no excitatory activity, may be more concentrated in inhibitory neurons than in excitatory neurons. Unfortunately, the distribution of NAA has not been studied sufficiently to permit any conclusions regarding this possibility.

The results of other studies indicate that NAA may serve additional roles. Clarke *et al.* (1975) have reported that NAA can stimulate the synthesis of protein in nerve tissues. Metabolic studies have demonstrated that NAA is selectively utilized for the synthesis of fatty acids in young animals, and in this way it may serve a role in myelinogenesis (D'Adamo and Yatsu, 1966).

7.3.   Peptides Derived from Glutamate and Aspartate

A number of di- and tripeptides that contain glutamate and/or aspartate have been isolated from extracts of mammalian CNS tissues. Except for glutathione, which is prevalent in most animal tissues, and N-acetylaspartylglutamic acid (NAAGA), these peptides are present in very small amounts (Sano *et al.,* 1966; Reichelt and Fonnum, 1969; Reichelt, 1970).

Because NAAGA carries a net charge of -3, it contributes to the intracellular pool of anions. However, the content of this peptide is not sufficient for it to serve as a major intracellular organic anion (Reichelt and Fonnum, 1969).

Several of the peptides are γ-glutamyl dipeptides composed of glutamate and any one of several other amino acids (Reichelt, 1970). The presence of these peptides in nerve tissues may reflect the existence of the γ-glutamyl cycle in the CNS (see the following section).

8.   THE POSSIBLE ROLE OF GLUTAMATE IN AMINO ACID TRANSPORT

The enzymes of the γ-glutamyl cycle (Figure 5) are known to be present in the CNS of mammals, and there is considerable evidence that this cyclic metabolic process functions in the transport of amino acids across cell membranes (Meister, 1973, 1975). In the transport model proposed by Meister (1973), the membrane-bound enzyme γ-glutamyl trans-

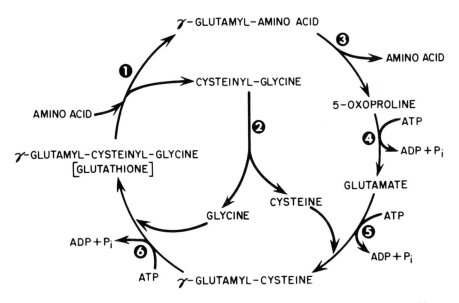

FIGURE 5. The γ-glutamyl cycle. The enzymes of the cycle are (1) γ-glutamyl transpeptidase; (2) cysteinyl glycinase; (3) γ-glutamyl cyclotransferase; (4) 5-oxoprolinase; (5) γ-glutamyl-cysteine synthetase; and (6) glutathione synthetase. Reproduced from Meister (1975) with permission.

peptidase catalyzes the transfer of the γ-glutamyl moiety of glutathione to an amino acid which is to be transported across the membrane, then the γ-glutamyl–amino acid complex migrates into the cell, whereupon the dipeptide is hydrolyzed by γ-glutamyl cyclotransferase to glutamate and the transported amino acid. According to this hypothesis glutamate functions as a transport carrier molecule.

9. FUTURE DIRECTIONS

Up until the mid-1960s most research on glutamate and aspartate was concerned with their roles in nitrogen and energy metabolism, and the metabolic compartmentation phenomenon. Since then interest in the putative neurotransmitter function has intensified greatly and now dominates the research conducted on these amino acids. This trend will no doubt continue in the coming years and we can anticipate that continued emphasis will be placed on (1) identifying those neurons which utilize glutamate and aspartate as transmitters, (2) finding selective and potent blockers of the excitatory action and the uptake (inactivation) of these amino acids, and (3) isolating and characterizing their synaptic receptors.

Although the controversy surrounding glutamate and aspartate, and the physiological significance of their excitatory activity, has declined in recent years, the possibility that the role of these amino acids in neuroexcitation transcends their putative neurotransmitter function must not be ignored in future studies. Another consideration that should be emphasized more in the coming years is the relationship between the metabolism of these amino acids and their role as neuroexcitatory agents. Recent observations by Van Gelder and Courtois (1972) are of interest in this regard.

The potential neurotoxicity of glutamate is now well recognized (Van Harreveld and Fifkova, 1970; Olney *et al.*, 1974; Reif-Lehrer, 1976). However, the possibility that biochemical defects involving these amino acids may be the cause of certain neurological and mental disorders has not been studied extensively. One report has appeared which indicates that the levels of glutamate and aspartate in blood plasma are significantly elevated in certain mentally retarded children (Hirsch *et al.*, 1969). If the concentrations of these two amino acids are also abnormally high in the extracellular fluids within the CNS, this condition could alter the excitability of neurons and be the causative factor of the mental retardation in these children.

In conclusion it seems reasonable to expect that in the coming years even more neuroscientists, especially those in the pharmacological and clinical disciplines, will develop an interest in glutamate and aspartate. Therefore, in the future, our knowledge of the roles of these amino acids should continue to advance at a rapid pace.

10. REFERENCES

Agrawal, H. C., Davis, J. M., and Himwich, W. A., 1968, Developmental changes in mouse brain: Weight, water content and free amino acids, *J. Neurochem.* **15**:917–923.

Altmann, H., Ten Bruggencate, G., Pickelmann, P., and Steinberg, R., 1976, Effects of glutamate, aspartate, and two presumed antagonists on feline rubrospinal neurones, *Pflugers Arch.* **364**:249–255.

Anwyl, R., and Usherwood, P. N. R., 1974, Voltage clamp studies of a glutamate synapse, *Nature* **252**:591–593.

Aprison, M. H., and Werman, R., 1965, The distribution of glycine in cat spinal cord and roots, *Life Sci.* **4**:2075–2083.

Aprison, M. H., and Werman, R., 1968, A combined neurochemical and neurophysiological approach to identification of central nervous system transmitters, in: *Neurosciences Research* (S. Ehrenpreis and O. S. Solnitzky, eds.), Vol. 1, pp. 143–174, Academic Press, New York.

Aprison, M. H., McBride, W. J., and Freeman, A. R., 1973, The distribution of several amino acids in specific ganglia and nerve bundles of the lobster, *J. Neurochem.* **21**:87–95.

Awapara, J., 1962, Free amino acids in invertebrates: A comparative study of their distribution and metabolism, in: *Amino Acid Pools* (J. T. Holden, ed.), pp. 158–175, Elsevier, Amsterdam.

Badger, T. M., and Tumbleson, M. E., 1975, Postnatal changes in free amino acid, DNA, RNA and protein concentrations of miniature swine brain, *J. Neurochem.* **24**:361–366.

Balázs, R., and Cremer, J. E. (eds.), 1972, *Metabolic Compartmentation in the Brain*, Wiley, New York, 383 pp.

Balcar, V. J., and Johnston, G. A. R. 1972, The structural specificity of the high affinity uptake of L-glutamate and L-aspartate by rat brain slices, *J. Neurochem.* **19**:2657–2666.

Baxter, C. F., 1970, The nature of gamma-aminobutyric acid, in: *Handbook of Neurochemistry* (A. Lajtha, ed.), Vol. 3, pp.,289–353, Plenum Press, New York.

Benjamin, A. M., and Quastel, J. H., 1972, Locations of amino acids in brain slices from the rat, *Biochem. J.* **128**:631–646.

Benjamin, A. M., and Quastel, H. H., 1974, Fate of glutamate in the brain, *J. Neurochem.* **23**:457–464.

Berl, S., and Clarke, D. D., 1969, Metabolic compartmentation of glutamate in the CNS, in: *Handbook of Neurochemistry* (A. Lajtha, ed.), Vol. 1, pp. 447–472, Plenum Press, New York.

Berl, S., Lajtha, A., and Waelsch, H., 1961, Amino acid and protein metabolism. VI. Cerebral compartments of glutamic acid metabolism, *J. Neurochem.* **9**:168–197.

Berl, S., Clarke, D. D., and Schneider, D. (eds.), 1976, *Metabolic Compartmentation and Neurotransmission,* Plenum Press, New York.

Borys, H. K., Weinreich, D., and McCaman, R. E., 1973, Determination of glutamate and glutamine in individual neurons of *Aplysia californica, J. Neurochem.* **21**:1349–1351.

Bradford, H. F., and Richards, C. D., 1976, Specific release of endogenous glutamate from piriform cortex stimulated *in vitro, Brain Res.* **105**:168–172.

Bradford, H. F., and Ward, H. K., 1976, On glutaminase activity in mammalian synaptosomes, *Brain Res.* **110**:115–125.

Brand, M. D., and Chappel, J. B., 1974, Glutamate and aspartate transport in rat brain mitochondria, *Biochem. J.* **140**:205–210.

Buniatian, H. C., 1970, Deamination of nucleotides and the role of their deamino forms in ammonia formation from amino acids, in: *Handbook of Neurochemistry* (A. Lajtha, ed.), Vol. 3, pp. 399–413, Plenum Press, New York.

Burton, R. F., 1973, The significance of ionic concentrations in the internal media of animals, *Biol. Rev.* **48**:195–231.

Carew, T. J., Pinsker, H., Rubinson, K., and Kandel, E. R., 1974, Physiological and biochemical properties of neuromuscular transmission between identified motoneurons and gill muscle in *Aplysia, J. Neurophysiol.* **37**:1020–1039.

Clarke, D. D., Greenfield, S., Dicker, E., Tirri, L. J., and Ronan, E. J., 1975, A relationship of *N*-acetylaspartate biosynthesis to neuronal protein synthesis, *J. Neurochem.* **24**:479–486.

Colquhoun, D., 1973, The relation between classical and cooperative models for drug action, in: *Drug Receptors* (H. P. Rang, ed.), pp. 149–187, University Park Press, Baltimore.

Cory, H. T., and Rose, S. P. R., 1969, Glucose and amino acid metabolism in octopus optic and vertical lobes *in vitro, J. Neurochem.* **16**:979–988.

Coulson, R. A., and Hernandez, T., 1971, Catabolic effects of cycloheximide in the living reptile, *Comp. Biochem. Physiol.* **40B**:741–749.

Crawford, I. L., and Connor, J. D., 1973, Localization and release of glutamic acid in relation to the hippocampal mossy fiber pathway, *Nature* **244**:442–443.

Cull-Candy, S. G., 1976, Two types of extrajunctional L-glutamate receptors in locust muscle fibers, *J. Physiol.* **255**:449–464.

Cull-Candy, S. G., Donnellan, J. F., James, R. W., and Lunt, G. G., 1976, 2-Amino-4-phosphonobutyric acid as a glutamate antagonist on locust muscle, *Nature* **262**:408–409.

Curtis, D. R., and Crawford, J. M., 1969, Central synaptic transmission-microelectrode studies, *Annu. Rev. Pharmacol.* **9**:209–240.

Curtis, D. R., and Johnston, G. A. R., 1974, Amino acid transmitters in the mammalian central nervous system, *Ergebn. Physiol.* **69**:97–188.

Curtis, D. R., and Watkins, J. C., 1960, The excitation and depression of spinal neurones by structurally related amino acids, *J. Neurochem.* **6**:117–141.

Curtis, D. R., Phillis, J. W., and Watkins, J. C., 1960, The chemical excitation of spinal neurones by certain acidic amino acids, *J. Physiol. (Lond.)* **150**:656–682.

Curtis, D. R., Duggan, A. W., Felix, D., Johnston, G. A. R., Tebecis, A. K., and Watkins, J. C., 1972, Excitation of mammalian neurones by acidic amino acids, *Brain Res.* **41**:283–301.

D'Adamo, A. F., Jr., and Yatsu, F. M., 1966, Acetate metabolism in the nervous system. *N*-Acetyl-L-aspartic acid and the biosynthesis of brain lipids, *J. Neurochem.* **13**:961–965.

Daoud, A., and Miller, R., 1976, Release of glutamate and other amino acids from arthropod nerve–muscle preparations, *J. Neurochem.* **26**:119–124.

Davidoff, R. A., Graham, L. T., Jr., Shank, R. P., Werman, R., and Aprison, M. H., 1967, Changes in amino acid concentrations associated with loss of spinal interneurons, *J. Neurochem.* **14**:1025–1031.

DeBelleroche, J. S., and Bradford, H. F., 1972, Metabolism of beds of mammalian cortical synaptosomes: Response to depolarizing influences, *J. Neurochem.* **19**:585–602.

DeFeudis, F. V., 1971, Effects of electrical stimulation on the efflux of L-glutamate from peripheral nerve *in vitro, Exp. Neurol.* **30**:291–296.

Deffner, G. G. J., 1961, The dialyzable free organic constituents of squid blood; a comparison with nerve axoplasm, *Biochim. Biophys. Acta* **47**:378–388.

De Robertis, E., and Fiszer DePlazas, S., 1976a, Differentiation of L-aspartate and L-glutamate high-affinity binding sites in a protein fraction isolated from rat cerebral cortex, *Nature* **260**:347–349.

De Robertis, E., and Fiszer DePlazas, S., 1976b, Isolation of hydrophobic proteins binding amino acids. Stereoselectivity of the binding of L-[^{14}C]glutamic acid in cerebral cortex, *J. Neurochem.* **26**:1237–1243.

Dowson, R. J., and Usherwood, P. N. R., 1972, The effect of low concentrations of L-glutamate and L-aspartate on transmitter release at the locust excitatory nerve–muscle synapse, *J. Physiol. (Lond.)* **229**:13P.

Drainville, G., and Gagnon, A., 1972, Osmoregulation in *Acanthamoeba castellanii* I. Variations of the concentrations of free intracellular amino acids and of the water content, *Comp. Biochem. Physiol.* **45A**:379–388.

Dudel, J., 1975, Potentiation and desensitization after glutamate-induced postsynaptic currents at the crayfish neuromusuclar junction, *Pflugers Arch.* **356**:317–327.

Duggan, A. W., 1974, The differential sensitivity to L-glutamate and L-aspartate of spinal interneurons and Renshaw cells, *Exp. Brain Res.* **19**:522–533.

Duggan, A. W., and Johnston, G. A. R., 1970, Glutamate and related amino acids in cat, dog, and rat spinal roots, *Comp Gen. Pharmacol.* **1**:127–128.

Dzubow, L. M., and Garfinkel, D., 1970, A simulation study of brain compartments, II. Atom-by-atom simulation of the metabolism of specifically labelled glucose and acetate, *Brain Res.* **23**:407–417.

Evans, P. D., 1973, Amino acid distribution in the nervous system of the crab, *Carcinus maenus* (L.), *J. Neurochem.* **21**:11–17.

Fishman, R. A., 1974, Cell volume, pumps, and neurologic function: Brain's adaptation to osmotic stress, in: *Brain Dysfunction in Metabolic Disorders* (F. Plum, ed.), *Res. Publ. Assoc. Nerv. Ment. Dis.,* Vol. 53, pp. 159–177, Raven Press, New York.

Fleming, M. C., and Lowry, O. H., 1966, The measurement of free and *N*-acetylated aspartic acids in the nervous system, *J. Neurochem.* **13**:779–783.

Florey, E., 1967, Neurotransmitters and modulators in the animal kingdom, *Fed. Proc. Fed. Am. Soc. Exp. Biol.* **26**:1164–1177.

Florkin, M., and Schoffeniels, E., 1965, Euryhalinity and the concept of physiological radiation, in: *Studies in Comparative Biochemistry* (K. A. Monday, ed.), pp. 6–40, Pergamon Press, Oxford.

Frank, E., 1974, The sensitivity to glutamate of denervated muscles of the crayfish, *J. Physiol. (Lond.)* **242**:371–382.

Freeman, A. R., 1976, Polyfunctional role of glutamic acid in excitatory synaptic transmission, *Prog. Neurobiol.* **6**:137–153.

Gent, J. P., Morgan, R., and Wolstencroft, J. H., 1974, Determination of the relative potency of two excitant amino acids, *Neuropharmacology* **13**:441–447.

Gerschenfeld, H. M., 1973, Chemical transmission in invertebrate central nervous systems and neuromuscular junctions, *Physiol. Rev.* **53**:1–119.

Gjessing, L. R., Gjesdahl, P., and Sjoastad, O., 1972, The free amino acids in human cerebrospinal fluid, *J. Neurochem.* **19**:1807–1808.

Gordon, M. S., 1965, Intracellular osmoregulation in skeletal muscle during salinity adaptation in two species of toads, *Biol. Bull.* **12**:218–229.

Graham, L. T., Jr., Shank, R. P., Werman, R., and Aprison, M. H., 1967, Distribution of some synaptic transmitter suspects in cat spinal cord: Glutamic acid, aspartic acid, γ-aminobutyric acid, glycine, and glutamine, *J. Neurochem.* **14**:465–472.

Haldeman, S., and McLennen, H., 1972, The antagonistic action of glutamic acid diethylester towards amino acid-induced and synaptic excitations of central neurones, *Brain Res.* **45**:393–400.

Haldeman, S., Huffman, R. D., Marshall, K. L., and McLennen, H., 1972, The antagonism of the glutamate-induced and synaptic excitations of thalamic neurones, *Brain Res.* **39**:419–425.

Hammerschlag, R., and Weinreich, D., 1972, Glutamic acid and primary afferent transmission, in: *Studies of Neurotransmitters at the Synaptic Level: Advances in Biochemical Psychopharmacology* (E. Costa, L. L. Iverson, and R. Paoletti, eds.), Vol. 6, pp. 165–180, Raven Press, New York.

Hammerschlag, R., Potter, L. T., and Vinci, J., 1971, *In vitro* uptake of ^{14}C-glutamate by rat spinal cord, *Trans. Am. Soc. Neurochem.* **2**:78.

Harvey, J. A., Scholfield, C. N., Graham, L. T., Jr., and Aprison, M. H., 1975, Putative transmitters in denervated olfactory cortex, *J. Neurochem.* **24**:445–449.

Henn, F. A., Goldstein, M. N., and Hamberger, A., 1974, Uptake of the neurotransmitter candidate glutamate by glia, *Nature* **149**:663–664.

Himwich, W., and Agrawal, H., 1969, Amino acids, in: *Handbook of Neurochemistry* (A. Lajtha, ed.), Vol. 1, pp. 33–52, Plenum Press, New York.

Hirsch, W., Mex, A., and Vogel, F., 1969, Metabolic traits in mentally retarded children as compared with normal populations: Monoaminodicarboxylic acids and their half amides and total amino acids, *J. Ment. Defic. Res.* **13**:130–142.

Höfelt, T., Elde, R., Johansson, O., Luft, R., Nilsson, G., and Arimura, A., 1976, Immunohistochemical evidence for separate populations of somatostatin-containing and substance P-containing primary afferent neurons in the rat, *Neuroscience* **1**:131–136.

Hösli, L., Andres, P. F., and Hösli, E., 1973, Ionic mechanisms underlying the depolarization of L-glutamate on rat and human spinal neurones in tissue culture, *Experientia* **29**:1244–1247.

Hösli, L., Andres, P. F., and Hösli, E., 1976, Ionic mechanisms associated with the depolarization by glutamate and aspartate on human and rat spinal neurons in tissue culture, *Pflugers Arch.* **363**:43–48.

Jacobson, K. B., 1959, Studies on the role of N-acetylaspartic acid in the mammalian brain, *J. Gen. Physiol.* **43**:323–333.

Jasper, H., and Koyama, I., 1969, Rate of release of amino acids from the cerebral cortex in the cat as affected by brainstem and thalamic stimulation, *Can. J. Physiol. Pharmacol.* **47**:889–905.

Jasper, H. H., Khan, R. T., and Elliott, K. A. C., 1965, Rate of release of amino acids from the cerebral cortex in the cat in relation to its state of activation, *Science* **147**:1448–1449.

Johnson, J., and Aprison, M. H., 1970, The distribution of glutamic acid, a transmitter candidate, and other amino acids in the dorsal sensory neuron of the cat, *Brain Res.* **24**:285–292.

Johnson, J., and Aprison, M. H., 1971, The distribution of glutamate and total free amino acids in thirteen specific regions of the cat central nervous system, *Brain Res.* **26**:141–148.

Johnston, G. A. R., Curtis, D. R., Davies, J., and McCulloch, R. M., 1974, Spinal interneurone excitation by conformationally restricted analogues of L-glutamic acid, *Nature* **248**:804–805.

Jones, M. E., Anderson, D., Anderson, C., and Hodes, S., 1961, Citrulline synthesis in rat tissues, *Arch. Biochem. Biophys.* **95**:499–507.

Kerkut, G. A., and Wheal, H. V., 1974, The excitatory effects of aspartate and glutamate on the crustacean neuromuscular junction, *Br. J. Pharmacol.* **51**:136P–137P.

Kittridge, J. S., Simonsen, D. G., Roberts, E., and Jelinek, B., 1962, Free amino acids of marine invertebrates, in: *Amino Acid Pools* (J. T. Holden, ed.), pp. 176–186, Elsevier, Amsterdam.

Kravitz, E. A., Slater, C. R., Takahashi, K., Bownds, M. D., and Grossfeld, R. M., 1970, Excitatory transmission in invertebrates—Glutamate as a potential neuromuscular transmitter compound, in: *Excitatory Synaptic Mechanisms* (P. Anderson and J. K. S. Jansen, eds.), pp. 85–93, Universitetsforlaget, Oslo.

Krnjević, K., 1974, Chemical nature of synaptic transmission in vertebrates, *Physiol. Rev.* **54**:418–540.

Krnjević, K., and Phillis, J. W., 1963, Iontophoretic studies of neurones in the mammalian cerberal cortex, *J. Physiol. (Lond.)* **165**:274–304.

Krnjević, K., and Schwartz, S., 1967, Some properties of unresponsive cells in the cerebral cortex, *Exp. Brain Res.* **3**:306–319.

Lajtha, A., 1968, Transport as a control mechanism of cerebral metabolite levels, in: *Brain*

Barrier Systems, Progress in Brain Research (A. Lajtha and D. Ford, eds.), Vol. 29, pp. 201–216, Elsevier, Amsterdam.

Lajtha, A., Berl, S., and Waelsch, H., 1959, Amino acid and protein metabolism of the brain— IV. The metabolism of glutamic acid, *J. Neurochem.* **3**:322–332.

Lang, M. A., and Gainer, H., 1969, Isosmotic intracellular regulation as a mechanism of volume control in crab muscle fibers, *Comp. Biochem. Physiol.* **30**:445–456.

Lea, T. J., and Usherwood, P. N. R., 1972, The site of action of ibotenic acid and the identification of two populations of glutamate receptors on insect muscle fibers, *Comp. Gen. Pharmacol.* **4**:333–350.

Levi, G., Kandera, J., and Lajtha, A., 1967, Control of cerebral metabolite levels. I. Amino acid uptake and levels in various species, *Arch. Biochem. Biophys.* **119**:303–311.

Lewis, P. R., 1952, The free amino acids of invertebrate nerve, *Biochem. J.* **52**:330–338.

Lin, S., and Cohen, H. P., 1973, Crayfish ventral nerve cord and hemolymph: Content of free amino acids and other metabolites, *Comp. Biochem. Physiol.* **45B**:249–263.

Logan, W. J., and Snyder, S. H., 1972, High affinity uptake systems for glycine, glutamic and aspartic acids in synaptosomes of rat central nervous system, *Brain Res.* **42**:413–431.

Lowagie, C., and Gerschenfeld, H. M., 1974, Glutamate antagonists at a crayfish neuromuscular junction, *Nature* **248**:421–422.

Lux, H. D., Loracher, C., and Neher, E., 1970, The action of ammonium on postsynaptic inhibition in cat spinal motoneurons, *Exp. Brain Res.* **11**:431–447.

Mahler, H. R., and Cotman, C. W., 1970, Insoluble proteins of the synaptic plasma membrane, in: *Protein Metabolism of the Nervous System* (A. Lajtha, ed.), pp. 151–184, Plenum Press, New York.

Mangan, J. L., and Whitaker, V. P., 1966, The distribution of free amino acids in subcellular fractions of guinea pig brain, *Biochem. J.* **98**:128–137.

Marks, N., Datta, R. K., and Lajtha, A., 1970, Distribution of amino acids and of exo- and endopeptidases along vertebrate and invertebrate nerves, *J. Neurochem.* **17**:53–63.

McBride, W. J., Shank, R. P., Freeman, A. R., and Aprison, M. H., 1974, Levels of free amino acids in excitatory, inhibitory and sensory axons of the walking limbs of the lobster, *Life Sci.* **14**:1109–1120.

McBride, W. J., Freeman, A. R., Graham, L. T., Jr., and Aprison, M. H., 1975, Content of amino acids in axons from the CNS of the lobster, *J. Neurobiol.* **6**:321–328.

McBride, W. J., Aprison, M. H., and Kusano, K., 1976, Contents of several amino acids in the cerebellum, brain stem and cerebrum of the "staggerer," "weaver" and "nervous" neurologically mutant mice, *J. Neurochem.* **26**:867–870.

McIntosh, J. C., and Cooper, J. R., 1965, Studies on the function of N-acetylaspartic acid in brain, *J. Neurochem.* **12**:825–835.

Meister, A., 1973, On the enzymology of amino acid transport, *Science* **180**:30–39.

Meister, A., 1975, Function of glutathione in kidney via the γ-glutamyl cycle, *Med. Clin. North Am.* **59**:649–666.

Michaelis, E. K., 1975, Partial purification and characterization of a glutamate-binding membrane glycoprotein from rat brain, *Biochem. Biophys. Res. Commun.* **65**:1004–1011.

Miledi, R., 1972, Synaptic potentials in nerve cells of the stellate ganglion of the squid, *J. Physiol. (Lond.)* **225**:501–514.

Minard, F. N., and Richter, D., 1968, Electroshock-induced seizures and the turnover of brain protein in the rat, *J. Neurochem.* **18**:1463–1468.

Minchin, M. C. W., and Iversen, L. L., 1974, Release of [³H]gamma-aminobutyric acid from glial cells in rat dorsal root ganglia, *J. Neurochem.* **23**:533–540.

Morgan, R., Vrbova, G., and Wolstencroft, J. H., 1972, Correlation between the retinal input to the lateral geniculate neurones and their relative response to glutamate and aspartate, *J. Physiol. (Lond.)* **224**:41P–42P.

Moore, B. W., 1965, A soluble protein characteristic of the nervous system, *Biochem. Biophys. Res. Commun.* **19**:739–744.

Moore, B. W., 1975, Brain-specific proteins: S-100 protein, 14-3-2 protein and glial fibrillary protein, in: *Advances in Neurochemistry* (B. W. Agranoff and M. H. Aprison, eds.), Vol. 1, pp. 137–155, Plenum Press, New York.

Murthy, M. R. V., and Roux, H., 1974, Reactions of free and tRNA bound glutamate and glutamine, *J. Neurochem.* **23**:645–649.

Nagy, A., Baker, R. R., Morris, S. J., and Whitaker, V. P., 1976, The preparation and characterization of synaptic vesicles of high purity, *Brain Res.* **109**:285–309.

Nistri, A., and Constanti, A., 1975, Effects of glutamate and glutamic acid diethyl ester on the lobster muscle fibre and the frog spinal cord, *Eur. J. Pharmacol.* **31**:377–379.

Okumura, N., Otsuka, S., and Aoyama, T., 1959, Studies on the free amino acids and related compounds in the brains of fish, amphibia, reptile, aves, and mammal by ion exchange chromatography, *J. Biochem. (Tokyo)* **46**:207–212.

Oldendorf, W., 1971, Brain uptake of radiolabelled amino acids, amines, and hexoses after arterial injection, *Am. J. Physiol.* **221**:1629–1639.

Olney, J. W., Rhee, V., and Ho, O. L., 1974, Kainic acid: A powerful neurotoxic analogue of glutamate, *Brain Res.* **77**:507–512.

Onodera, K., and Takeuchi, A., 1975, Ionic mechanism of the excitatory synaptic membrane of the crayfish neuromuscular junction, *J. Physiol. (Lond.)* **252**:295–318.

Osborne, R. H., and Bradford, H. F., 1975, The influence of sodium, potassium, and lanthanum on amino acid release from spinal-medullary synaptosomes, *J. Neurochem.* **25**:35–41.

Osborne, R. H., Bradford, H. F., and Jones, D. G., 1973, Patterns of amino acid release from nerve-endings isolated from spinal cord and medulla, *J. Neurochem.* **21**:407–419.

Otsuka, M., 1977, Substance P and sensory transmitter, in: *Advances in Neurochemistry* (B. W. Agranoff and M. H. Aprison, eds.), Vol. 2, pp. 193–208, Plenum Press, New York.

Otsuka, M., Konishi, S., and Takahasi, T., 1975, Hypothalamic substance P as a candidate for transmitter of primary afferent neurons, *Fed. Proc.* **34**:1922–1928.

Perry, T. L., Hansen, S., Berry, K., Mok, C., and Lesk, D., 1971, Free amino acids and related compounds in biopsies of human brain, *J. Neurochem.* **18**:521–528.

Peterkofsky, A., 1973, Involvement of glutamic acid and glutamine in protein synthesis and maturation, in: *The Enzymes of Glutamine Metabolism* (S. Prusiner and E. R. Stadtman, eds.), pp. 331–342, Academic Press, New York.

Pierce, S. K., Jr., and Greenberg, M. J., 1973, The initiation and control of free amino acid regulation of cell volume in salinity-stressed marine bivalves, *J. Exp. Biol.* **59**:435–440.

Potts, W. T. W., and Parry, G., 1964, *Osmotic and Ionic Regulation in Animals,* Pergamon Press, Oxford.

Quastel, J. H., 1974, Amino acids and the brain, *Biochem. Soc. Trans.* **2**:765–780.

Quastel, J. H., and Wheatley, A. H. M., 1932, Oxidations by the brain, *Biochem. J.* **26**:725–744.

Raiteri, M., Federico, R., Coletti, A., and Levi, G., 1975, Release and exchange studies relating to the synaptosomal uptake of GABA, *J. Neurochem.* **24**:1243–1250.

Rassin, D. K., 1972, Amino acids as putative transmitters: Failure to bind to synaptic vesicles of guinea pig cerebral cortex, *J. Neurochem.* **19**:139–148.

Ratner, S., Morell, H., and Caravalho, E., 1960, Enzymes of arginine metabolism in brain, *Arch. Biochem. Biophys.* **91**:280–289.

Reichelt, K. L., 1970, The isolation of gamma-glutamyl peptides from monkey brain, *J. Neurochem.* **17**:19–25.

Reichelt, K. L., and Fonnum, F., 1969, Subcellular localization of N-acetylaspartyl-glutamate and glutathione in brain, *J. Neurochem.* **16**:1409–1416.

Reiffenstein, R. J., and Neal, M. J., 1974, Uptake, storage, and release of γ-aminobutyrate in normal and chronically denervated cat cerebral cortex, *Can. J. Physiol. Pharmacol.* **52**:286–290.

Reif-Lehrer, L., 1976, Possible significance of adverse reactions to glutamate in humans, *Fed. Proc.* **35**:2205–2211.

Roberts, E., Baxter, C. F., Van Harreveld, A., Wiersma, C. A. G., Adey, W. R., and Killam, K. F. (eds.), 1960, *Inhibition in the Nervous System and Gamma-Aminobutyric Acid,* Pergamon Press, Oxford.

Roberts, E., Chase, T. N., and Tower, D. B. (eds.), 1976, *GABA in Nervous System Function,* Raven Press, New York.

Roberts, P. J., 1974a, Amino acid release from isolated rat dorsal root ganglia, *Brain Res.* **74**:327–332.

Roberts, P. J., 1974b, Glutamate receptors in the rat central nervous system, *Nature* **252**:399–401.

Roberts, P. J., and Watkins, J. C., 1975, Structural requirements for the inhibition for L-glutamate uptake by glia and nerve endings, *Brain Res.* **85**:120–125.

Sadasivudu, B., and Hanumantharao, T. I., 1974, Studies on the distribution of urea cycle enzymes in different regions of the rat brain, *J. Neurochem.* **23**:267–269.

Sano, I., Kakimoto, Y., Kanazawa, A., Nakajima, T., and Shimizu, H., 1966, Identification of glutamylpeptides in brain, *J. Neurochem.* **13**:711–719.

Schmidt-Nielsen, B., 1975, Comparative physiology of cellular ion and volume regulation, *J. Exp. Zool.* **194**:207–219.

Schoffeniels, E., 1964, Cellular aspects of active transport, in: *Comparative Biochemistry* (M. Florkin and H. S. Mason, eds.), Vol. 7, pp. 137–202, Academic Press, New York.

Schoffeniels, E., 1970, Isosmotic intracellular regulation in "Maja squinado" risso and "Penaeus aztecus" yves, *Arch. Int. Physiol. Biochim.* **78**:461–466.

Schoffeniels, E., and Gilles, R., 1970, Osmoregulation in aquatic arthropods, in: *Chemical Zoology* (M. Florkin and B. T. Sheer, eds.), pp. 255–286, Academic Press, New York.

Schultz, V., and Lowenstein, J. M., 1976, Purine nucleotide cycle—Evidence for the occurrence in brain, *J. Biol. Chem.* **251**:485–492.

Shank, R. P., and Aprison, M. H., 1970, The metabolism *in vivo* of glycine and serine in eight areas of the rat central nervous system, *J. Neurochem.* **17**:1461–1475.

Shank, R. P., and Aprison, M. H., 1977, Glutamine uptake and metabolism by the isolated toad brain: Evidence pertaining to its proposed role as a transmitter precursor, *J. Neurochem.* **28**:1189–1196.

Shank, R. P., and Baxter, C. F., 1973, Metabolism of glucose, amino acids, and some related metabolites in the brain of toads (*Bufo boreas*) adapted to fresh water or hyperosmotic environments, *J. Neurochem.* **21**:301–313.

Shank, R. P., and Baxter, C. F., 1975, Uptake and metabolism of glutamate by isolated toad brains containing different levels of endogenous amino acids, *J. Neurochem.* **24**:641–646.

Shank, R. P., and Freeman, A. R., 1975, Cooperative interaction of glutamate and aspartate with receptors in the neuromuscular excitatory membrane in walking limbs of the lobster, *J. Neurobiol.* **6**:289–303.

Shank, R. P., and Freeman, A. R., 1976, Agonistic and antagonistic activity of glutamate analogs on neuromuscular excitation in the walking limbs of lobster, *J. Neurobiol.* **7**:23–26.

Shank, R. P., Whiten, J. T., and Baxter, C. F., 1973, Glutamate uptake by isolated toad brain, *Science* **181**:860–862.

Shank, R. P., Freeman, A. R., McBride, W. J., and Aprison, M. H., 1975, Glutamate and aspartate as mediators of neuromuscular excitation in the lobster, *Comp. Biochem. Physiol.* **50C**:127–132.

Shinozaki, H., and Shibuya, I., 1974, Potentiation of glutamate-induced depolarization by kainic acid in the crayfish opener muscle, *Neuropharmacology* **13**:1057–1065.

Silber, R. H., and Schmitt, F. O., 1940, The role of free amino acids in electrolyte balance of nerve, *J. Cell. Comp. Physiol.* **16**:247–254.

Simon, J. R., Contrera, J. F., and Kuhar, M. J., 1976, Binding of ³H-kainic acid, an analogue of L-glutamate of brain membranes, *J. Neurochem.* **26**:141–148.

Snyder, S. H., Young, A. B., Bennett, J. P., and Mulder, A. H., 1973, Synaptic biochemistry of amino acids, *Fed. Proc.* **32**:2039–2047.

Sorenson, M. M., 1973, The free amino acids in peripheral nerves and in isolated inhibitory and excitatory nerves of *Cancer magister, J. Neurochem.* **20**:1231–1245.

Spencer, H. J., 1976, Antagonism of cortical excitation of striatal neurons by glutamic acid diethyl ester: Evidence for glutamic acid as an excitatory transmitter in the rat striatum, *Brain Res.* **102**:91–101.

Takahashi, T., and Otsuka, M., 1975, Regional distribution of substance P in the spinal cord and nerve roots of the cat and the effects of dorsal roots section, *Brain Res.* **87**:1–11.

Takeuchi, A., and Onodera, K., 1973, Reversal potenials of the excitatory transmitter and L-glutamate at the crayfish neuromuscular junction, *Nature New Biol.* **242**:124–126.

Takeuchi, A., and Takeuchi, N., 1972, Actions of transmitter substances on neuromuscular junctions of vertebrates and invertebrates, *Adv. Biophys.* **3**:45–95.

Tallan, H. H., 1962, A survey of the amino acids and related compounds in nervous tissue, in: *Amino Acid Pools* (J. T. Holden, ed.), pp. 471–485, Elsevier, Amsterdam.

Taraskevich, P. S., 1971, Reversal potentials of L-glutamate and the excitatory transmitter at the neuromuscular junction of the crayfish, *Biochem. Biophys. Acta* **241**:700–702.

Thurston, J. H., Hauhart, R. E., Jones, E. M., and Alter, J. L., 1975, Effect of salt and water loading on carbohydrate and energy metabolism and levels of selected amino acids in the brains of young mice, *J. Neurochem.* **24**:953–957.

Tower, D. B., and Wherrett, J. R., 1971, Glutamyl and aspartyl moieties of cerebral proteins: Enrichment in membrane-containing microsomal subfractions, *J. Neurochem.* **18**:1043–1051.

Triggle, D. J., 1971, *Neurotransmitter–Receptor Interactions,* Academic Press, New York.

Tsukada, Y., Nagata, Y., Hirano, S., and Matsutani, T., 1963, Active transport of amino acids into cerebral slices, *J. Neurochem.* **10**:241–256.

Van den Berg, C. J., 1970, Glutamate and glutamine, in: *Handbook of Neurochemistry* (A. Lajtha, ed.), Vol. 3, pp. 355–379, Plenum Press, New York.

Van den Berg, C. J., Reignierse, G. L. A., Blochuis, G. G. C., Kron, M. C., Ronda, G., Clarke, D. D., and Garfinkel, D., 1976, A model of glutamate metabolism in brain: A biochemical analysis of a heterogeneous structure, in: *Metabolic Compartmentation and Neurotransmission—Relation to Brain Structure and Function* (S. Berl, D. D. Clarke, and S. Schneider, eds.), pp. 515–544, Plenum Pres, New York.

Van Gelder, N. M., and Courtois, A., 1972, Close correlation between changing content of specific amino acids in epileptogenic cortex of cats, and severity of epilepsy, *Brain Res.* **43**:477–484.

Van Harreveld, A., and Fifkova, E., 1970, Glutamate release from the retina during spreading depression, *J. Neurobiol.* **2**:13–29.

Virkar, R. A., and Webb, K. L., 1970, Free amino acid composition of the soft-shell clam, *Mya arenaria* in relation to salinity of the medium, *Comp. Biochem. Physiol.* **32**:775–783.

Wajda, I. J., 1970, Transglutaminase changes in the brain and other tissues during allergic encephalomyelitis, in: *Protein Metabolism of the Nervous System* (A. Lajtha, ed.), pp. 671–684, Plenum Press, New York.

Weil-Malherbe, H., 1950, Significance of glutamic acid for the metabolism of nervous tissue, *Physiol. Rev.* **30**:549–568.

Weil-Malherbe, H., 1975, Further studies on ammonia formation in brain slices: The effect of hadacidin, *Neuropharmacology* **14**:175–180.

Weinreich, D., and Hammerschlag, R., 1975, Nerve impulse-enhanced release of amino acids from nonsynaptic regions of peripheral and central nerve trunks of bullfrog, *Brain Res.* **84**:137–142.

Wheal, H. V., and Kerkut, G. A., 1975, The effect of diethyl ester L-glutamate on evoked excitatory junction potentials at the crustacean neuromuscular junction, *Brain Res.* **82**:338–340.

Wheeler, D. D., Boyarsky, L. L., and Brooks, W. H., 1966, The release of amino acids from nerve during stimulation, *J. Cell. Physiol.* **67**:141–148.

Wherrett, J. R., and Tower, D. B., 1971, Glutamyl and aspartyl amide moieties of cerebral proteins: Metabolic aspects *in vitro, J. Neurochem.* **18**:1027–1042.

Wolfgram, F., and Kotorii, 1968a, The composition of myeling proteins of the central nervous system, *J. Neurochem.* **18**:1281–1290.

Wolfgram, F., and Kotorii, 1968b, The composition of the myelin proteins of the peripheral nervous system, *J. Neurochem.* **18**:1291–1296.

Yamamoto, C., and Matsui, S., 1976, Effect of stimulation of excitatory nerve tract on release of glutamic acid from olfactory cortex slices *in vitro, J. Neurochem.* **26**:487–491.

Yarowsky, P. J., and Carpenter, D. P., 1976, Aspartate: Distinct receptors on aplysia neurons, *Science* **192**:807–809.

Young, A. B., Oster-Granite, M. L., Herndon, R. M., and Snyder, S. H., 1974, Glutamic acid: Selective depletion by viral-induced granule cell loss in hamster cerebellum, *Brain Res.* **73**:1–13.

Zieglgansberger, W., and Puil, E. A., 1973, Actions of glutamate on spinal neurones, *Exp. Brain Res.* **17**:35–49.

BIOCHEMICAL ASPECTS OF TRANSMISSION AT INHIBITORY SYNAPSES:
The Role of Glycine

M. H. APRISON AND E. C. DALY

Section of Applied and Theoretical Neurobiology
The Institute of Psychiatric Research and
Departments of Biochemistry and Psychiatry
Indiana University Medical Center
Indianapolis, Indiana

1. INTRODUCTION

1.1. Background and Task

The biochemical aspects of the neurophysiology of transmission have been clarified during the years since the late 1950s. Thus, it is interesting to recall that during this period many biochemists became aware for the first time that most neurons in the central nervous system of higher vertebrates do not touch. With the aid of the electron microscope, the neuroanatomists have shown that a space of approximately 200 Å separates the terminal endings of the axon of one neuron and the cellular membranes of the next neuron. This space is called the synaptic cleft and can vary from 100 to 500 Å depending on the tissue and the location; this whole minute region in the nervous system (i.e., the terminal ending of one neuron, the cellular membrane of the second neuron in juxtaposition to the specific nerve ending, and the synaptic cleft) is called a synapse. Various organic compounds can be released from the axonal endings of the presynaptic cell into the synaptic cleft. The compounds which reach and can affect the conductance across the postsynaptic membrane at this region of the synapse in a specific manner are called transmitters and the whole process is called transmission. This latter process is chemical in nature.

Evidence from electron microscopic and subcellular fractionation studies of the nervous tissue indicates that some transmitters but not all (i.e., the amino acid transmitters) are associated with spherical structures approximately 200–500 A in diameter. These special structures are packed in the presynaptic nerve terminals and are called synaptic vesicles; they are rarely seen in the cvtoplasm of the synaptic region of the postsynaptic neuron. There is also evidence of another type of synaptic vesicle, more flattened and elongated, which is approximately 100–200 A wide and 300–600 A long. The two types of vesicles have not been found in the same nerve ending.

Although the release mechanisms for transmitters are not well understood, data indicate that a critical calcium ion concentration at or within the presynaptic membrane is necessary for the release of the specific transmitter. After its release, the "free" transmitter diffuses across the 200 Å synaptic cleft and reacts with a specific receptor located in the postsynaptic membrane. This action gives rise to the postsynaptic response, i.e., the increase in conductance due to the movement of specific ions. Depending on the particular transmitter and receptor, the postsynaptic response, as measured by neurophysiological techniques, may result in excitation or inhibition of the postsynaptic neuron. Thus some transmitters are excitatory in their actions while others are inhibitory.

During the initiation of excitation, the increase in conduction is primarily due to sodium ions which "flow" down their concentration gradients from outside to inside the neuron. As a result of this action, the membrane is partially depolarized and is more likely to fire. On the other hand, during inhibition the increase in conductance is primarily due to chloride ions which also flow from outside to inside. In this case, the membrane is partially hyperpolarized and stabilized, making it less likely to fire. In some cases of inhibition, potassium ions account for the increased conductance flowing from inside the neuron to the outside, whereas in other cases, the movement of both Cl^- and K^+ may be associated with the inhibition. Postsynaptic inhibition is accompanied by a membrane hyperpolarization and an inhibitory postsynaptic potential (IPSP). When the membrane potential is lowered from the resting state, i.e., depolarized, the IPSPs are increased. The reverse is true when the membrane potential is increased. At the equilibrium potential of the IPSP, the IPSP is essentially zero. If the membrane potential is increased further, reversal occurs, i.e., IPSP becomes depolarizing.

From these brief comments it becomes clear that the final identification of central nervous system (CNS) transmitters must come from both neurochemical and neurophysiological data, and the experiments that produce these data invariably have been based on neuroanatomical considerations and information. Therefore, it is not surprising that beginning in the mid-1960s, several neurochemical and neurophysiological groups began to work together in this area of research where our knowledge of neuroanatomical relationships has been clarified. In this period, numerous techniques have been developed for the chemical quantification of transmitter suspects in small specific areas of the CNS as well as for testing their pharmacological actions on neurons having well-defined inputs. Thus, there have been some significant advances in our understanding of the ionic mechanisms of excitation and inhibition. In addition, important experimental techniques have been developed which permitted the clarification of specific inhibitory pathways in the vertebrate CNS. In the case of the inhibitory transmitters, considerable neurochemical (distribution of substrates and enzyme activities), neurophysiological (hyperpolarization and conductance changes), and neuropharmacological data (antagonism by strychnine, bicuculline, and picrotoxin) have now been published which indicate that two nonessential amino acids derived metabolically from glucose in the CNS—glycine and γ-aminobutyric acid (GABA)—may serve in such roles at different sites within the vertebrate neuroaxis. Although several other compounds may also function as inhibitory transmitters, the most convincing data at present are available for glycine and GABA. This chapter focuses on the neurochemical data for the spinal cord and brain which support these conclusions in the case of glycine; however, owing to the volume of literature some selectivity was necessary.

The question is often asked by students: "How did glycine become a candidate for the postsynaptic inhibitory transmitter in the cat spinal cord when it is known to have a number of important *metabolic* roles?" (See Fig. 1.) The reason for this question stems from the fact that it is difficult to imagine how one would identify a compound as a neurotransmitter in a specific region or at specific synapses of the CNS when it is known that there are more than 10 billion neurons located in the CNS, and that there are a huge number of synaptic contacts between these neurons. What is equally difficult to understand is how a compound known to participate in a

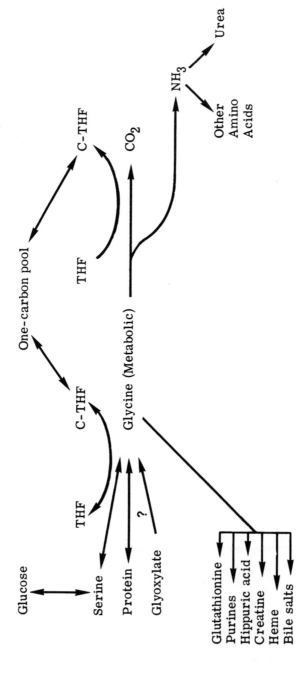

FIGURE 1. Fate of glycine in the metabolic pool.

number of metabolic steps could also play a role as a transmitter. Yet, in 1965, Aprison and Werman published a *biochemical* study on the distribution of glycine in the gray and white matter of the feline spinal cord as well as the spinal roots and concluded that the pattern of distribution for this amino acid was compatible with its possible role as the major postsynaptic spinal inhibitory transmitter. What "thinking pattern" and what kind of data led these investigators to suggest this additional role for glycine, structurally the simplest of all the amino acids?

1.2. A Research Approach

Although the inhibitory properties of glycine had been reported in a number of neurophysiological studies by 1965 (Purpura *et al.*, 1959; Curtis and Watkins, 1960; Krnjević and Phillis, 1963), a number of investigators also noted that several other amino acids such as GABA, glutamate, and aspartate could inhibit or excite many neurons in the CNS. In fact, since these specific amino acids seemed to affect most neurons, it was concluded that these compounds acted nonspecifically on neurons in vertebrates (Crawford and Curtis, 1964; Curtis, 1963; Curtis *et al.*, 1959, 1960; Curtis and Watkins, 1963, 1965). Some of these investigators also studied the action of inhibitory amino acids on spinal neurons and reported that these compounds did not include the spinal postsynaptic inhibitory transmitter. When tested by iontophoresis on the postsynaptic membrane, the generality of action of an excitatory or an inhibitory amino acid on almost all neurons was used as an argument to support the contention of its nonspecific action. These arguments included glycine. However, such a position cannot be used as evidence against the role of glycine or any other amino acid as an inhibitory transmitter unless it is known that the presynaptic endings of the specific synapses under study do not release the compounds as transmitters. This fact had not been established and hence should not have been used as evidence against the idea. Even the suggestion that these amino acids produced no hyperpolarization was contradicted by the data published later by Kuno and Muneoka (1962), Obata (1965), Krnjević and Schwartz (1966), and Werman *et al.* (1966). During this period some investigators had failed to show that strychnine acted as an antagonist of glycine and GABA. However, these data also should not have been used as evidence against these inhibitory amino acids since it had not been proven at that time that this drug acted primarily on the postsynaptic inhibitory membrane. Considering these concepts and reports, Aprison and Werman devised a new combined neurochemical and neurophysiological approach to identification of transmitters in the CNS.

1.2.1. Three Criteria for Identification of Transmitters in the CNS

Although there is a tendency among neurophysiologists and neuro-pharmacologists to stress the neurophysiological approach in studies involving the identification of CNS transmitters, it is generally accepted by most experts in neurobiology today that in such studies the final proof of identification must come from *both* neurochemical and neurophysiological data. Thus, it is not surprising that in the course of their early work on identifying spinal cord transmitters, Werman and Aprison (1968) concluded that compelling evidence for the identification of a suspected biological compound as a transmitter in the CNS would be provided by a combination of three pieces of neurochemical and neurophysiological data. Their experiments were designed to test whether the putative transmitter (1) was present in the presynaptic neurons of the synapses studied (neurochemical data), (2) reproduced the ionic membrane processes evoked by transmitter action (neurophysiological data), and (3) could be collected from the extracellular fluid in response to stimulation of the presynaptic nerve (combined neurophysiological and neurochemical data). These three pieces of data are often referred to as the Presynaptic Criterion, the Criterion of Identity of Action, and the Release Criterion.

The historical development of this problem indicates that the investigators had to determine which area or specific sites in the CNS should be studied. In view of the advanced state of physiology concerning the lumbosacral spinal cord of the cat (Eccles, 1964), this area appeared to be an ideal site to search for transmitters in the CNS. Based on anatomical and physiological considerations, hypothetical distributions of the excitatory and inhibitory transmitters in the lumbosacral spinal cord were predicted by Aprison and Werman (1965). Physiological studies had indicated that inhibition is mediated through interneurons (Eccles, 1964). There were sufficient data available which showed that a small neuron (interneuron) is interpolated in inhibitory pathways from dorsal root fibers to spinal motoneurons. Since the soma and the short axons of such interneurons lie in the gray matter of the spinal cord, it was reasonable to expect a higher concentration of the inhibitory transmitter to be found in the gray matter and lower levels to be found in white matter and spinal roots. On the other hand, the excitatory transmitter released from primary afferent terminals should be manufactured and concentrated in cells of the dorsal root and in areas of the spinal cord that are rich in the dorsal primary afferent collaterals and terminals, i.e., dorsal gray matter and dorsal medial columns of the white matter (see Fig. 2). It was only necessary to do biochemical analyses of the dorsal and ventral gray matter, dorsal and ventral white matter, and

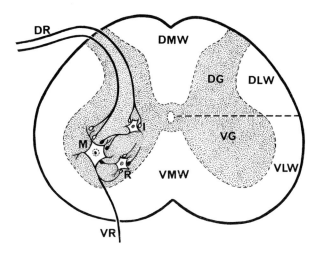

FIGURE 2. Diagram of cross section of cat spinal cord at L_7. Abbreviations: DG, dorsal gray; DMW, dorsal medial white; DR, dorsal root; DLW, dorsal lateral white; VG, ventral gray; VMW, ventral medial white; VR, ventral root; VLW, ventral lateral white; M, motoneuron; I, interneuron; R, Renshaw cell.

dorsal and ventral roots, once it was determined which compound or compounds were to be measured in these samples. Aprison and Werman chose to study amino acids in these specific areas. This decision was based on three factors: (1) known pharmacological actions of some amino acids, (2) evidence existing at that time that GABA and glutamate were putative inhibitory and excitatory transmitters at the crustacean neuromuscular jucntion, and (3) the "hunch" that such a successful solution to the problem of synaptic transmission in more primitive animals was probably not lost in evolution. This reasoning led to the experiments reported in 1965 and reviewed in Section 2.1.

2. THE PRESYNAPTIC CRITERION

2.1. Distribution of Glycine in Specific Areas of the Lumbosacral Spinal Cord of the Cat

The search for transmitter candidates with distributions compatible with those expected for synaptic transmission was begun by using the technique of ion exchange column chromatography. Samples from supernatants of pooled homogenates from spinal gray, dorsal, and ventral roots treated with picric acid were run on high-resolution columns (Aprison and Werman, 1965). An immediate result of this experiment was finding the high content of glycine in spinal gray matter (4.47 μmol/g) compared to both dorsal roots (0.28 μmol/g) and ventral roots (0.32 μmol/g). With the knowledge that Curtis and Watkins (1960) had shown glycine to inhibit the firing of spinal neurons (at that time this observation was considered to be a nonspecific effect), Aprison and Werman (1965) extended their neurochemical studies to discrete areas of the spinal cord employing newly perfected specific micromethods for the measurement of several amino acids (Graham and Aprison, 1966).

The data in Table 1 show the distribution of glycine and GABA in four areas of the spinal cord of the cat as well as in the dorsal and ventral roots as measured by specific biochemical methods (Graham *et al.*, 1967). Both glycine and GABA have the distribution postulated for the inhibitory transmitter. The order of decreasing content of glycine (in μmol/g) was as follows: ventral gray (7) > dorsal gray (5.6) > ventral white (4.4) > dorsal white (3.0) > dorsal root (0.6) = ventral root (0.6). This unusual variation in the content of glycine in the six areas of the cat spinal cord was later confirmed by Johnston (1968), and is also shown in Table 1. In addition, the uneven distribution of glycine in the rabbit spinal cord has now been reported by Berger *et al.* (1977a); the pattern is similar to that found in cat spinal cord. The content of GABA (in μmol/g) followed a different pattern: dorsal gray (2.2) > ventral gray (1.0) > ventral white (0.4) = dorsal white (0.4) > ventral root (0.08) > dorsal root (0.06). This distribution for GABA

TABLE 1.   Content of Glycine and GABA in Dorsal and Ventral Roots and Four Areas of the Lumbosacral Spinal Cord of the Cat

		Content (μmol/g)[a]		
Tissue analyzed		Glycine[b]	Glycine[c]	GABA[b]
Dorsal white	(DW)	3.04 ± 0.26	2.92 ± 0.10	0.43 ± 0.05
Dorsal gray	(DG)	5.65 ± 0.18	5.42 ± 0.14	2.18 ± 0.25
Ventral gray	(VG)	7.08 ± 0.31	6.51 ± 0.17	1.04 ± 0.10
Ventral white	(VW)	4.39 ± 0.26	4.55 ± 0.09	0.44 ± 0.06
Dorsal root	(DR)	0.64 ± 0.04	0.61 ± 0.06	0.06 ± 0.01
Ventral root	(VR)	0.64 ± 0.00	0.60 ± 0.10	0.08 ± 0.01

[a] Mean ± SEM.
[b] Graham *et al.* (1967).
[c] Johnston (1968).

(and glycine) for cat spinal cord was confirmed by Miyata and Otsuka (1975). These data suggest more than metabolic roles for glycine and GABA in the spinal cord.

2.2. Distribution of Glycine in Specific Areas of the Lumbosacral Spinal Cord of the Cat after Ligation of the Thoracic Aorta

Since it was not possible on the basis of distribution alone to tell whether either glycine or GABA or both was likely to be an inhibitory transmitter associated with interneurons in the spinal cord, a different approach was necessary. It was important to see if a loss of inhibitory interneurons would be accompanied by a change in the content of glycine or GABA. Such a loss can be produced by clamping the thoracic aorta just below the exit of the left subclavian artery for periods of 15–60 min (Tureen, 1936; Murayama and Smith, 1965). Utilizing such a technique to produce a loss of spinal interneurons, it was shown that glycine, but not GABA, is concentrated in these interneurons located in ventral and dorsal (more central) gray (Davidoff et al., 1967a,b). Cats were sacrificed at different times between 11 and 35 days after surgery and the seventh lumbar spinal segment was removed, frozen, and dissected. The tissue was analyzed for cell loss and its content of glycine, GABA, glutamate, aspartate, and glutamine. One slice was preserved in formalin, embedded in paraffin, serially sectioned at 5 μm, and stained with toluidine blue for histological study and cell count. The number of neurons in either the right or left half of five nonserial (random) histological sections of the L_7 segment from each of the experimental animals and the normal cats were also counted. Neurons were identified by the presence of nucleoli and were divided into two groups on the basis of size: (1) large neurons with at least one dimension of 20 μm or greater (considered to contain most motoneurons as well as some large interneurons), and (2) small neurons less than 20 μm in diameter (considered to consist mainly of interneurons) (Gelfan and Tarlov, 1963).

The mean count of small neurons was significantly decreased by aortic occlusion and the histological study revealed that the most severe losses of neurons occurred in the central portions of the spinal gray which are the areas of the cord with the highest density of interneurons (Aitken and Bridger, 1961). The large motoneurons, clustered in the peripheral portions of the ventral horn, were relatively unaffected.

A significant decrease of the mean content of glycine in both dorsal and ventral gray and ventral white matter was observed after the loss of interneurons, whereas the mean count of GABA did not differ appreciably from that of normal animals (see Table 2). Moreover, a significant linear correlation was found between the content of glycine in dorsal and ventral gray matter and in the number of remaining small neurons (dorsal gray, $r = 0.71$, $P < 0.05$; ventral gray, $r = 0.75$, $P < 0.02$). If the regression lines were extrapolated to the point at which the small neuron count becomes zero and these values were subtracted from the content of glycine in dorsal and ventral gray in the normal and experimental animals, a 50% loss of small neurons was found to be paralleled by reductions of 40 and 45% in the content of glycine in dorsal and ventral gray matter (Davidoff *et al.*, 1967*b*).

Examination of the histological sections showed no evidence of glial cell proliferation, cavity formation, or edema. It was therefore not possible to explain the reduction in glycine other than by concluding that the interneurons "removed" by aortic occlusion contained glycine at levels significantly higher than those found in other spinal elements. This was confirmed by the statistical correlation between the content of glycine and the count of small neurons.

The possibility that the surgical procedure produced a nonspecific loss of amino acids was ruled out by the finding that the content of GABA did not change during the change in neuronal count nor with the degree of neurological deficit. Furthermore, the content of glutamine was unchanged

TABLE 2. Content of Inhibitory Amino Acids, Excitatory Amino Acids, and Glutamine Following Loss of Interneurons

			Content of amino acid (μmol/g)[a]	
	Condition (*n*)		Dorsal gray	Ventral gray
Glycine	Normal	(9)	5.65 ± 0.55	7.08 ± 0.98
	Experimental	(9)	4.05 ± 1.20^{b}	4.95 ± 1.40^{b}
GABA	Normal	(8)	2.23 ± 0.66	1.07 ± 0.25
	Experimental	(8)	2.12 ± 0.38	1.33 ± 0.45
Glutamate	Normal	(8)	6.48 ± 0.40	5.39 ± 0.48
	Experimental	(8)	4.72 ± 0.90^{b}	4.48 ± 0.72^{b}
Aspartate	Normal	(8)	2.05 ± 0.45	3.06 ± 0.48
	Experimental	(8)	1.54 ± 0.58^{c}	2.41 ± 0.76^{c}
Glutamine	Normal	(3)	5.30 ± 0.69	5.35 ± 0.19
	Experimental	(8)	5.09 ± 1.38	5.01 ± 1.32

[a] Mean $\pm$ SD.
[b] Significant at $P < 0.005$.
[c] Significant at $P < 0.05$.

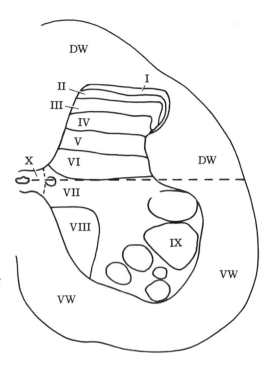

FIGURE 3. Schematic drawing of the laminations of the spinal gray matter at the seventh lumbar spinal segment in cat (DW, dorsal white; VW, ventral white). After Rexed (1954).

in the animals with decreased numbers of interneurons (Davidoff *et al.*, 1967*b*).

Although glutamate levels in the experimental samples were significantly decreased in both dorsal and ventral gray, no correlation was found between its content in these areas and the neuronal count. However, the content of aspartate was also decreased in gray matter, but a significant correlation was found between the content of aspartate in gray matter and the count of small neurons (Davidoff *et al.*, 1967*b*). The physiological significance of this result has been discussed elsewhere (Aprison and Werman, 1968) (see also Chapter 4).

The results of these experiments employing the technique of aortic occlusion are consistent with the idea that glycine and not GABA is concentrated in the interneurons located in Rexed's laminae V–IX (see Fig. 3). At the conclusion of these studies it was suggested that GABA probably functions as an inhibitory transmitter at receptor sites located in the Rexed's laminae I–IV (Davidoff *et al.*, 1967*b*). More recent work showing the immunocytochemical localization of glutamate decarboxylase (McLaughlin *et al.*, 1975) and the distribution studies by Miyata and

Otsuka (1975) employing 200- or 500-μm-square blocks of frozen spinal cord confirms this idea and supports the suggestion that GABA is the presynaptic inhibitory transmitter which is highly concentrated in the interneurons of the dorsal horn.

2.3. Autoradiographic Localization Studies with [³H]Glycine

Employing the technique of autoradiography, Hökfelt and Ljungdahl (1971) as well as Matus and Dennison (1971) demonstrated that after slices of spinal cord from rats were incubated with [³H]glycine, the labeled amino acid appeared associated predominantly with many but *not all* nerve terminals. At the light microscopic level, a higher concentration of grains was noted over gray matter than over white matter. Dotlike and fiberlike accumulations of grains were reported over the neuropil on many but not all neurons in the gray matter. Strong accumulations were reported over small cell bodies in the area corresponding to lamina VI and the dorsal part of lamina VII. At the ultrastructural level, Hökfelt and Ljungdahl (1971) reported that labeled glycine not only accumulated in certain boutons, but also in thin myelinated axons and glial elements. The latter may represent the glial uptake mechanism suggested for inactivation of glycine and gluta- mate. Matus and Dennison (1972) noted that the electron microscopic autoradiographs showed accumulations of grains in about 60% of nerve endings containing "flat" vesicles but not with boutons containing round vesicles. The latter usually have a diameter of about 400 Å whereas the flat or ellipsoidal vesicles are smaller in size. In addition, no labeling above background occurred in myelinated axons. The association of [³H]glycine with flat vesicles in certain boutons was confirmed by Ljungdahl and Hökfelt (1973). Thus Uchizono's 1965 hypothesis, namely that ellipsoidal or flat vesicles are associated with the presynaptic nerve ending of the inhibitory synapse whereas round vesicles are in presynaptic nerve endings of excitatory synapses, was of considerable interest since it appeared that the shape of the vesicles present in terminals may be correlated with the physiological role of the synapse. Therefore, the uptake of [³H]glycine into nerve endings containing ellipsoidal or flat vesicles was indeed of great importance.

Since Matus and Dennison (1972) found that only 60% of the nerve endings containing flat vesicles showed accumulations of grains, these data support the suggestion that other inhibitory transmitters (i.e., taurine, alanine, peptides, etc.) may be associated with the remaining 40% of these axonal endings. Recently Lane *et al.* (1977) reported a unique distribution of taurine in canine spinal cord. Thus, this area of research is only beginning.

Other interesting research approaches in this area have recently appeared. Dennison *et al.* (1976) studied the localization of radioactivity after perfusion of [³H]glycine through the central canal of the lumbosacral cord of spinalized cats. They found 82% of the synapses accumulating activity contained flat vesicles. Price *et al.* (1976) used direct microinjection of [³H]glycine to label synapses in rat ventral horn cells *in vivo*. Identification of these synapses was made by electron microscopic autoradiography. These investigators found that (1) the grain density was greatest in the synaptic terminals, (2) a high proportion of axosomatic and proximal axodendritic synapses take up [³H]glycine, and (3) many of the labeled terminals have elliptical and pleomorphic vesicles. Price's group reported that [³H]glycine was taken up into 40% of synapses in the neuropil of ventral horns, in contrast with the *in vitro* studies of Iversen and Bloom (1972) which showed selective uptake into approximately 28% of nerve terminals in homogenates of whole spinal cord. One explanation of the higher value of Price *et al.* (1976) was the fact that they studied synapses only in the ventral horn rather than the whole spinal cord.

2.4. Presence of Glycine in Specific Presynaptic Nerve Terminals

In Section 2, three findings were presented which provide evidence that glycine is localized in the nerve endings of the interneurons of spinal gray matter. These findings are that (1) the uneven distribution of glycine in spinal gray matter corresponded to the regions containing the majority of interneurons, (2) the fall in glycine levels in central and ventral gray matter after ligation of the thoracic aorta was correlated with the selective loss of interneurons, and (3) the accumulations of labeled glycine occurred in nerve endings containing flat vesicles as seen in electron microscopic autoradiograms after perfusion of the central canal, direct microinjection, or incubation of slices of spinal cord with [³H]glycine. Since the nerve terminals on the presynaptic side of the inhibitory synapses on the motoneurons in the lumbosacral spinal cord of the cat are the axonal endings of the interneurons, the presynaptic criterion appears to be satisfied.

Perhaps it would not be presumptuous for the authors to point out that if the *neurochemical* studies had not been done in the early and mid-1960s, the renewed interest in amino acids as transmitters, and more specifically the discovery that glycine is probably the postsynaptic inhibitory neurotransmitter, would have been delayed. One can certainly ask the question, "Would neurophysiologists working in the area of identification of transmitters have added glycine to their microelectrodes if the literature pointed out only that the inhibitory effects of glycine (and several other amino acids) were nonspecific?'' The authors believe the young investigator should be on the alert when the Presynaptic Criterion is suggested not to be as important as the others (Snyder *et al.*, 1973*a*). In truth, it fits well with the other two, and the *three together* provide a powerful set of criteria to use in the final identification of a putative transmitter (Werman and Aprison, 1968; Aprison and Werman, 1968).

3. THE CRITERION OF IDENTITY OF ACTION

3.1. Neurophysiological Data from Spinal Cord

As discussed earlier, the inhibitory properties of glycine were known in the early 1960s but these actions were considered nonspecific. When glycine molecules were passed by iontophoresis onto the surface of motoneurons, the firing rate of these neurons was inhibited. In an early survey of the effects of many amino acids on the firing rate of spinal neurons, Curtis and Watkins (1960) rated glycine as only a weak inhibitory agent. However, after noting the glycine distribution data for the lumbosacral spinal cord, Werman and co-workers (1966) immediately repeated these extracellular iontophoretic studies and found that not only was glycine comparable to GABA in inhibiting spinal neurons, but in many cases it was a better inhibitor. In order to study these inhibitory actions of glycine, a parallel microelectrode containing glycine trailed by 40–100 μm a double-barreled microelectrode for intracellular recording and current delivery. In this manner, glycine was released by iontophoresis into the extraneuronal space while recording intracellularly. Iontophoretic administration of glycine regularly produced an increase in membrane potential and a fall in membrane resistance. The hyperpolarization of motoneurons by glycine was rapid in onset and was readily reversible; it was increased when iontophoretic currents were increased (see Fig. 4, A_1–A_4). Glycine inhibited spike electrogenesis and decreased the amplitude of both excitatory and inhibitory (IPSP) postsynaptic potentials in a graded fashion. In all motoneurons tested, extracellular glycine increased the ionic conductance (increase in chloride permeability), a phenomenon associated with postsynaptic inhibition (see Fig. 4, B_1–B_2). The increased conductance was directly related to the dose of glycine. Intracellular glycine was ineffective.

When studying an IPSP in an L_7 motoneuron, Werman *et al.* (1967, 1968) showed that a supramaximal dose of glycine caused complete abolition of the IPSP, i.e., the IPSP reached its equilibrium potential of glycine-produced hyperpolarization and the inhibitory process. When the equilibrium potential was changed by passing hyperpolarizing current, a depolarizing IPSP was recorded (see Fig. 4, C_1–C_3). These data confirmed the

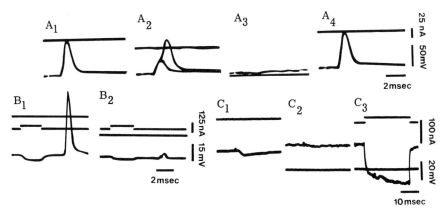

FIGURE 4. The effects of glycine on membrane potential, action potential, and membrane conductance in L_7 motoneurons and evidence for the equivalence of equilibrium potentials for the IPSP and the polarization produced by glycine. Current calibration refers to glycine iontophoretic current. A_1, Antidromic spike (before application of glycine); A_2, two superimposed traces, 1 and 2 sec after the onset of 31 nA glycine; A_3, 2 sec after onset of 90 nA glycine; A_4, 12 sec after turning off glycine; B_1, control conductance measured with 35-nA current pulse and antidromic spike; B_2, during 189 nA glycine. C_1 shows a control IPSP in L_7 motoneurons elicited by stimulation of dorsal root L_6; C_2 shows the marked reduction of the IPSP during application of 193 nA of glycine; C_3 shows that while the glycine current was maintained, delivery of a 35-nA pulse of inward current caused the IPSP to reverse, i.e., in the depolarizing direction. Reprinted with permission from Aprison (1978).

equivalence of the equilibrium potentials of the glycine-produced hyperpolarization and the inhibitory process. Thus, data were available which showed that both glycine and the inhibitory transmitter released by stimulating presynaptic cells evoked identical ionic responses in the membrane of motoneurons (Werman et al., 1967, 1968).

The observations on motoneurons were soon confirmed by Curtis et al. (1968a). The group from Canberra also reported that iontophoretically administered glycine, β-alanine, and GABA hyperpolarized spinal motoneurons in cats. These authors found that the reversal potential for these hyperpolarizations was similar to that of the inhibitory postsynaptic potentials. Comparable observations have also been reported for spinal interneurons (Ten Bruggencate and Engberg, 1968; Curtis et al., 1968a).

3.2. Neurophysiological Data from Other CNS Areas

It is beyond the scope of this chapter to discuss the neurophysiological studies involving other synapses in the CNS. The interested student of neurobiology is referred directly to the following references for discussion of work on (1) the *cuneate nucleus* (Galindo *et al.*, 1967; Davidson and Southwick, 1971; Kelly and Renaud, 1971, 1973*b*; Hill *et al.*, 1973, 1976); (2) the *brain stem cells* (Davis and Huffmann, 1969; Hösli and Haas, 1972; Hösli *et al.*, 1971*a*; Tebēcis and DiMaria, 1972; Tebēcis *et al.*, 1971; Ten Bruggencate and Engberg, 1971; Ten Bruggencate and Sonnhof, 1972); (3) *cortical neurons* (Krnjević and Phillis, 1963; Kelly and Krnjević, 1969; Biscoe *et al.*, 1972); and (4) *cerebellar neurons* (Kawamura and Provini, 1970; Geller and Woodward, 1974).

It should be pointed out that the electrophysiological studies of glycine on cortical and cerebellar neurons indicate that its potency on these cells was much less than that of GABA. Recently Krnjević *et al.* (1977) estimated that the postsynaptic action of glycine was less than 1/12th the action of GABA in the cat cerebal cortex whereas in the spinal cord, glycine was more than five times as potent as GABA. These data and the neurochemical data to be referred to later support the suggestion that glycine probably does not act as an inhibitory transmitter in cerebral cortex and cerebellum unless it does so in a small group of specialized cells that might be missed in studies involving relatively large areas (Aprison, 1971).

3.3. The Postsynaptic Inhibitory Transmitter in the Cat Lumbosacral Spinal Cord

Review of the data in the preceding subsections of Section 3 indicates that the action of glycine on the synaptic membrane of the motoneuron in the spinal cord is remarkably similar to that of the transmitter released by stimulating inhibitory interneurons. Thus, the Criterion of Identity of Action appears to be satisfied for these synapses of cat spinal cord.

4. THE RELEASE CRITERION

4.1. The Problem

It had been known in the early 1960s that a number of amino acids including glycine are accumulated in brain slices to levels above those in the incubation medium and that the uptake involves a carrier-mediated process which is dependent on available energy (Tsukada *et al.*, 1963; Blasberg and Lajtha, 1965). These data suggested to many biochemists that these amino acids would be used solely in metabolic processes. During this period it was also reported that the concentration of glycine in cerebrospinal fluid (CSF) was very low (Aprison and Werman, 1965; Humoller *et al.*, 1966; Dickinson and Hamilton, 1966). When the ratio of glycine in CSF to glycine in blood was calculated, it was found that glycine has one of the lowest ratios among the amino acids measured in these two fluids. Why was this ratio so low? Did it imply another role for glycine—a functional role? On the basis of such data, Aprison and Werman (1965, 1968) and Werman and Aprison (1968) suggested that once released, a neurotransmitter would have to be rapidly removed from a synaptic cleft and the region of the receptor. Such a process could be an uptake system similar to that noted in the *in vitro* studies with brain slices and/or involving passage of the amino acid into the circulatory system. Such a process also would readily account for the extremely low CSF/blood ratio for glycine if the movement of glycine molecules from CSF to blood was markedly greater than from blood to CSF.

These concepts immediately point to several problems of trying to demonstrate release of a neurotransmitter from its functional compartment in nerve endings after the electrophysiological stimulation of appropriate neural circuits. First, a rapid and efficient uptake system operating for glycine would tend to reduce markedly the probability of demonstrating its presence in the synaptic cleft after stimulation of proper inputs to that synapse(s). An inhibitor of glycine uptake would greatly facilitate the consistent demonstration of a stimulus-dependent release of glycine. Such a specific inhibitor is not yet available; work directed toward identifying such a compound would be of great value!

Another major problem is the inability to ascertain if the amount of glycine released comes only from the functional transmitter compartment or pool and not the metabolic pool. One approach to solving this problem has been in the use of radioactive glycine. However, even if radioactive glycine is used, one cannot be entirely certain that it is being exclusively taken up and released from glycinergic nerve terminals. Furthermore, even if it is solely within the glycinergic nerve ending, there may be at least two and possibly more glycine compartments (Aprison *et al.,* 1975; Aprison, 1978), and the investigator cannot be certain that the glycine molecules are being released from the functional pool. On the other hand, autoradio-graphic localization data (discussed in Section 2.3) indicate that [^{3}H]glycine is mainly if not exclusively taken up by specific nerve terminals in the gray matter of the spinal cord. These presynaptic terminals seem to contain flat or ellipsoidal synaptic vesicles (Matus and Dennison, 1972; Ljungdahl and Hökfelt, 1973) which are currently thought to be associated with inhibitory synapses. Thus, one can at least be fairly certain that the labeled amino acid is within the glycinergic terminals.

Before discussing in detail the data on release of glycine from various types of preparations, we shall now review some data from uptake studies. These studies indicate that glycinergic terminals in specific areas of the CNS possess a unique property.

4.2.   Studies on the Uptake of Glycine by Nerve Endings

From the considerations just noted, it became apparent that investigators had to design unique experiments to clarify three possible mechanisms for the termination of the action of released transmitter in the immediate vicinity of the glycinergic synapse: (1) uptake into the presynaptic cell, the postsynaptic cell, surrounding glia, or any combination of these cells; (2) diffusion out of the synaptic cleft through the extraneuronal fluid to some other site; and/or (3) catabolism by a degradative enzyme. Following the suggestion by Aprison and Werman (1968) that item (1) was probably the major mechanism of glycine removal from the postsynaptic receptor at glycinergic synapses, a number of studies were published which support this idea. Neal and Pickles (1969) and Neal (1969) reported that labeled glycine was rapidly taken up by tissue slices prepared from rat spinal cord. Neal (1971) extended the earlier studies to show that [^{14}C]glycine is taken up by slices of tissue prepared from various brain areas of the rat as well as from spinal cord and gray matter. Neal (1969, 1971) reported that the K_m of glycine uptake by rat spinal cord was 31 μM. However, these studies did not demonstrate whether the accumulation of labeled glycine represented net uptake or exchange with the endogenous glycine in the tissue.

Since many amino acids have been shown to be transported or taken up by brain slices, Johnston and Iversen (1971) and Logan and Snyder (1971, 1972) reasoned that those amino acids which were shown to be putative transmitters may have an uptake system with higher affinity than amino acids which were not candidates for the role of transmitters. One could easily argue that a high-affinity uptake system would probably be required for efficient removal of the amino acids (putative transmitters) from the synaptic cleft (see Curtis et al., 1976a). Johnston and Iversen (1971) and Logan and Snyder (1972) reported the presence of both a high- and low-affinity transport system for labeled glycine in preparations from the spinal cord of the rat; it is very interesting that only the low-affinity transport system was detected in the cerebral cortex. A similar high and low uptake system has been reported in the cat spinal cord by Balcar and Johnston (1973). Using nuclei-free homogenates of rat CNS tissues, Logan and Snyder (1972) reported that glycine was accumulated by a single-component low-affinity uptake in the cerebral cortex ($K_m = 760 \ \mu M$), whereas in the spinal cord, double reciprocal plots for glycine uptake produced curves that could be resolved graphically into two components. The high-affinity system in spinal cord had a K_m of 26 μM and the low-affinity system had a K_m of 923 μM.

In 1972, Bennett et al. reported that Na$^+$ is required for activity of the high-affinity uptake system in the rat spinal cord. They used synaptosomal preparations in their investigations of the accumulation of glutamic acid, aspartic acid, and glycine. All three amino acids were taken up by separate Na^+-dependent high-affinity systems in the spinal cord. In synaptosomes prepared from the cerebral cortex, the former two amino acids were taken up by separate Na^+-dependent high-affinity systems, whereas glycine was taken up by a low-affinity system only.

Voaden *et al.* (1974), studying the isolated retina of the frog, reported that GABA accumulated within both the amacrine and horizontal cells. However, in the dark adapted retina labeled glycine specifically entered a single population of cells, the amacrine cells. The uptake processes were both Na^+ dependent, being reduced by 85% in its absence. Glycine uptake appeared to be mediated by a high-affinity system with a K_m of 16.7 μM.

Data for the K_m in low- and high-affinity systems are summarized in Table 3. Neurochemical studies support the fact that the high-affinity uptake system is Na^+ dependent whereas the low-affinity uptake system is only slightly influenced by this cation.

Aprison and McBride (1973) studied the uptake of [U-^{14}C]glycine and *unlabeled* glycine into crude preparations of synaptosomes containing pinched-off nerve endings isolated from the telencephalon and spinal cord. Studies with unlabeled glycine were included in order to circumvent the objection that an exchange reaction between labeled exogenous and unlabeled endogenous glycine molecules might be occurring instead of net uptake in the studies referred to earlier. In studies with labeled glycine, Aprison and McBride (1973) found that during the first 3 min the rates of [U-^{14}C]glycine ($8 \times 10^{-7} M$) uptake by synaptosomal preparations (P$_2$) from

TABLE 3.   Uptake of Labeled Glycine: K_m Values

	K_m (μM)			
	Rat[a]	Rat[b]	Cat[c]	Frog[d,e]
Cerebral cortex				
Low-affinity	250	760	—	—
High-affinity	—	—	—	5[f]
Spinal cord				
Low-affinity	—	923	121	—
High-affinity	36	26	14	26
Retina				
High affinity	—	—	—	17

[a] Johnston and Iversen (1971).
[b] Logan and Snyder (1972).
[c] Balcar and Johnston (1973).
[d] Voaden *et al.* (1974).
[e] Davidoff and Adair (1976).
[f] 5 μM refers to the cerebrum. Other data presented by Davidoff and Adair (1976) are for the optic tectum (12.1 μM) and medulla (35 μM).

TABLE 4.   Net Accumulation of Glycine in a Crude Synaptosomal Fraction
Isolated from the Telencephalon and Spinal Cord of the Rat

Concentration (mM) glycine in incubation medium	Net uptake of glycine[a] (nmol/mg protein/min)		Ratio (SC/Tel)
	Spinal cord	Telencephalon	
0.0375	1.20 ± 0.05	0.22 ± 0.06	5.4
0.075	2.00 ± 0.31	0.70 ± 0.03	2.8
0.150	3.36 ± 0.20	1.65 ± 0.26	2.0

[a] Mean ± SEM.
Source: From Aprison and McBride (1973).

the spinal cord and telencephalon were estimated to be 0.100 and 0.0243 nmol/mg protein/min, respectively. The addition of either 10^{-5} M ouabain or 10^{-3} M DNP significantly inhibited this accumulation of [U-^{14}C]glycine. Approximately 85% of the radioactivity taken up by the incubated P_2 fraction was found in the subfraction of P_2 containing synaptosomes. In the second group of experiments, a net accumulation of unlabeled glycine was observed when the crude synaptosomal fraction was incubated at 37°C in the presence of 0.0375, 0.075, and 0.15 mM glycine (see Table 4). This uptake of unlabeled glycine appeared to occur against a large concentration gradient. In the presence of 37.5 μM glycine, the rate of uptake was more than five times greater in preparations from the spinal cord than in similar preparations from the telencephalon. At still lower concentrations of glycine, the difference between the uptake into P_2 from spinal cord and telencephalon may be even greater.

Thus, the data and conclusions from several laboratories on the subject of uptake of glycine are in agreement. It is now widely accepted that termination of the glycine inhibitory response at the glycinergic synapse is due mainly to its removal by an efficient reuptake process.

4.3.   *In Situ* Release Studies

4.3.1.   *Spinal Cord Preparations*

Measurement of the release of endogenous glycine in cat spinal cord after stimulation of peripheral nerves at various rates has been attempted employing two types of preparations in the authors' laboratory. One type of experimental approach was to prepare a closed dural sac containing the lumbar cord of the cat after fine polyethylene tubing was inserted into the subdural space from both ends. Tight ligatures were placed around the sacral and thoracic dura and cord. The preparation looked like a "condenser." Fluid (saline with and without Ca^{2+}) was introduced into the polyethylene tubing at the sacral end and allowed to pass over and around the spinal cord at very slow rates. It was removed through the tubing at the thoracic end, and then emptied into a fraction collector which permitted fixed volumes to be collected in serial test tubes. In the other approach, after laminectomy and incision of the dura, a plastic chamber was prepared and fixed to the cord surface; the area was immediately superfused with 0.9% NaCl or with artificial CSF at slow rates. Tubes were collected as just described.

In both experimental situations, a viable spinal cord preparation capable of transmitting reflex action from peripheral nerves to ventral roots was produced (M. H. Aprison, R. A. Davidoff, and R. Werman, unpublished results). A slow efflux of amino acids including glycine, glutamate, glutamine, and aspartate into the perfusate occurred during a period as long as 10 hr. The comparatively high background level of amino acids, which was variable from perfusion period to perfusion period, made it difficult to demonstrate convincingly significant increments in glycine release during nerve stimulation. Although significant release was measured in approximately 25% of preliminary experiments, the fact that the amino acids released into the perfusate were those present in highest concentration in cat plasma suggested that much of this material may have diffused into the subarachnoid space from blood in the pial vessels.

Aprison then shifted to a different experimental technique—the use of a "push–pull" cannula and [^{14}C]glycine to label specific nerve endings, thereby obtaining a more sensitive and hopefully selective method. The problem arising from the diffusion of amino acids from blood would perhaps be circumvented by the direct radioactive labeling of the transmitter pool within the nerve terminals. This technique proved to be a useful approach since the detection of labeled transmitter released in response to stimulation of nerves was possible owing to the sensitivity of radioactive techniques. Following introduction into the tissue or subarachnoid space labeled glycine was rapidly taken up by cat and rat spinal cord and was shown to be present in both "free" and "bound" forms (compounds such as protein) as reported by Koenig (1958) and Shank and Aprison (1970a).

A cat preparation was used in the first experiments and consisted of an exposed cord (L_5–S_2) under oil which was temperature-controlled. The skin flaps of the laminectomy incision were arranged to form a pouch which was filled with mineral oil. Body temperature and the temperature of oil pool were maintained at $37 \pm 0.1°C$ by an automatic direct-current-operating temperature-control device (Richardson *et al.*, 1965). Movement of the spinal cord was minimized by rigid clamping of the spinal column and the pelvis. Following dural incision, specific roots were transected and mounted on silver hooks. The L_5, L_6 dorsal roots were placed on one set of stimulating electrodes, L_7, S_1 dorsal roots on another, and ventral S_1, L_7 on recording electrodes. The neuronal activity was continuously monitored with standard neurophysiological recording equipment. A small incision was made in the pia and the cannula was carefully inserted into the spinal cord with as little pressure as possible. With the aid of a micromanipulator, the end of the cannula was placed in the region of the interneuronal pool just dorsal to the motoneurons. Methylene blue studies indicated that leakage often occurred around the cannula. The placing and sealing of the cannula in the spinal cord were very important and failure to do this properly contributed to the number of unsuccessful experiments. This problem had to be corrected by carefully sealing the cannula in the cord. In a few experiments this was done using Eastman 910 compound. The interneuronal pool in cord of a live cat then was labeled with [^{14}C]glycine by passing a solution containing the labeled amino acid through the implanted cannula. Since [^{3}H]methoxyinulin is not taken up into cells but remains in the intraneuronal compartment, it also was added to the [^{14}C]glycine solution for control purposes.

After the surgical and neurophysiological manipulations were completed, artificial cat CSF was passed through the cannula with the aid of a Harvard pump. Dorsal roots were stimulated at specific times. Samples were collected and an aliquot from each tube was monitored for total radioactivity (^{14}C and ^{3}H). Another aliquot from each sample was used to separate the amino acids in the perfusate. This was done by first converting the amino acids to the dinitrophenyl derivatives and then separating each derivative by thin-layer chromatography (TLC) on ChromAR sheets. The yellow spots were eluted and then the amount of label was measured (Shank and Aprison, 1970b). Again, only about 15–20% of the experiments were successful in showing a release of labeled glycine during stimulation of the dorsal roots (Aprison and Werman, unpublished results).

In 1971, Jordan and Webster loaded the spinal cord of a cat with [^{14}C]glycine and then perfused the central canal with artificial CSF containing 10^{-5} M p-hydroxymercuribenzoate. These investigators reported that in four out of six experiments an increased release *in vivo* occurred after stimulation (5-HZ) of femoral and sciatic nerves. Although p-hydroxymercuribenzoate is not considered a specific blocker of glycine, Neal and Pickles (1969) reported that this compound reduced the uptake of [^{14}C]glycine into slices of the spinal cord from rat. Cutler (1975) reported that when p-chloromercuribenzoate (0.1 mM) was used in the medium to perfuse a rat spinal cord *in vivo* (through the subarachnoid space), glycine release occurred consistently after stimulation of the sciatic nerve.

In 1976, Fagg and co-workers reported preliminary experiments in which they studied the *in vivo* release of endogenous amino acids including glycine from the cat spinal cord. They perfused the central canal (L_4–S_1) of the cat spinal cord with artificial CSF (0.06 ml/min) after the animals were spinalized at C_1 under halothane anesthesia and immobilized with gallamine triethiodide. Bipolar platinum electrodes, 5 mm apart at the tip, were inserted into the cord at C_2 to deliver the stimuli. When 10^{-4} *M* *p*-chloromercuriphenylsulfonate (pCMS) was added to the artificial CSF to inhibit uptake of amino acids, a significant increase in efflux of leucine, aspartate, GABA, glutamate, lysine, and proline in addition to glycine was noted. Further increases in all these amino acids except lysine and proline resulted from stimulation of descending spinal tracts with pCMS in the perfusion medium. Fagg *et al.* (1976) report that stimulation in the absence of pCMS did not consistently increase the efflux of any of these amino acids. These authors suggest a note of caution when they conclude that their data show that the stimulated release of glutamate, glycine, GABA, and alanine could be related to proposed transmitter roles (Graham *et al.,* 1967; Curtis and Johnston, 1974), whereas the release of leucine could not. The presence of amino acids in the effluent that do not affect the postsynaptic receptor directly, but are released along with the natural transmitter, may be indirect evidence against vesicular release. Thus, if cytoplasmic release occurs, it may not be unusual to find one or more nontransmitter amino acids released along with the transmitter in response to a proper stimulus.

4.3.2. Medulla Oblongata and Optic Tectum Preparations

In 1974, Roberts reported that *in vivo* stimulation of the medial lemniscus in the rat resulted in a significant increase in the release of glycine and GABA into a very small Perspex cylinder (25 μl) which had been surgically placed on the surface of the medulla over the region of the cuneate and gracile nuclei. Since stimulation of the medial lemniscus produced inhibition of the cuneothalamic relay system (Andersen *et al.,* 1962; Davidson and Suckling, 1967), these data were very important because they support the suggestion that glycine may be the inhibitory transmitter released from some of the interneurons of the cuneate nucleus. Thus, in addition to Roberts's results, three different sets of data support such a role for glycine at this site: (1) the neurochemical measures which show that the highest glycine levels in brain are in the medulla oblongata (Aprison *et al.,* 1969);

(2) the neurophysiological measurements which show that glycine inhibits the firing of cuneate neurons (see Section 3.2 for references); and (3) the neuropharmacological data which indicate that there is a strychnine antagonism of the glycine effect in this region but not of that of GABA (Kelly and Renaud, 1973*a,b*; Hill *et al.*, 1976).

Reubi and Cúenod (1976) have investigated the pathway in the pigeon which originates in the nucleus isthmi pars parvocellularis (Ipc) and terminates in the optic tectum. These investigators perfused the upper strata of the optic tectum with a push–pull cannula and demonstrated the release of both [^{14}C]glycine and [^{14}C]GABA but not [^{14}C]leucine or [^{14}C]urea after electrical stimulation of the Ipc. No release occurred if other sites were stimulated. Reubi and Cúenod (1976) suggest that the Ipc neuronal terminals in the optic tectum take up glycine and release it upon stimulation of the Ipc nucleus. Glycine levels are higher in this area of the brain than in the cerebral cortex or cerebellum (Aprison *et al.*, 1969).

4.3.3. Retinal Preparation

In Section 5, neurochemical data are reviewed which suggest that glycine may be an inhibitory transmitter released from interneurons located in the retina. However, in this section the authors wish to discuss the evidence of *in situ* release of glycine from the retina before the other data are presented.

Ehinger and Lindberg-Bauer (1976) prepared adult cats so the head was placed in a position such that the vertex cornea of one eye pointed upward. This eye was opened by removal of the cornea and anterior uvea; after carefully removing all the vitreous fluid, the eyecup was filled with a solution (superfusion fluid) containing 0.9% NaCl and [^{3}H]glycine. The preparation was then placed in darkness or very dim red light. Two cannulas, 10 mm apart, were placed in front of the retina and the superfusion fluid was pumped into one and out the other. This system provided a 10-mm-long preretinal stream through the fluid filling the eyecup. After superfusion for 15 min, the eyecup was drained and washed, and the fluid changed to one containing 0.9% NaCl and 1.3 m*M*glycine. The superfusion was continued with this solution in the dark for 30 min. Then light flashes (2 sec^{-1}) were given for 10 min. *In vivo* release of [^{3}H]glycine from the retina occurred after the light (flash) stimulation. Continuous light did not cause an increase in efflux of radioactivity. The site of uptake of [^{3}H]glycine into retina was shown by these investigators to be almost exclusively in amacrine cells. In addition, most of the radioactivity released was identified as glycine. The light-evoked release of labeled glycine from retina was dependent on temperature and Ca^{2+}. When the retinas were preloaded with [³H]valine instead of [³H]glycine, it was not possible to detect any light-inducible efflux of radioactivity.

4.4. Release Studies with *in Vitro* Preparations

4.4.1. *Hemisectioned and Intact Spinal Cord*

It is not surprising that the *in vivo* experiments designed to show release of a neurotransmitter such as glycine from spinal cord yield few positive results. These experiments are very difficult since any movement of the brain or spinal cord relative to the cannula which is caused by direct stimulation of the tissues can cause false peaks to appear. Furthermore, it is currently not easy to prevent the reuptake of glycine by cells after release. Perhaps for these reasons, a number of investigators turned to *in vitro* preparations which appeared not to be subject to such technical limitations.

On the basis of the distribution of the content of glycine within the spinal cord of seven vertebrates (Aprison *et al.*, 1969), the isolated amphibian spinal cord (Mitchell and Phillis, 1962; Tebēcis and Phillis, 1969) seemed to be a useful preparation since the biochemical data support the transmitter role of glycine in this tissue. Aprison (1970*a*,*b*) conducted some of these experiments in which the spinal cord of the toad was isolated, hemisectioned, and placed in a modified Lucite bath for transmitter release studies. Stimulation of dorsal roots at very low rates caused a release of [¹⁴C]glycine but not of labeled inulin (see Fig. 5). The ¹⁴C-labeled amino acids in the tissue bath before stimulation, during stimulation, and after stimulation were separated by TLC (Shank and Aprison, 1970*b*). Increased radioactivity in both glycine and serine was found associated with the fractions collected during stimulation (see Fig. 5). These experiments yielded data showing a correlation between the amount of [¹⁴C]glycine released (area under the peak) and the number of stimuli applied to the dorsal roots (Aprison, 1970*b*). Owing to the probable rapid reuptake of released [¹⁴C]glycine, success with this preparation was still not as predictable as one would have preferred.

In 1972, Roberts and Mitchell reported that after incubation of the tissue in the presence of the labeled compound for 40 min, [¹⁴C]glycine could be released consistently from isolated frog or toad hemicords by direct stimulation of the rostral portion of the spinal cords. These investigators did not find release when dorsal or ventral roots were stimulated (150 Hz, 3 msec, 2 mA). After stimulating the rostral cord, Roberts and Mitchell

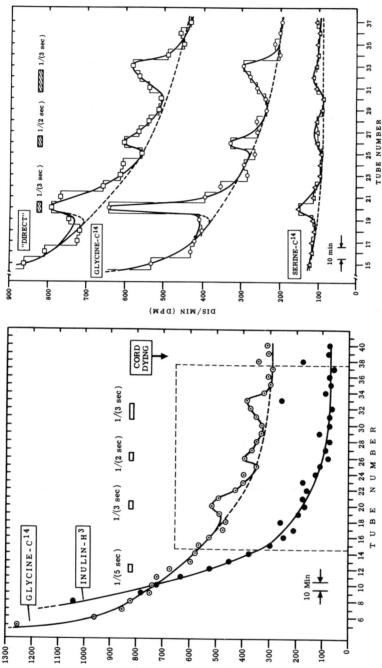

FIGURE 5. Left side: Time course of efflux of [³H]inulin and [¹⁴C]glycine from hemisectioned toad spinal cord at rest and during stimulation. The rate of stimulation and the duration are shown. The samples within the dotted lines (Nos. 15–37) were used for chemical analysis. Right side: Time course of efflux of [¹⁴C]glycine and [¹⁴C]serine from hemisectioned toad spinal cord at rest and during stimulation. Analysis of samples 15–37 showed that only glycine and serine of the amino acids assayed were radioactive. These data are replotted here along with the original data (direct). Reprinted with permission from Aprison et al. (1975) and Aprison (1978).

also observed a release of [³H]GABA, [¹⁴C]glutamate, and L-[¹⁴C]aspartate, but not of [¹⁴C]serine, L-[-¹⁴C]threonine, [³H]leucine, [¹⁴C]mannitol, or [¹⁴C]urea. Roberts and Mitchell (1972) have reported that after stimulation of the intact rostral cord at a variety of frequencies (5–100 Hz), release of labeled glycine is proportional to the number of applied stimuli. These authors speculate that such stimulation excited the glycinergic interneurons either directly or indirectly via descending inhibitory fibers.

It is not clear why dorsal root stimulation did not produce a release of amino acids. Further, it is surprising that these investigators did not find biochemical evidence of greater metabolism of the labeled amino acids after the hemicords were incubated for 40 min in the presence of either [¹⁴C]glycine, L-[¹⁴C]serine, or L-[¹⁴C]glutamate. In view of the positive results after stimulation of the rostral cord, one would have expected [¹⁴C]glycine to be released in their experiments in which incubations were carried out in the presence of [¹⁴C]serine, since serine is readily converted to glycine (McBride *et al.*, 1973; Shank and Aprison, 1970*a*).

4.4.2. Slices of Spinal Cord and Brain

Hopkin and Neal (1970, 1971) reported that electrical stimulation and elevated K^+ concentrations caused an efflux of [¹⁴C]glycine from slices of rat spinal cord. After slices of spinal cord were incubated for 15 min, [¹⁴C]glycine was added to give a final concentration of $6 \times 10^{-7}\ M$ and allowed to be taken up into the slices during the next 30 min. The slices were recovered and transferred to a small perfusion chamber. There the slices were stimulated either electrically via two silver electrodes by applying rectangular pulses of 100 Hz (5-msec duration, 20 mA) or by the addition of high K^+ to the medium, yielding a final concentration of 40 mM. In either case, the increase in efflux of glycine was not reduced by the absence of Ca^{2+} in the medium. Hopkin and Neal (1971) also reported the efflux of [³H]GABA and [¹⁴C]glutamate from rat spinal cord slices after electrical stimulation, but not [³H]alanine or [¹⁴C]urea.

Two reports appeared in 1971 and one in 1972 which described some factors influencing both the spontaneous efflux and the electrically induced efflux of [¹⁴C]glycine and [³H]GABA from rat spinal cord slices. Cutler *et al.* (1971, 1972) found that a relatively specific transport mechanism mediated the efflux of [¹⁴C]glycine from preloaded spinal cord slices. These investigators reported that after incubation of pooled slices in 10 ml of glycine-free medium for 30 min, the rate of loss of endogenous glycine and that of [¹⁴C]glycine were quite similar; these results suggested that there was uniform isotopic labeling of the endogenous glycine pools in nerve cells within the tissue. Cutler's group noted that the rate of spontaneous efflux of [^{14}C]glycine was increased by the addition of unlabeled glycine to the superfusion medium and concluded that exchange diffusion occurred. Thus, extracellular glycine exchanged with intracellular [^{14}C]glycine, but did not affect the rates of efflux of labeled GABA, proline, L-lysine, or cycloleucine. Ouabain increased the rate of efflux of [^{14}C]glycine and [^{3}H]GABA, but did not affect [^{14}C]urea efflux. Furthermore, Cutler and co-workers found that the carrier mechanism for spontaneous efflux was saturable in the presence of high intracellular glycine concentrations.

Hammerstad et al. (1971) and Cutler et al. (1972) confirmed the report of Hopkin and Neal (1970) that [^{14}C]glycine is released upon stimulation of rat spinal cord slices. Hammerstad et al. (1971) found there was a greater than twofold increase in the efflux of [^{14}C]glycine and [^{3}H]GABA from spinal cord slices upon electrical stimulation but could demonstrate only a negligible increase in the release of [^{3}H]lysine or [^{14}C]urea. The maximum increase in release was usually noted 2–6 min after stimulation.

These authors also studied the specificity of electrically stimulated efflux. They found after preloading the spinal cord slices with various labeled amino acids prior to stimulation that [^{14}C]taurine was released to the same extent as [^{14}C]glycine and [^{3}H]GABA, whereas [^{3}H]lysine, [^{3}H]proline, and [1-^{14}C]aminocyclopentanecarboxylic acid (cycloleucine) were released in extremely small quantities. Hammerstad et al. (1971) also reported that there were no statistically significant differences in the release of glycine and GABA from electrically stimulated slices of cerebral cortex, cerebellum, or spinal cord of the rat. Since evidence suggests that glycine and GABA are inhibitory transmitters in different areas of the CNS, these results are surprising; the data on the cortical and cerebellar slices conflict with some other studies reported in this section. Potassium in concentrations of 30–60 mM or sodium in low levels (i.e., 28 mM) in the superfusion medium did not influence the electrically stimulated release of glycine or GABA from slices of spinal cord. Hammerstad and co-workers also noted that when incubation of the slices in standard medium was followed by superfusion with Ca^{2+}-free medium, no effect was found on the stimulated release of these two amino acids. However, when the slices were incubated and superfused in Ca^{2+}-free medium containing 2 mM EDTA, there was a marked fall in the amount of electrically stimulated release of glycine and GABA. Finally, these authors also studied the effect of strychnine, ouabain, and cyanide on release of these two amino acids after electrical stimulation of spinal cord slices. Strychnine (1 mM), which abolishes the depressant action of glycine on spinal and medullary neurons, had no effect on the release of glycine from the spinal cord slices subjected to electrical stimulation, whereas superfusion with 0.4 mM ouabain completely abolished the release of both glycine and GABA. When the superfusate contained 1 mM cyanide, a differential effect on the release was noted; release of labeled glycine was inhibited by approximately 50% whereas no effect on labeled GABA release was observed.

Mulder and Snyder (1974) have studied the release of exogenous (labeled) amino acids from slices of CNS tissues following potassium depolarization. They report glycine was released from slices of rat spinal cord but not from the cerebral cortex, whereas much less release from either CNS area was noted with alanine, arginine, histidine, lysine, serine, and phenylalanine. In addition, depletion of sodium during labeling of slices with radioactive amino acids resulted in the markedly decreased release of these compounds during the test period. Because of the evidence for a high-affinity uptake of glycine, as well as its sodium dependence, Mulder and Snyder (1974) concluded that potassium-induced release of glycine from spinal cord may involve a specific functional compartment which is labeled with [^{14}C]glycine.

Davies *et al.* (1975) reported on the postnatal changes in potassium-stimulated (44.75 mM), Ca^{2+}-dependent (1.77 mM) release of [^{3}H]glycine and [U-^{14}C]GABA from slices of rat cerebral cortex and spinal cord. They showed that radioactive glycine and GABA were released but not 2-aminoisobutyric acid when the K$^+$ concentration was increased from 4.75 to 44.75 mM in the perfusing medium. This solution was passed through their special apparatus which was used to perfuse the minitissue slices from rats of varying ages. The K$^+$-stimulated, Ca^{2+}-dependent release of glycine from slices of adult spinal cord was approximately twice that observed from slices of adult cerebral cortex. Since "high affinity" uptake of glycine into slices of adult cerebral cortex cannot be demonstrated (Johnston and Iversen, 1971), and since neurophysiological data do not support glycine as an inhibitory transmitter in the cerebral cortex, it is interesting that Davies *et al.* (1975) can show K$^+$-stimulated release of radioactive glycine from slices of adult cerebral cortex. Apparently radioactive glycine enters a compartment which can be released by K$^+$ stimulation.

Beart and Bilal (1976) incubated slices of adult rat spinal cord in Krebs bicarbonate medium containing either [^{14}C]glucose, [^{14}C]pyruvate, [^{14}C]serine, or [^{14}C]glyoxylate for 45 min. They noted that 44 mM K$^+$ stimulated the release of [^{14}C]glycine synthesized from [^{14}C]glucose and [^{14}C]serine. These investigators found that the specific activity of glycine released upon incubation of the slices with [^{14}C]glyoxylate and [^{14}C]pyruvate was lower and suggest that these data can be interpreted to reflect compartmentation of glycine within nerve terminals.

Davidoff and Adair (1976) studied the transport and release of [^{3}H]glycine and [^{3}H]GABA in the cerebrum, optic tectum, medulla, and spinal cord of the frog. They found a rapid accumulation of both amino acids from the surrounding medium in these tissues. Significant release of [^{3}H]glycine and [^{3}H]GABA, but not [^{3}H]leucine, was reported after raising the K^+ concentration of the medium used to superfuse the four CNS areas of the frog from 2 to 40 mM for 60 min. This release was Ca^{2+}-dependent.

4.4.3. Synaptosomes

It is now known that synaptosomes possess many of the metabolic properties of intact nervous tissue (Bradford, 1969; Bradford and Thomas, 1969) and respond to stimulation in a manner similar to tissue slices (Bradford, 1970; De Belleroche and Bradford, 1972; Osborne et al., 1973). Further, there appears to be no significant morphological change after electrical stimulation of these preparations (Jones and Bradford, 1971) and it has been suggested that stimulation causes a depolarization of the synaptosomal membrane (Bradford et al., 1973). Therefore, it is not surprising that some investigators turned to the use of synaptosomes in studying the release of transmitters.

Bradford and co-workers were among the first to show the evoked release of endogenous amino acids after electrical or potassium stimulation in preparations of isolated synaptosomes in vitro. There was a significant Ca^{2+}-dependent release of endogenous glycine from synaptosomes isolated from the medulla and spinal cord of the rat (Osborne et al., 1973), whereas there was not a significant release from synaptosomes isolated from cerebral cortex (Bradford, 1970; De Belleroche and Bradford, 1972; Bradford et al., 1973) or hypothalamus (Edwardson et al., 1972; Bradford et al., 1973). More recently, K^+-induced, Ca^{2+}-dependent release of exogenous glycine from synaptosomes isolated from the spinal cord of the rat has been reported (Nelson-Krause and Howard, 1976).

The specificity of the release of glycine from spinal cord and medulla synaptosomes is further suggested from studies with synaptosomes isolated from rats treated with tetanus toxin (Osborne et al., 1973; Osborne and Bradford, 1973). Although there was no change in the synaptosomal content of glycine, there was a significant decrease in its evoked release after stimulation. These findings correlate well with the unaltered levels of glycine in the whole spinal cord after tetanus toxin treatment (Johnston et al., 1969; Fedineć and Shank, 1971; but see Semba and Kano, 1969) and the postulated presynaptic site of blockage of the natural inhibitory transmitter in the spinal cord by the toxin (Brooks et al., 1957; Curtis and DeGroat, 1968; Gushchin et al., 1969) (see Section 5.5).

4.5. Present Status

It may now be clear to the reader that the evidence for the role of glycine in neurotransmission based on the Release Criterion is weaker than the evidence for the other two criteria because of the difficulty in designing the experiments. Certainly the remoteness of the collection site from the stimulated synapses, the relatively insensitive methods to measure endogenous glycine, and the lack of a specific antagonist for the potent uptake of glycine all add to this problem. On the other hand, after an electrical stimulation, release of labeled glycine has been reported (1) from preloaded hemisectioned spinal cord from the toad, (2) from slices of spinal cord from the rat, and (3) from synaptosomes isolated from the medulla and spinal cord. Release of exogenous glycine and some other putative amino acid transmitters from slices of cord also has been reported following potassium depolarization. Thus, all the studies reviewed in Section 4 are suggestive of the release of endogenous glycine by a specific, calcium-dependent mechanism initiated by presynaptic depolarization. The conditions in most of these studies are not sufficiently physiological or definitive to satisfy fully this third criterion for the identification of glycine as a neurotransmitter, at least not until the studies measuring the release of endogenous glycine under physiological conditions are confirmed.

5. OTHER NEUROBIOLOGICAL SUPPORTIVE STUDIES

5.1. Distribution of Glycine in Other Areas of the CNS: Vertebrates

Employing the same neurochemical–anatomical approach used in the studies on the spinal cord of the cat to locate areas of high glycine content, Aprison *et al.* (1969) determined the distribution of glycine in ten areas of the neuraxis in seven vertebrates (cat, rat, caiman, pigeon, bullfrog, catfish, and boa constrictor). These data showed that for each species, the medulla oblongata and spinal cord contained higher levels of glycine than any other area of the brain. In any one species the mean content of glycine in the medulla oblongata was three to seven times higher than the mean content in either the cerebral hemispheres or the cerebellum (Aprison *et al.,* 1969). The data on the different regions of the spinal cord showed that the mean content of glycine in the cervical and lumbar enlargements of the cat, rat, pigeon, and caiman was higher than in the midthoracic cord. It is interesting that in the case of the snake and the catfish, animals without limbs, glycine was uniformly distributed along the spinal cord (Aprison *et al.,* 1969). The data on the vertebrates support the observation that the content of glycine is higher in the regions of the spinal cord which innervate the limbs (cervical and lumbar enlargements), and lower in the thoracic region, which has less musculature to supply (see Table 5). Thus, in the case of the caiman, which has powerful hind limbs and tail, the content of glycine was highest in lumbar and sacral spinal cord. In the pigeon, which has a strong wing musculature, the level of glycine was highest in the cervical cord.

The distribution data for glycine in specific areas of the brain indicated that the medulla oblongata might contain glycinergic synapses (Aprison *et al.,* 1968, 1969). The neurophysiological evidence and release studies reviewed earlier confirmed this suggestion. Thus, in the case of the medulla, another example is available in which the *neurochemical evidence* strongly pointed to an area of the neuraxis in which glycine may function as a transmitter. The success of the neurophysiological and release experiments appear to confirm the validity of the approach made by Aprison and Werman (1965) in suggesting that areas in which glycine is concentrated may be areas containing some neurons capable of utilizing glycine as a transmitter. Certainly the *uneven* content of glycine from the telencephalon

TABLE 5. Content of Glycine (μmol/g) in the Vertebrate CNS

Region	Cat[a]	Rat [b]	Rat [a]	Caiman[a]	Pigeon[a]	Bullfrog[a]	Rabbit[c]	Human[d]
Cerebrum	1.27	0.83	0.95	1.16	1.21	0.71	2.56	1.4[e]
Diencephalon	1.60	—	1.00	1.17	1.32	0.81	2.58	2.4[f]
Midbrain	1.97	1.45	1.55	1.19	1.45	1.37	2.30	—
Medulla	3.42	3.63[g]	3.81	4.03	4.79	3.41	3.86	—
Cerebellum	0.83	1.04	0.62	1.00	1.18	1.08	3.69	1.7[h]
Cervical cord	3.76	—	4.14	4.65	4.80	3.89	—	2.5[i]
Thoracic cord	2.13	—	3.43	3.83	3.20	3.66	—	2.2[i]
Lumbar cord	4.52	—	4.30	5.32	4.53	4.08	—	2.9[i]
Sacral cord	4.53	—	4.08	4.91	—	—	—	—

[a] Aprison *et al.* (1969).
[b] Shaw and Heine (1965).
[c] Wiechert and Schroter (1964).
[d] Boehme *et al.* (1973).
[e] Frontal cortex.
[f] Thalamus.
[g] Pons plus medulla.
[h] Cerebellar cortex.
[i] Average of data on white and gray matter in Table 1 of reference *d*.

TABLE 6. Distribution of Glycine in Five Areas from Three Segments of the Human Spinal Cord

	Glycine content (μmol/g)[a]				
Segment	DW	DG	VG	VW	Lateral column
Cervical	2.31 ± 0.29	2.40 ± 0.31	3.14 ± 0.33	2.28 ± 0.23	2.55 ± 0.33
Thoracic	2.11 ± 0.36	2.18 ± 0.24	2.72 ± 0.47	2.04 ± 0.31	2.13 ± 0.33
Lumbar	2.30 ± 0.31	2.85 ± 0.38	3.65 ± 0.29	2.94 ± 0.27	3.05 ± 0.43

[a] Mean ± SEM (μmol/g); $N = 20$.
Source: From Boehme et al. (1973).

to the sacral spinal cord would be difficult to explain if the sole role of this amino acid was that of a substrate in intermediary metabolism.

Boehme et al. (1973) measured the content of glycine in five areas of the cervical, thoracic, and lumbar human spinal cord and found that the highest levels were in the lumbar ventral gray (see Table 6). Recently Boehme et al. (1976) confirmed their earlier study of 1973 and reported that the content of glycine was highest in the gray matter of the lumbar segments. A comparison of the distribution data of glycine in specific gray and white areas of the human spinal cord to those comparable areas in the cat spinal cord (Table 7) is of interest. The absolute levels of glycine in ventral gray, dorsal gray, and the ventral white matter are lower in the human spinal cord than in comparable areas of the cat. However, the relative differences between these areas within each species are in the same order. It might be of interest to compare the number of interneurons and their synaptic junctions in the various gray areas from a number of vertebrates including man, to the amount of glycine in each region.

TABLE 7. Distribution of Glycine in Six Areas from Five Segments of Cat Spinal Cord[a]

	Glycine content[b]					
Segment	DMW	DLW	DG	VG	VMW	VLW
Cervical enlargement	0.88 ± 0.15	2.11 ± 0.23	5.34 ± 0.34	6.90 ± 0.47	3.35 ± 0.24	4.36 ± 0.34
Upper thoracic	0.80 ± 0.20	1.84 ± 0.28	4.61 ± 0.66	6.10 ± 0.43	2.86 ± 0.46	2.81 ± 0.35
Middle thoracic	0.92 ± 0.20	1.55 ± 0.06	4.24 ± 0.36	5.44 ± 0.32	2.53 ± 0.31	2.33 ± 0.26
Lower thoracic	1.19 ± 0.12	3.05 ± 0.50	4.88 ± 0.62	6.69 ± 0.43	3.47 ± 0.16	3.87 ± 0.25
Lumbar enlargement	1.15 ± 0.16	4.60 ± 0.13	5.59 ± 0.26	6.75 ± 0.27	3.52 ± 0.23	5.55 ± 0.24

[a] Data taken from Aprison et al. (1969)
[b] Mean values are given in μmol/g wet weight ± SEM; $N = 4$ except for lumbar enlargement where $N = 8$.

The distribution of glycine in several areas of the cerebral cortex from the cat and human is shown in Table 8. When compared to the levels in ventral gray of the spinal cord, the content of glycine is very low in these cortical areas. The content of glycine is also very low in the cerebellum (Table 5). Neurophysiological studies of the effect of glycine on cortical neurons indicated that its potency on these cells was less than that of GABA and other longer-chain amino acids (Krnjević and Phillis, 1963). Further studies on cortical neurons (Kelly and Krnjević, 1969; Biscoe *et al.*, 1972; Krnjević *et al.*, 1977) have confirmed these earlier findings. Cerebellar neurons also appear to be less sensitive to glycine than they are to GABA (Kawamura and Provini, 1970). The very weak effects of glycine on the cortical and cerebellar neurons therefore are in agreement with the neurochemical data and these results support the suggestion that glycine probably does not act as an inhibitory transmitter in these two areas of the CNS unless it does so in a small group of specialized cells (see Section 3.2).

The content of glycine has been reported to be elevated in the retina (Starr, 1973) and it appeared to be concentrated in the inner layers (Cohen *et al.*, 1973). Kennedy *et al.* (1977) recently measured the distribution of several putative and nonputative transmitter amino acids including glycine, GABA, taurine, glutamate, and aspartate within anatomically defined layers of the retina in the rat. Glycine was found to have a distribution similar to that of GABA. The highest levels occurred in the amacrine cell, inner-plexiform, and ganglion cell layers. Berger *et al.* (1977*b*) have measured glycine and three other putative transmitter amino acids in discrete layers

TABLE 8.   Content of Glycine in Different Areas of the
Cat and Human Cerebral Hemispheres

| | Glycine content (μmol/g)[a] | |
Area	Cat[b]	Human
Frontal gray	1.31 ± 0.09	1.40 ± 0.17[c]
Parietal gray	1.34 ± 0.07	—
Temporal gray	1.41 ± 0.14	1.95 ± 0.31[d]
Occipital gray	1.28 ± 0.07	1.80 ± 0.25[d]
Subcortical white	0.75 ± 0.03	1.50 ± 0.16[c,e]

[a] Mean ± SEM.
[b] Data on cat cortical areas taken from Aprison *et al.* (1969); $N = 6$.
[c] Data on human cortical areas taken from Boehme *et al.* (1973); $N = 14$–16.
[d] Data on human temporal and occipital cortex taken from Perry *et al.* (1971*a*); $N = 5$. The values for these tissues were reported to be lower in biopsied samples (Perry *et al.*, 1971*b*).
[e] Frontal white matter.

of the rhesus monkey retina. The peak levels of glycine were found to be near the border as well as throughout the inner nuclear and inner reticular layers. Autoradiographic and uptake studies with labeled glycine indicate it accumulates in the region of the horizontal and amacrine cells (Voaden et al., 1974). As noted earlier, glycine has been shown to be released from the retina after light stimulation (Ehinger and Lindberg-Bauer, 1976). Perhaps the release is coming from a subpopulation of amacrine cells. The retina, like specific areas of the spinal cord but unlike the cerebral cortex, possesses a high-affinity uptake system for glycine (Neal et al., 1973). Furthermore, it is known that glycine depresses the spontaneous and evoked activity of retinal neurons and hyperpolarizes horizontal cells (Ames and Pollen, 1969; Murakami et al., 1972). Thus, all the neurochemical and neurophysiological data on this area of the CNS support the suggestion that glycine is released from interneurons and acts as an inhibitory transmitter in the retina.

5.2. Comparative Distribution of Glycine in Nervous Tissue of Invertebrates

Values for the content of glycine in several different nervous tissues in *Aplysia,* squid, cuttlefish, crab, lobster, and bee are shown in Table 9. The high value of glycine found in the ganglia of the lobster *(Homarus americanus)* is very interesting. In fact, after measuring the level of alanine, proline, GABA, glutamate, and aspartate in addition to glycine in (1) the brain or supraesophageal ganglion, (2) the next five thoracic ganglia, and (3) the nerve bundles connecting these ganglia, Aprison et al. (1973) reported glycine to be present at the highest level of any of the amino acids in the lobster. GABA and aspartate were also unevenly distributed in these tissues. In the abdominal ganglion of *Aplysia (A. californica)* the content of glycine was three to ten times that found in the other ganglia (Iliffe et al., 1977). These investigators report that this may be due in large part to the concentration of glycine in neurons labeled R_3–R_{14} in the abdominal ganglion. These specific neurons have a content of glycine that is 20 times higher than that in the somata of most of the other neurons in this invertebrate.

Whether glycine has any transmitter function in the invertebrate nervous system is not clear at this time. Lewis (1952), commenting on the high levels of glycine and alanine in lobster leg nerves, suggested that their function in these structures may be to maintain the proper external osmotic pressure. Similarly, aspartate and glutamate may simply serve as anions to balance the high internal levels of K^+.

TABLE 9.   Content of Glycine in Invertebrates

Organism	Tissue	Content[a]	Reference
Aplysia	Abdominal ganglia	1.0	Iliffe et al., 1977
	Buccal ganglia	0.21	
	Cerebral ganglia	0.25	
Bee	Brain	5.3	Frontali, 1964
Crab	Leg nerve	<5	Lewis, 1952
Cuttlefish	Axon	<5	Lewis, 1952
Lobster	Leg nerve	35	Lewis, 1952
	Ventral nerve cord	32.4	Gilles and Schoffeniels, 1964
	Supraesophageal ganglion	80	Aprison et al., 1973
	Thoracic ganglia 1–5	63–76	Aprison et al., 1973
	Excitatory axon	76[b]	McBride et al., 1974
	Inhibitory axon	47[b]	McBride et al., 1974
	Sensory fiber	40[b]	McBride et al., 1974
Squid	Giant axon	14.0	Koechlin, 1955
	Axoplasm	11.6	Deffner, 1961

[a] μmol/g.
[b] mmol/liter of axoplasm.

Since the content of glycine is found to be highest in the phylogenetically older parts of the CNS in the vertebrates, it is interesting to speculate that as our knowledge in the field of neurotransmission continues to develop and expand, glycine as well as some of the other amino acids may indeed be found to have a functional role in addition to their obvious metabolic roles at some level of development or evolution below that of the vertebrates.

5.3.   CSF/Blood Ratios and Clearance of Glycine from the CSF

In 1967, Davson reviewed the data which led to the conclusion that the concentrations of most ions and metabolites in CSF are controlled by transport mechanisms which regulate the fluxes of compounds between brain, CSF, and blood. Such transport systems have been shown to mediate the efflux of amino acids from brain to blood (Lajtha and Toth, 1961, 1963), and from CSF to blood (Snodgrass et al., 1969; Murray and Cutler, 1970). Blasberg and Lajtha (1965, 1966) also showed that such transport systems operated in brain slices and suggested that such systems served to transport amino acids into neurons. These systems no doubt play an important role in the regulation of the content of amino acids in the CNS.

Except for possibly glutamine in the rat (see Franklin *et al.,* 1975, Table 1), the concentrations of most amino acids including glycine are higher in plasma than in CSF. Data published by Aprison and Werman (1965), Dickinson and Hamilton (1966), Humoller *et al.* (1966), Snodgrass *et al.* (1969), Franklin *et al.* (1975), and McGale *et al.* (1977) permit the calculation of the concentration ratio of glycine in CSF to that in blood (serum or plasma). Such ratios for glycine and several other amino acids in different species are shown in Table 10. Values for the ratio of glycine levels are among the lowest. If they were not, it would indicate that large amounts of glycine were present in the extraneuronal spaces which might well interfere with normal function of the spinal cord and/or brain. These data may be explained by (1) rapid movement of glycine from CSF to blood, (2) a restriction of its entry into the CSF, or (3) both processes. Studies already published have shown that the glycine concentration in spinal fluid changed only slightly when the blood level was elevated (Christensen *et al.,* 1947; Wiechert, 1963). However, Krieger *et al.* (1977) have shown an acute rise in CSF of glycine after an oral load.

The observation that the concentration of glycine in CSF is much lower than the level in serum or plasma is of great interest and physiological

TABLE 10. Concentration Ratio of Glycine and Several Other Amino Acids in CSF to That in Blood

Amino acid	Species	CSF (nmol/ml)	Plasma (nmol/ml)	Ratio (CSF/ plasma)
Glycine	Cat [a]	15	348	0.043
	Cat [b]	18	367	0.049
	Rat [c]	15	221	0.068
	Human [d]	6.6	232	0.028
Alanine	Cat [b]	52	497	0.105
	Rat [c]	47	430	0.109
	Human [d]	23	345	0.067
Taurine	Rat [c]	42	432	0.097
	Human [d]	6.3	66.3	0.095
Serine	Cat [b]	26	125	0.208
	Rat [c]	80	196	0.408
	Human [d]	38	166	0.229
Lysine	Cat [b]	58	224	0.259
	Rat [c]	87	290	0.300
	Human [d]	19	174	0.110

[a] Aprison and Werman (1965).
[b] Snodgrass *et al.* (1969).
[c] Franklin *et al.* (1975).
[d] Dickinson and Hamilton (1966).

importance. Such data would suggest that glycine, a molecule that can inhibit motoneurons, would under normal conditions be rapidly transported out of extraneuronal fluid as originally suggested by Aprison and Werman (1965, 1968). In fact, carrier-mediated transport of glycine and other amino acids from CSF to plasma has been suggested to explain the low concentration ratios. Since there is a relationship between the concentration of amino acids in CSF and their concentration in the brain extraneuronal fluid, one would expect a greater flux of glycine from CSF to blood than from blood to CSF. Murray and Cutler (1970) using cats and Dudzinski and Cutler (1974) using rats addressed themselves to this problem and measured the directional or bidirectional flux of glycine between spinal fluid and plasma. These investigators found that (1) glycine was transported out of the spinal fluid by a saturable process (in the rat, a transport velocity of 26.5 nmol/min was reported), (2) [^{14}C]glycine clearance from spinal fluid was five times greater than its clearance from plasma, (3) the rate of clearance from the spinal subarachnoid compartments was five to seven times higher than that from the ventricular compartment in the cat, and (4) the rate of transport of glycine out of the spinal fluid was unaffected by GABA, β-alanine, and taurine, three amino acids shown to be present in varying amounts in different areas of the spinal cord and which have depressant actions when iontophoresed onto spinal neurons. The glycine transport capacity reported for the rat by Dudzinski and Cutler (1974) is sufficient to remove all the glycine from the spinal fluid in less than 1 min. Franklin *et al.* (1975) also found that the concentration of glycine in the spinal fluid of the rat is regulated by bidirectional transport systems between blood and spinal fluid. It is also interesting that McGale *et al.* (1977) found a significantly higher concentration of glycine (and serine) in ventricular CSF as compared to lumbar CSF; these data support the greater clearance of glycine from the lumbar region.

The demonstration of the presence of a rapid clearance system for compounds like glycine also points to the problem of demonstrating consistent release of preloaded [^{14}C]glycine in an *in vivo* experiment. However, the physiological meaning for the existence of such a process fits well with the role of glycine as the major postsynaptic inhibitory transmitter in the lumbosacral spinal cord.

5.4. Strychnine Antagonism and Glycine Receptor Studies

Perhaps it is apparent to the reader that a criterion requiring pharmacological identity or blockage was *not* listed in Section 1 along with the original three criteria. The reason is simple. This proposed criterion applies to drugs acting at the postsynaptic receptor site. It is not possible to use the action of a drug to identify a transmitter in the CNS without prior knowledge of the identity of the neurotransmitter, since the investigator cannot be certain of the *site of action* of the compound in such an experiment. On the other hand, if it is already known that a drug acts at the receptor in the postsynaptic membrane at one site, and the drug interacts in the same manner with both the natural transmitter and the suspected transmitter at the postsynaptic membrane when tested at another site, such data can be used in a *supportive* manner in the identification process at the second site. In the case of the transmitter action of glycine, strychnine is thought to be such a drug. Thus, it is now accepted that although higher concentrations of the alkaloid can result in nonspecific alterations of membrane properties (Curtis *et al.*, 1971; Werman, 1972; Freeman, 1973; Straughan, 1974; Gahwiler, 1976), the primary effects of strychnine are postsynaptic. Strychnine is also known to antagonize the physiological effects of certain other amino acids on spinal (Curtis *et al.*, 1968*a,b*) and brainstem neurons (Haas and Hösli, 1973*a*). However, quantitative aspects of the antagonism between strychnine and glycine have been challenged (Roper *et al.*, 1969; Curtis and Johnston, 1970; Roper and Diamond, 1970; Diamond *et al.*, 1973). The possiblity that there are two types of receptors for glycine, strychnine-sensitive and strychnine-resistant, has been postulated (Ryall *et al.*, 1972; Barker *et al.*, 1975).

The studies by Eccles and co-workers (Bradley *et al.*, 1953; Eccles *et al.*, 1954; Coombs *et al.*, 1955) and Curtis (1959, 1962, 1963) explained the well-known convulsant properties of strychnine by a blockage of spinal postsynaptic inhibition. Almost all spinal postsynaptic inhibitions are blocked by strychnine and strychninelike drugs, whereas strychnine does not affect presynaptic inhibitions or excitatory postsynaptic potentials (Curtis, 1963; Curtis and Johnston, 1974). Consequently, strychnine sensitivity has become an importont supportive criterion for the screening of transmitter candidates at inhibitory synapses in the spinal cord.

The case for glycine's role in inhibitory transmission in the spinal cord was greatly strengthened by the finding that strychnine blocked the depressant effect of glycine but not the effects of GABA on spinal neurons (Curtis *et al.*, 1968*a,b*, 1971). Furthermore, Curtis and co-workers reported that the drug is competitive with glycine. Although these observations have been confirmed by Larson (1969) and DeGroat (1970), there is a report by Davidoff *et al.* (1969) which suggests that the effect was noncompetitive.

If glycine is the transmitter at strychnine-sensitive synapses, the data in the literature are best explained by a reversible and specific interaction between strychnine and the spinal postsynaptic receptor for glycine (Larson, 1969; Curtis *et al.*, 1971). However, somewhat of a controversy exists on whether mutual inhibition (inhibition of Renshaw cells by Renshaw cells) in the spinal cord is strychnine-sensitive. Since strychnine sensivitity is characteristic of both recurrent inhibition (inhibition of motor neurons by Renshaw cells) (Eccles *et al.*, 1954; Curtis, 1963; Larson, 1969) and inhibition of group IA interneurons by Renshaw cells (Ryall *et al.*, 1972; Belcher *et al.*, 1976), one would predict on the basis of Dale's hypothesis that the same transmitter is released by the Renshaw cell during mutual inhibition, and, therefore, this inhibition should be strychnine-sensitive. Ryall *et al.* (1972) and Belcher *et al.* (1976) have reported that the mutual inhibition is strychnine-resistant and postulate the existence of two glycine receptors, one strychnine-sensitive and the other strychnine-resistant. This situation would be analogous to the two types of cholinergic receptors, muscarinic (motor neuron on muscle end plate) and nicotinic (motor neuron collateral on Renshaw cell) (Ryall *et al.*, 1972). However, Curtis *et al.* (1976c) have found mutual inhibition to be strychnine-sensitive, making the postulation of two types of glycine receptor unnecessary.

The sensitivity of both glycine and the natural transmitter to strychnine in the brainstem supports the role of glycine as a neurotransmitter in some neuronal pathways in the (1) *reticular formation* (Tebēcis and DiMaria, 1972; Tebēcis and Ishikawa, 1973; Haas and Hösli, 1973b), (2) *hypoglossal nucleus* (Morimoto *et al.*, 1968; Duggan *et al.*, 1973), and (3) *cuneate nucleus* (Boyd *et al.*, 1966; Banna and Jabbur, 1969; Kelly and Renaud, 1973b; but see Kelly and Renaud, 1973c). The natural inhibitory transmitter within the semicircular canal of the ear (Precht *et al.*, 1973) and the amacrine cell region of the retina (Straschill, 1968; Ames and Pollen, 1969; Burkhardt, 1972; Korol and Owens, 1974; however, see Belcheva and Vitanova, 1974) also appears to be sensitive to strychnine. On the other hand, strychnine sensitivity has not been found to be a feature of more rostral postsynaptic inhibitions such as those in the (1) *cerebral cortex* (Crawford *et al.*, 1963; Krnjević *et al.*, 1966; Biscoe and Curtis, 1967), (2) *hippocampus* (Andersen *et al.*, 1963), (3) *cerebellum* (Andersen *et al.*, 1963; Crawford *et al.*, 1963; Obata *et al.*, 1970; Kawamura and Provini, 1970; Bisti *et al.*, 1971), (4) *thalamus* (Duggan and McLennan, 1971), (5) *hypothalamus* (Nicoll and Barker, 1971; Yagi and Sawaki, 1975), and (6) *olfactory bulb* (Felix and McLennan, 1971). In all these studies the pharmacological evidence for glycine as a neurotransmitter is consistent with the more direct physiological and biochemical evidence.

In 1973, Young and Snyder reported that [³H]strychnine could bind to synaptic membrane fractions isolated from the spinal cord and brainstem, and this binding appeared to represent a specific interaction between strychnine and the same postsynaptic receptor to which glycine normally bound to produce its inhibitory action. The distribution of specific strychnine binding in the rat spinal cord and areas of the brain approximately parallels the distribution of endogenous glycine in these parts as reported by Shank and Aprison (1970*a*).

Snyder and his co-workers were able to demonstrate that (1) there is higher [^{3}H]strychnine binding in the spinal cord and medulla than in other brain areas (Young and Snyder, 1973); (2) the binding of [^{3}H]strychnine in the spinal cord and medulla is associated with the synaptic membrane fraction (Young and Snyder, 1974*a*); (3) glycine and strychnine appear to bind to two *separate sites* of the same receptor which are capable of mutually influencing each other (Young and Snyder, 1974*b*); (4) both the high-affinity uptake system of glycine and the [^{3}H]strychnine binding develop between days 14 and 21 in the chick embryo (Zukin *et al.,* 1975)—data which are consistent with the time of emergence of electrophysiologically observable inhibition in the chick embryo spinal cord (Stokes and Bignall, 1974; Oppenheim and Reitzel, 1975); and (5) the binding of strychnine is reversed by glycine *and* the four amino acids, taurine, serine, alanine, and β-alanine, whose physiological effects after iontophoresis are also antagonized by strychnine (Snyder *et al.,* 1973*b*; Young and Snyder, 1973).

The ability of a series of anions to inhibit [^{3}H]strychnine binding to synaptic membranes isolated from spinal cord correlates closely with their neurophysiologic capacity to reverse inhibitory postsynaptic potentials in the spinal cord of the rat (Young and Snyder, 1974*b*). These results suggest that the inhibition of strychnine binding by these anions may be closely associated with the ionic conductance mechanism for chloride in the glycine receptor. The data also suggest that glycine and strychnine appear to bind to distinct sites which interact in a cooperative manner, i.e., the two compounds may affect the same receptor complex but function primarily at *distinct sites within it,* thereby interacting cooperatively with each other. Thus, it is suggested that glycine binds at the "glycine recognition" site and strychnine binds at a distinct site which may represent the chloride ionic gate mechanism. Perhaps such an observation might explain the report of noncompetitive inhibition of glycine's hyperpolarizing actions by strychnine at some synapses (Davidoff *et al.,* 1969).

Young *et al.* (1974), Snyder and Enna (1975), and Snyder (1975) also reported that benzodiazepines have an *in vitro* potency similar to that of glycine in displacing [^{3}H]strychnine from the receptor. These authors found that the clinical efficacy of these drugs parallels their potency of antagonism of strychnine binding. These *in vitro* data suggesting an interaction between the benzodiazepines and the glycinergic system are not supported by *in vivo* studies conducted by Curtis *et al.* (1976*b,d*) and Dray and Straughan (1976). In the former experiments with cats, diazepam given intravenously did not affect strychnine antagonism of glycine's action on spinal neurons. In the latter experiments with mice, diazepam given intravenously also failed to have any effect on the action of strychnine. Thus, caution must be exercised in the extrapolation of the *in vitro* data to *in vivo* conditions.

Whether or not [^{3}H]strychnine binding is an accurate measure of the distribution of the glycine receptors, the observations that strychnine blocks inhibition by glycine in specific areas of the CNS are very important. As is discussed in Section 9.1, the *concepts* that glycine can act as a postsynaptic inhibitory transmitter and that strychnine can block this type of inhibition by an interaction in the receptor have already been used to help a patient (Gitzelmann *et al.,* 1977). The use of strychnine may also be important in distinguishing between the actions of glycine and those of GABA. Thus, Straughan (1974) points out that blockade of transmitter action by strychnine at a specific site can at times be the only evidence for the identification of the transmitter if the conductance changes of GABA and glycine are the same. This is possible because the antagonism of glycine by strychnine appears to be more specific than the antagonism of GABA by bicuculline or picrotoxin (Hill *et al.,* 1976).

5.5. Studies with Tetanus Toxin

The clinical manifestations of tetanus have been known for centuries and the disease has been one of man's most dreaded afflictions. Even today the disease is approximately 50% fatal. Tetanus in its generalized form proceeds through various stages to a hyperexcitability of the CNS resulting in convulsive muscular spasms and respiratory impairment. Death usually results from pulmonary infection secondary to hypoventilation and aspiration. The disease is caused by *Clostridium tetani,* an anaerobic gram-positive, spore-forming rod that is found ubiquitously in nature. This bacterium only enters the body after breakdown of the skin and remains localized to the site of entrance. The devastating effects of tetanus are a result of the production of the exotoxin tetanospasmin and its migration to and interaction with the CNS. This toxin is second only to botulinum toxin in its lethality. Its potency has been extrapolated from animal studies to be such that approximately 1 kg could kill the entire population of the world! Yet, the disease process itself is completely reversible—those who do survive the intoxication suffer no direct residual effects.

Brooks *et al.* (1957) first showed the effects of tetanus toxin on blocking the postsynaptic inhibition of Renshaw cells in the spinal cord. Numerous other studies have shown the effect of tetanus toxin on blocking both postsynaptic and presynaptic inhibitions in the spinal cord (Curtis, 1959; Wilson *et al.,* 1960; Curtis and DeGroat, 1968; Guschchin *et al.,*

1969; Curtis *et al.*, 1973; Kryzhanovsky and Sheykhon, 1973; Benecke *et al.*, 1977). With the assumption that glycine and GABA are transmitters in spinal cord, pharmacological studies have postulated a presynaptic site of action of tetanus toxin in blocking neurotransmission (Curtis and DeGroat, 1968; Guschin *et al.*, 1969; Curtis *et al.*, 1973). Osborne *et al.* (1973) found a significant decrease in the electrically stimulated release of glycine, GABA, and aspartate from synaptosomes isolated from the spinal cord and medulla of animals poisoned with tetanus toxin. Krzyhanovsky (1975) has postulated that the presynaptic action of tetanus toxin is nonspecific in that it does not depend on the nature of the transmitter released. Ultrastructural studies have shown an increase in synaptic vesicles in the presynaptic nerve terminal at both the neuromuscular junction and axosomatic synapses in the spinal cord. In the latter, flattened synaptic vesicles appeared to be selectively increased (Kryzhanovsky, 1973).

Although the hyperexcitable state in tetanus intoxication appears to be the result of inhibition of central synapses in the motor system, the toxin also affects the neuromuscular junction (Kaeser and Saner, 1970; Zacks and Sheff, 1970; Kryzhanovsky, 1973), the autonomic nervous system (Corbett and Harris, 1973), and peripheral organs including the lungs and heart (Kryzhanovsky, 1975). These actions would undoubtedly contribute to the clinical picture of tetanus.

Owing to the important role of amino acids in synaptic transmission within the spinal cord, a number of studies have looked at their levels in spinal cord from animals with experimentally induced tetanus. Semba and Kano (1969) reported a significant decrease of glycine in the gray matter of the spinal cord but unchanged levels in the white matter. However, Johnston *et al.* (1969) and Fedineć and Shank (1971) found no change in the content of glycine. The latter authors found no change in the content of any amino acid but the former authors found a marked increase in aspartate both in the dorsal and ventral gray and dorsal white matter. The reported increase in aspartate is difficult to explain, but the unaltered levels of glycine and GABA are consistent with the proposed presynaptic blockade of transmitter release produced by tetanus toxin.

The binding of tetanus toxin to CNS tissue is due to the ganglioside content of the tissue and depends on its sialic acid content (van Heyningen, 1974). In subcellular fractionation studies, the toxin is preferentially bound to synaptosomes (Mellanby *et al.*, 1965), and after hypoosmotic shock of the synaptosomes, the presynaptic membrane fraction retains the greatest binding capacity (Mellanby and Whittaker, 1968). The tetanus toxin molecule appears to consist of three distinct moieties: (1) antigenic component, (2) toxic component, and (3) binding component (Habermann and Wellhöner, 1974).

The fact that tetanus toxin binds to nervous tissue has been known since the beginning of the century, but the pathway from the site of local infection to the CNS has been a subject of controversy. There is currently general agreement that the toxin reaches the CNS by ascent of peripheral nerves (Fedineć, 1967; Habermann and Wellhöner, 1974; King and Fedineć, 1974; Kryzhanovsky, 1975; Price et al., 1975).

Both toxin and toxoid bind to CNS, the latter only weakly, whereas liver tissue does not bind either (Habermann, 1973). When toxin binding was studied in vitro utilizing tissue slices, more receptors were found in the cerebrum than in the spinal cord. The binding in the spinal cord was almost exclusively limited to gray matter (Habermann, 1973). However, when ^{125}I-labeled tetanus toxin is injected into the gastrocnemius muscle of rats 40–50 hr before killing, the toxin appears to be enriched sixfold in the gray matter as compared to the white matter of the spinal cord on the injected side (Habermann et al., 1973). When the distribution of the labeled toxin was studied by autoradiography, the label was highest in the ventral gray matter with some concentration around neuronal cell bodies (Dimfel and Habermann, 1973). The apparent abundance of toxin receptors in the cerebrum is probably of limited significance owing to the lack of peripheral nerves arising in this area.

The postulated presynaptic mechanism of action of tetanus toxin and its retrograde ascent of peripheral nerves would require migration of the molecule across at least two synapses (the peripheral neuromuscular junction and at least one central synapse with the motoneuron being the postsynaptic element). Electron microscopic autoradiography of the spinal cord after peripheral intramuscular injection of labeled toxin showed label accumulated in the presynaptic elements surrounding motoneurons. Moreover, there was good temporal correlation between the appearance of the presynaptic label and the clinical signs of tetanus intoxication (Schwab and Thoenen, 1976). The transsynaptic migration of tetanus toxin exhibits some specificity in that these authors found label in the presynaptic elements of the superior cervical ganglion after injection of the labeled toxin into the submandibular gland or anterior eye chamber but not after injection of labeled nerve growth factor (Schwab and Thoenen, 1977).

After intraspinal injection of labeled toxin, the radioactivity localizes in the presynaptic elements of axosomatic synapses of spinal gray matter (Price et al., 1977). This is the same compartment that accumulates [3H]glycine after intraspinal injection (Price et al., 1976) (see Section 2.3).

In a brief abstract it was reported that intraperitoneal administration of glycine or oxyaminoacetic acid (a GABA transaminase inhibitor used to increase CNS GABA levels) could increase the survival time of mice with experimental tetanus (Hadzović and Brankov, 1974). Although no details were given, it was reported that only the effect of oxyaminoacetic acid was significant. It would be of great interest to determine whether peripherally induced adjustments in the CNS levels of glycine or GABA could influence the disinhibition of physiological spinal inhibitory processes as studied in the reports cited at the beginning of this section. The therapeutic implications are clear if such adjustment could be shown both safe and efficacious in clinical situations. Adjustment of glycine and/or GABA levels would not be curative in tetanus, but would offer a more specific modality of supportive care to the clinician.

6. METABOLIC STUDIES

6.1. Precursor and Flux Studies

Since glycine is a nonessential amino acid, glycine levels in the CNS could be maintained by (1) the transport of glycine from the periphery, (2) synthesis from endogenous compounds supplied to the CNS, (3) resynthesis from catabolic products, or (4) most likely a combination of these possibilities. Since glucose enters the CNS at rates far greater than other metabolites, it would ultimately serve as the principal source of the carbon units of glycine in CNS tissues. This possibility was tested by studying the rate at which label was incorporated into glycine and several other amino acids in CNS tissues of the rat after intraperitoneal administration of [U-^{14}C]glucose. Glycine received label at a slower rate than other amino acids studied, but calculations of the rate of carbon flux from glucose to glycine indicated that glucose might serve as an important source of carbon units for glycine via serine (Shank and Aprison, 1970a).

In animals there are a number of possible pathways leading from glucose to glycine (Figure 6). In the first two pathways (I, II) serine is the immediate precursor of glycine, and in the last two pathways (IV, V) glyoxylate is the immediate precursor of glycine. Pathways I and II involve the synthesis of serine via phosphorylated and nonphosphorylated pathways, respectively. The final conversion of serine to glycine in either pathway would be mediated by serine hydroxymethyltransferase (EC 2.1.2.1) (SHMT). In pathway III, glycine is formed by the condensation of NH_3, CO_2, and N^5, N^{10}-methylenetetrahydrofolate (C-THF). The C-THF may be formed from the third carbon of serine during the SHMT reaction. Pathway IV involves the nonoxidative decarboxylation of hydroxypyruvate to glycoaldehyde, and its subsequent oxidation to glyoxylate. The conversion of glyoxylate to glycine is mediated by glycine:2-oxoglutarate aminotransferase (glycine transaminase) (EC 2.6.1.4). In pathway V, glyox-

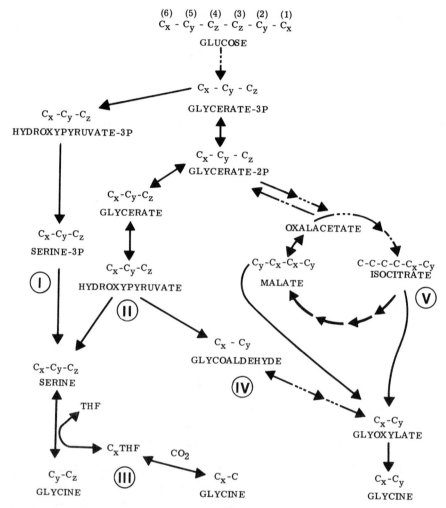

FIGURE 6. Pathways of carbon flow from glucose to glycine. Reprinted with permission from Aprison *et al.* (1975).

ylate is formed by the action of isocitrate lyase and then transaminated to glycine as in the previous pathway.

Bridgers (1965) has demonstrated that the phosphorylated pathway of serine synthesis (pathway I, Figure 6) is predominant in mouse brain extracts. He has also suggested that the control point in serine synthesis is the phosphoserine phosphohydrolase reaction (Bridgers, 1967). Uhr and

Sneddon (1971, 1972) have suggested that the nonphosphorylated pathway of serine synthesis (pathway II, Figure 6) may be operative in the CNS of the cat and rat. They have found that D-glyceric acid dehydrogenase (first enzyme of the nonphosphorylated pathway) is correlated with the glycine content in various areas of the cat CNS (Uhr and Sneddon, 1972). They also found an *in vitro* inhibition of this enzyme by glycine and have suggested feedback inhibition by the end product of the synthetic pathway (Uhr and Sneddon, 1971). However, the presence of the nonphosphorylated pathway within the CNS has been challenged (Feld and Sallach, 1974).

Aprison and co-workers have suggested that the SHMT within the CNS is the biosynthetic enzyme for glycine (Aprison *et al.*, 1970; Shank and Aprison, 1970a). Their suggestion was based on reports of the presence of SHMT activity in brain extracts (Bridgers, 1968) and the labeling patterns of glycine and serine found (1) after incubation of tissue slices with radioactive glucose *in vitro* (Sky-Peck *et al.*, 1966) and (2) after injections of radioactive glucose and serine *in vivo* (Shank and Aprison, 1970a) (Table 11). The ratios of specific radioactivities of serine to glycine after intraperitoneal injection of [U-^{14}C]serine were nearly identical, as were the ratios after intracisternal injection of [3,4-^{14}C]glucose and [U-^{14}C]serine (Shank and Aprison, 1970a) (see Table 11). These data suggest that glucose and serine are metabolized to glycine by a common mechanism, i.e., SHMT. Based on the approximation formula of Shank and Aprison (1970a) for measuring *in vivo* flux rates, there appeared to be no correlation between the glycine levels in various regions of the CNS and its rate of synthesis from serine. However, this lack of correlation may be a result of using either the approximation formula or whole tissue samples and measuring the conversion of serine to glycine in the combined total metabolic pools of neurons and glia.

Banos *et al.* (1975) found that serine is taken up by the brain as rapidly as essential amino acids, and thus may be essential for the brain although not essential for the body as a whole. This rapid influx of serine may also be a significant source for the glycine within the CNS (Shank and Aprison, 1970a; Banos *et al.*, 1975). One laboratory has reported elevated glycine levels within the CNS after prolonged systemic administration of serine (Filipovic *et al.*, 1976).

Although the glycine cleavage system (GCS) is generally thought to be a catabolic pathway (the main pathway of glycine catabolism in liver) (Kikuchi, 1973), the system is reversible and may also function as a synthetic pathway (pathway III, Figure 6). However, the data of Shank and Aprison (1970a) do not suggest a significant incorporation of the third carbon of serine into glycine after intracisternal injection of [3-^{14}C]serine

TABLE 11. Mean Specific Radioactivity of Glycine and Serine in the Rat Medulla after Intraperitoneal or Intracisternal Injection of ^{14}C-Labeled Metabolites

Labeled metabolite	Route of injection	Quantity injected[a] (nmol; μCi)	Time after injection (min)	Glycine (dpm/nmol)	Serine (dpm/nmol)	Ser/Gly[b]
[U-^{14}C]Glucose[c]	Intraperitoneal	290; 43.8	20	0.36	7.39	20
[3,4-^{14}C]Glucose[d]	Intracisternal	2000; 2	30	0.49	4.59	9
[1-^{14}C]Glucose[d]	Intracisternal	333; 3[e]	30	0.10	4.95	50
[U-^{14}C]Glycine[c]	Intraperitoneal	290; 43.8	20	3.83	11.3	3
[U-^{14}C]Glycine[c]	Intracisternal	2.9; 0.44	20	421	310	0.7
[U-^{14}C]Serine[c]	Intraperitoneal	290; 43.8	20	2.34	49.2	21
[U-^{14}C]Serine[c]	Intracisternal	2.9; 0.44	20	76.0	793[f]	10
[3-^{14}C]Serine[c]	Intracisternal	73; 0.44	20	2.35	1870	796
[U-^{14}C]Glyoxylate[c]	Intracisternal	30; 0.18	20	3.50	—	—
[1,5-^{14}C]Citrate[d,g]	Intracisternal	250; 5	30	0.69	3.66	5

[a] Values calculated from references using (1) average specific radioactivity of metabolite and μCi injected, or (2) average specific radioactivity of metabolite, average weight of rats used, and microcuries injected per 100 g weight.

[b] Ratio of specific radioactivity of serine to glycine.

[c] Data from Shank and Aprison (1970a).

[d] Data from Shank et al. (1973).

[e] The actual values were reduced by one-third to make them comparable to the data for [3,4-^{14}C]glucose.

[f] The actual value of serine was reduced by one-third on account of the small, if not nonexistent, conversion of [3-^{14}C]serine to glycine (see table) and to make the data comparable to those after [3,4-^{14}C]glucose injection since [3,4-^{14}C]glucose does not label the serine molecule in the C-3 position (see Figure 6).

[g] Sample consisted of medulla oblongata and upper cervical segments of spinal cord.

(Table 11). Consequently, this pathway does not appear to be important for the synthesis of glycine within the CNS.

Johnston and co-workers have proposed an alternative enzyme, glycine transaminase (GT), for glycine synthesis within the CNS (Johnston and Vitali, 1969a,b; Johnston et al., 1970). The nonoxidative decarboxylation of hydroxypyruvate in brain extracts (Hedrick and Sallach, 1964) and the presence of D-glyceric acid dehydrogenase in the CNS (Uhr and Sneddon, 1971, 1972) support the possibility of pathway IV in glycine synthesis. Although the formation of glyoxylate from the cleavage of isocitrate by the enzyme isocitrate lyase (pathway V) is widespread in plants and bacteria, this reaction is generally thought not to occur in the animal kingdom. However, Kondrashova and Rodionova (1971) have reported its presence in rat and pigeon liver mitochondria especially during low-energy states. Johnston et al. (1970) have briefly alluded to preliminary evidence for the enzyme in extracts of rat spinal cord.

Factors that favor a role for glyoxylate in the metabolism of glycine within the CNS are (1) the large increase of glyoxylate and glycine in experimental thiamine deficiency (Liang, 1962; Gaitonde et al., 1975); (2) the presence of the glycine transaminase in CNS tissues (Johnston and Vitali, 1969a,b; Johnston et al., 1970; Benuck et al., 1971, 1972; Daly and Aprison, 1974); and (3) the high levels of hydroxypyruvate decarboxylase activity (forming glycoaldehyde from hydroxypyruvate, pathway IV, Figure 6) found in the CNS (Hedrick and Sallach, 1964). Factors that argue against a major role for glyoxylate in glycine metabolism within the CNS are (1) the low levels of glyoxylate in the CNS—approximately 10 nmol/g (Liang, 1962; Johnston et al., 1970; Shank et al., 1973); (2) the toxic effect of glyoxylate on nerve cells (Laborit et al., 1971; Lamothe et al., 1971; Schwander and Lamarche, 1972); (3) the possible nonspecificity of the glycine transaminase (Shank and Aprison, 1970a); (4) the apparent lack of a readily available precursor of glyoxylate within the CNS (Shank et al., 1973; Aprison et al., 1975); and (5) the very slow influx of glyoxylate from the blood into the CNS (Romano and Cerra, 1967).

[14C]Glyoxylate can label glycine in both in vivo (Shank and Aprison, 1970a) and in vitro P_2 preparations (W. J. McBride, E. Daly, and M. H. Aprison, unpublished data). However, the flux of label from glyoxylate to glycine and consequently the significance of this conversion cannot be estimated owing to the lack of methods to measure the specific radioactivity of the precursor glyoxylate within the tissue. Shank et al. (1973) attempted to estimate the significance of the conversion of glyoxylate to glycine by administering labeled metabolites from which glycine should be derived selectively through a pathway involving glyoxylate as opposed to serine (Figure 6, Table 11). Their data suggest a fivefold greater labeling of glycine after intracisternal injection of [3,4-^{14}C]glucose than after [1-^{14}C]glucose injection (Table 11). The former compound would label glycine via serine and the latter compound would label glycine either by the reverse of the GCS or via glyoxylate (Figure 6). Since the GCS does not appear to be important in the synthesis of glycine, this labeling of glycine from [1-^{14}C]glucose may indicate the presence of glyoxylate pathways. Also [1,5-^{14}C]citrate labeled glycine approximately twofold greater than would be expected from the serine/glycine ratios obtained after injection of [^{14}C]glucose or [^{14}C]serine (Shank *et al.*, 1973) (see Table 11). Interestingly, citrate appeared to be metabolized via a different compartment within the CNS on the basis of the glutamate/glutamine ratios (Shank *et al.*, 1973). [^{14}C]Aspartate, [^{14}C]ethanolamine, and [^{14}C]glycerate labeled glycine in a manner consistent with the serine pathways (Aprison *et al.*, 1975).

The data of Shank *et al.* (1973) concerning the labeling of glycine after [1-^{14}C]glucose and [1,5-^{14}C]citrate do not eliminate the possibility that a significant but small portion of glycine may be synthesized via glyoxylate. Besides the unknown effect that compartmentation may have on the interpretation of their data, the possibility exists that the large quantities of metabolites injected into the cisterna magna in the study of Shank et al. (Table 11) may have upset the metabolic steady state of the CNS tissues. Support for this possibility was obtained in preliminary experiments after the injection of much smaller quantities of metabolites into the cisterna magna (E. C. Daly and M. H. Aprison, unpublished data). Twenty minutes after the intracisternal injection of 56 nmol (0.41 μCi) of [1,5-^{14}C]citrate, the specific radioactivities of serine and glycine in the medulla–pons were 0.3 and 0 dpm/nmol, respectively ($N = 6$). Thirty minutes after the intracisternal injection of 8.8 nmol (0.42 μCi) of [1-^{14}C]glucose, the specific radioactivities of serine and glycine in the medulla–pons were 1.80 and 0 dpm/nmol, respectively; after 15 min the values were 3.28 and 0, respectively ($N = 1$). Thirty minutes after the intracisternal injection of 35 nmol (0.48 μCi) of [3,4-^{14}C]glucose the specific radioactivities were 1.56 and 0.42 dpm/nmol, respectively ($N = 1$). The concentration of metabolite injected in the study by Shank *et al.* (1973) was approximately 25–400 mM, whereas the concentration in these preliminary experiments (E. C. Daly and M. H. Aprison, unpublished data) was approximately 1–6 mM. Although the injection of such small quantities of compounds stresses the sensitivity of the assay (Shank and Aprison, 1970b) owing to the large amounts of endogenous glycine present in the medulla, these experiments suggest that the role of glyoxylate in glycine synthesis may have been overestimated by Shank *et al.* (1973) and that this role may be minor, if not insignificant, given the possible precursors studied.

6.2. *In Vitro* Experiments with P_2 Preparations

In the course of studying the metabolism of serine and glycine in subcellular fractions, the contents of various free amino acids were determined in the P_2 (crude synaptosomal) fractions isolated from different regions of the rat brain (McBride *et al.*, 1973). The content of glycine is highest in the P_2 fractions prepared from the medulla and spinal cord (Table 12) in agreement with the high levels found in extracts of homogenates from these regions (Shank and Aprison, 1970*a*). The content of glutamate was highest in the P_2 fractions of all areas studied, but glycine was present in the second highest amounts in P_2 fractions from the medulla and spinal cord (McBride *et al.*, 1973). Osborne *et al.* (1973) also found the content of glycine to be very high in synaptosomes prepared from the medulla and spinal cord.

The isolated P_2 fractions were suspended in buffered glucose–salt media and incubated with 8×10^{-7} M [U-^{14}C]glycine or [U-^{14}C]serine and an estimate was made of their rates of interconversion (McBride *et al.*, 1973). The rate of conversion of [^{14}C]serine to [^{14}C]glycine was greatest in the cerebellum and lowest in the medulla and telencephalon. An intermediate rate was found in the spinal cord (Table 12). The rate of conversion of [^{14}C]glycine to [^{14}C]serine was lowest in the cerebellum and approximately the same in the other three areas. This active conversion of serine to

TABLE 12. The Content of Serine and Glycine and Estimation of the Rate of Their Interconversion in Crude Synaptosomal Fractions (P_2) Isolated from Various Regions of the Rat CNS[a]

CNS area	Gly (nmol/mg protein)	Ser (nmol/mg protein)	Flux (pmol/min/mg protein)		Ratio
			Ser → Gly	Gly → Ser	Ser → Gly/Gly → Ser
Telencephalon	5.74	2.56	54	21	2.6
Cerebellum	3.48	1.76	159	7.1	22
Medulla	14.60	0.74	55	23	2.4
Spinal cord	11.80	0.79	71	22	3.2

[a] Values recalculated from the data of McBride *et al.* (1973). Flux values were calculated from the approximation formula described by Shank and Aprison (1970*a*) and the data for the content of glycine in the P_2 fractions and the average specific radioactivities of the precursor and product reported in the original paper. Compensation was made for the fact that the third carbon of serine is not converted to glycine (the contribution of the GCS to glycine synthesis was assumed to be negligible as described in the text). Therefore, the specific radioactivity of the serine isolated at the end of the incubations employing [U-^{14}C]serine as substrate was reduced by one-third.

glycine in the cerebellum was unexpected in view of the low levels of glycine and no known role of glycine in neurotransmission in this region. As was suggested in the original report, this active conversion may be important in the generation of one-carbon units for metabolic needs (McBride *et al.*, 1973). However, strict interpretations of these data cannot be made on account of the measured activity being subject to possible artifacts created by the homogenization and incubation procedures. These possible artifacts may alter the integrity of the enzymatic systems and/or endogenous cofactors involved in the interconversion of serine and glycine.

6.3. *In Vitro* Enzymatic Studies

6.3.1. *Serine Hydroxymethyltransferase Activities*

The *in vitro* results of Sky-Peck *et al.* (1966), the *in vivo* studies of Shank and Aprison (1970*a*) and Shank *et al.* (1973), and the studies with P_2 fractions reported by McBride *et al.* (1973) suggest that the serine hydroxymethyltransferase (SHMT) within the CNS plays a major role in maintaining glycine levels. Bridgers (1968) originally reported the enzymatic activity in mouse brain. This study utilized extracts of whole brain as a source of enzyme and did not investigate possible variations in the level of SHMT among different regions of the CNS. Likewise, Ordoñez and Wurtman (1973) measured the enzymatic activity in dialyzed soluble phosphate buffer extracts of rat brain. Broderick *et al.* (1972) purified SHMT 150-fold from soluble phosphate buffer extracts of fresh-frozen bovine brain. Since the SHMT within the CNS is largely localized in particulate fractions after homogenization in 0.32 *M* sucrose (see later), the efficiency of extraction is uncertain in the latter two studies. Moreover, since the enzymatic activities appear to have been measured with suboptimal concentrations of reactants based on the studies of Daly and Aprison (1974), the levels of enzyme reported in these studies probably do not reflect true tissue levels.

Owing to the large regional differences in glycine content within the CNS and its role in neurotransmission, two laboratories have studied the regional distribution of SHMT within the CNS (Davies and Johnston, 1973; Daly and Aprison, 1974). Davies and Johnston (1973) reported levels of SHMT activity between 2.32 and 2.64 μmol/hr/g wet weight in five regions of the rat CNS (cerebral cortex, cerebellum, medulla–pons, diencephalon–mesencephalon, and spinal cord). These authors found no correlation between glycine content and SHMT activity in these regions. However, they did find significantly higher levels of SHMT in cat spinal gray matter as compared to white matter. In addition, the ventral gray matter had significantly higher levels than the dorsal gray matter (Davies and Johnston, 1973). These findings are at least qualitatively correlated to the content of glycine in the spinal cord (see Section 2.1).

Daly and Aprison (1974) have also studied the regional distribution of SHMT in five similar regions of the rat CNS (Table 13). Values varied between 3.49 and 5.08 μmol/hr/g and except for the level found in the cerebellum, the SHMT appeared to be correlated with the glycine content in the various areas (Table 13). When the SHMT activity was expressed per milligram of protein in the homogenates, there was a linear correlation except for the cerebellar data (Figure 7). Levels of succinate dehydrogenase (SDH) have been shown to estimate the relative number of mitochondria in a sample of nervous tissue (Gregson and Williams, 1969). When the SDH levels in the five areas studied (Table 13) are used to adjust the SHMT activity per relative number of mitochondria (the SHMT within the CNS appears to be a mitochondrial enzyme—see later), there was an excellent correlation between the SHMT activity and the glycine content in the five regions (Figure 7). It is interesting that the cerebellum had a high level of SHMT activity as was suggested by the studies using P_2 fractions discussed earlier (McBride et al., 1973). From the data in Table 13 it can be seen that the cerebellum has a greater relative number of mitochondria than the other areas. More dramatically, the cerebellum contains approximately five to

TABLE 13. Distribution of Glycine, Serine Hydroxymethyltransferase, Succinate Dehydrogenase, Glycine Transaminase, Glycine Cleavage System, and DNA in Five Regions of the Rat CNS

	Telencephalon	Midbrain	Cerebellum	Medulla–Pons	Spinal cord
Glycine[a] (μmol/g tissue)	0.83	1.50	0.68	4.15	4.20
SHMT[a] (μmol/hr/g tissue)	3.49	3.74	4.80	5.08	4.35
SHMT[a] (nmol/hr/mg protein)	28.4	30.9	40.6	45.9	44.6
SDH[a] (μmol/hr/mg protein)	2.70	2.63	3.27	2.30	1.86
GT[a] (nmol/hr/mg protein)	162	162	158	166	133
GCS[b] (nmol/hr/mg protein)	4.35	0.88	2.06	0.39	0.07
DNA[c] (mg/g tissue)	0.86	0.94	4.57	0.83	0.48

[a] Values from Daly and Aprison (1974).
[b] Values from Daly et al. (1976).
[c] E. C. Daly and M. H. Aprison (unpublished data).

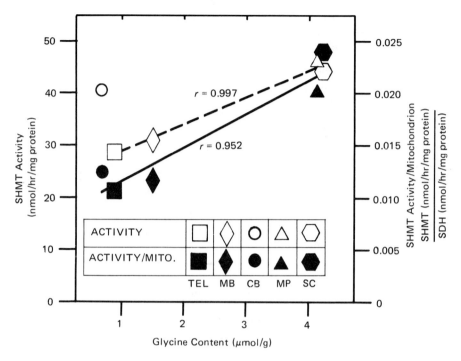

FIGURE 7. Correlation between the activity of serine hydroxymethyltransferase (SHMT) and the content of glycine in various areas of the rat CNS. In one correlation, the enzyme activity is expressed as nanomoles per hour per milligram of protein, and in the other correlation a ratio of SHMT to succinate dehydrogenase (SDH) is used. The SHMT activity has been given with respect to the SDH activity in order to correct or weight the former measure for the relative number of mitochondria present in the five areas of the CNS (Gregson and Williams, 1969). The points were fitted to the lines by a linear regression program and the correlation coefficients are given with the lines. In the first case, the data for the cerebellum were not used to calculate the line for SHMT versus glycine content. Both correlation coefficients are significant ($P < 0.05$). Reprinted with permission from Daly and Aprison (1974).

ten times the amount of DNA than the other regions. This increased content of DNA is most likely a reflection of the greater number of cells per gram of tissue in the cerebellum than in the other regions.

The correlation of SHMT activity with glycine levels suggests the possibility that the enzyme might be rate-limiting in the synthesis of glycine. Therefore, SHMT may be important in regulating the content of glycine in CNS tissues. However, extrapolation of the correlation line in Figure 7 to zero glycine content predicts that a significant portion of the enzymatic activity may serve another metabolic purpose. This finding is not unexpected in view of the reversible nature of the enzyme (McBride *et al.*,

1973) and the importance of this interconversion in one-carbon metabolism in the CNS (Bridgers, 1968). The high levels of SHMT activity found in the cerebellum (McBride *et al.,* 1973; Daly and Aprison, 1974) may be a reflection of the greater cell density in this structure and the subsequent greater demand for one-carbon units. Support for this idea is found in maturation studies where there appears to be a correlation between SHMT levels and growth rate of the CNS (Bridgers, 1968; Gaull *et al.,* 1973; Davies and Johnston, 1974). It is interesting to speculate that the SHMT activity is relatively constant from cell to cell in the CNS for its role in maintaining metabolic homeostasis and that the increased levels of the enzyme in the medulla-pons and spinal cord reflect its role in maintaining the "extra" glycine used for neurotransmission in these areas. Consequently, if one accepts the idea that the extra glycine found in the high-glycine regions of the CNS represents a functional pool(s), then serine appears to be a precursor of glycine in both the metabolic and functional compartments.

The studies of Davies and Johnston (1973) and Daly and Aprison (1974) do not agree upon the correlation of SHMT levels and glycine content within the rat CNS. Possible explanations for this discrepancy may be (1) the different concentrations of serine used in the two studies, (2) dialysis of the extracts for 5 hr in the former study, (3) freezing of samples before homogenization in the latter study, and (4) the different sources and concentrations of tetrahydrofolate used in the two studies (Daly and Aprison, 1974).

Some controversy also exists on the subcellular localization of SHMT within the CNS. Davies and Johnston (1973) reported a bimodal distribution of SHMT between soluble and particulate matter in subcellular fractions of rat CNS, whereas Daly and Aprison (1974) reported a nearly exclusive localization of SHMT in particulate fractions (96–99%). The enzymatic activity was closely associated with mitochondria. This discrepancy is most likely due to the differences in recovery of the enzymatic activity from the sucrose gradients in the two studies (approximately 33 and 80%, respectively). Our studies indicate that passage of the particulate matter through the high concentrations of sucrose on the gradient hinders the solubilization of enzymatic activity at time of assay. Repeated cycles of freezing and thawing the resuspended fractions after isolation, as well as increasing the concentrations of nonionic detergent (Triton X-100) in the assay system, tend to overcome this effect (Daly and Aprison, 1974).

The nearly exclusive particulate localization of SHMT within the CNS (Daly and Aprison, 1974) has been confirmed by two separate laboratories (Burton and Sallach, 1975; Rassin and Gaull, 1975). Indirect evidence suggests that SHMT may be associated with synaptosomes that band below

1.2 M sucrose in the usual procedure (Gray and Whittaker, 1962) employed in subcellular fractionation (Daly and Aprison, 1974; McClain *et al.*, 1975; Rassin and Gaull, 1975). It is well known that there exists a subpopulation of synaptosomes that band below 1.2 M sucrose during subcellular fractionation—the so-called noncholinergic synaptosomes (De Robertis *et al.*, 1962). It is interesting that there is direct evidence that glycine appears concentrated in "heavy" synaptosomes isolated from the medulla and spinal cord (Osborne *et al.*, 1973). Experiments are needed to verify the interesting possibility of an association between glycine and SHMT in "heavy" synaptosomes.

The lack of a soluble SHMT activity may be unique to the CNS since approximately 50% of the SHMT in liver of the rat is soluble (Nakano *et al.*, 1968). Yoshida and Kikuchi (1973) also found the brain to contain extremely small amounts of soluble SHMT activity. In fact, the soluble SHMT activity in brain was the lowest of the nine tissues examined. The compartmentation of SHMT exclusively in mitochondria may imply important and unique regulatory functions for glycine and/or one-carbon metabolism within the brain.

6.3.2. Glycine Transaminase Activities

The suggestion that glyoxylate may serve as a precursor of glycine within the CNS was first made by Johnston and Vitali (1969*a*) when they noted the presence of a transaminating activity between glutamate and glyoxylate in acetone powder extracts prepared from rat spinal cord. The activity was localized in the soluble and mitochondrial fractions prepared from sucrose homogenates of rat cerebral cortex (Johnston and Vitali, 1969*b*). The results of Benuck *et al.* (1972) using rat whole brain confirm this bimodal distribution. After subcellular fractionation of cat spinal cord, the enzymatic activity was predominantly localized in the soluble fraction although a significant amount (11%) was also found in the mitochondrial fraction (Johnston *et al.*, 1970). The glycine transaminase activity was higher in the spinal gray matter than in white matter.

Benuck *et al.* (1971) found 11 amino acids capable of participating in a transamination reaction with glyoxylate in dialyzed homogenates of rat whole brain. Glutamate and ornithine were found to be the best substrates for the reaction. Arginine, glutamine, and tyrosine were approximately two-thirds as active; aspartate, alanine, GABA, methionine, and phenylalanine approximately one-third as active; and tryptophan approximately one-sixth as active as glutamate and ornithine as substrates for transamination with glyoxylate. Johnston and Vitali (1969*b*) found glutamine to be 93% as active as glutamate and alanine 29% as active. These latter authors found no activity when aspartate was used as substrate. Therefore, there appear to be a number of transamination reactions with glyoxylate present within the CNS. Whether these activities represent separate enzymes or multiple reactions of a few enzymes has not been studied. However, the possibility of at least different isoenzymes is suggested by the finding that the glutamine:glyoxylate transaminase activity appears to be localized primarily in the mitochondrial fraction (Johnston and Vitali, 1969b; Benuck et al., 1972), whereas the glutamate:glyoxylate transaminase activity appears to be present in both the mitochondrial and soluble fractions (see above).

Benuck et al. (1972) reported the glutamate:glyoxylate transaminase activity approximately equal in the midbrain and the cortical gray matter of the rat. There was a trend toward lower activity in the spinal cord and higher activity in the corpus collosum. We have also measured this enzymatic activity after adjusting the reaction conditions for maximal activity (Daly and Aprison, 1974) (see Table 13). The levels of the transaminase were the same in the telencephalon, midbrain, cerebellum, and medulla–pons of the rat, and the spinal cord contained a significantly lower amount of activity. This distribution of glycine transaminase among the five regions does not correlate with the glycine content and is distinctly different from that found for SHMT (Table 13, Figure 7). Maturation studies indicate a tendency for the transaminase activity to increase during postnatal development (Benuck et al., 1971; Davies and Johnston, 1974).

Although the glycine transaminase activities within specific regions of the CNS are not correlated with the glycine content, this finding does not exclude the enzyme from playing a role in glycine synthesis since the low levels of glyoxylate found in the CNS (Liang, 1962; Johnston et al., 1970) may necessitate a large excess of this enzyme. The activity of glycine transaminase in vitro suggests that this enzyme could be capable of catalyzing the synthesis of a significant portion of the glycine within CNS tissues. However, since the affinity between glycine transaminase and glyoxylate is weak (apparent K_m = 10–15 mM) (E. C. Daly, N. S. Nadi, and M. H. Aprison, unpublished data), the enzyme is probably not saturated in vivo. If a yet undiscovered pathway that utilizes glyoxylate as the immediate precursor of glycine is found, the lack of any correlation between the transaminase activity and glycine content would suggest that the enzyme is not rate limiting and therefore may not be instrumental in regulating the content of glycine in CNS tissues.

6.3.3. Glycine Cleavage System

Four possible pathways have been shown to exist for the removal of glycine within/from the CNS: (1) an active carrier-mediated mechanism for transporting glycine from the CSF to blood exists—at least in the spinal subarachnoid space (see Section 5.3); (2) SHMT is readily reversible and may function in glycine degradation as well as synthesis; (3) D-amino acid oxidase is present within the CNS and can utilize glycine as substrate (DeMarchi and Johnston, 1969); and (4) the glycine cleavage system (GCS), which appears to be a major degradative mechanism in peripheral tissues (Yoshida and Kikuchi, 1973), is present within the CNS. Owing to the potent reuptake system present within the CNS (see Section 4.2), a degradative enzyme for glycine probably does not function in the same capacity during synaptic transmission as acetylcholinesterase does in cholinergic transmission.

In liver, the GCS has been found to be a complex of four proteins (Kikuchi, 1973) and together with a portion of the SHMT is located within the inner membrane fraction of mitochondria (Motokawa and Kikuchi, 1971). The properties of the GCS within the CNS (Bruin *et al.*, 1973; Uhr, 1973; Daly *et al.*, 1976) appear to be similar to those described for the system in liver (Sato *et al.*, 1969; Kikuchi, 1973). The enzymatic activity is exclusively located in mitochondria and is not a typical amino acid decarboxylase in that it is dependent on both NAD and tetrahydrofolate. The liberation of the carboxyl carbon of glycine is closely associated with the formation of serine via the condensation reaction between the α-carbon (attached to tetrahydrofolate) and a second molecule of glycine catalyzed by SHMT. The detailed experiments with liver mitochondria describing the membrane-bound nature of the four protein complexes have not been performed with CNS tissues. However, it should be noted that Triton X-100 completely abolished the GCS activity in CNS homogenates and this fact suggested to Daly *et al.* (1976) that the detergent causes disruption of membrane associations which are essential for enzymatic activity.

Bruin *et al.* (1973) found the total GCS activity to be the highest in the cerebrum of six species of animals. However, the specific activities for the enzyme in digitonin-treated mitochondrial fractions were greatest in the cerebellum. The cerebrum had a higher specific activity than the medulla pons except in the dog. Uhr (1973) found higher enzyme levels in homogenates of the rostral portions of of the CNS than in the medulla–pons and spinal cord of the sheep and cat. These findings were unexpected for three reasons (Daly *et al.*, 1976): (1) there are higher levels of glycine in the caudal portion of the CNS, (2) the GCS is important in the degradation of glycine in peripheral organs, and (3) there was a reported association between neurological disease localized to ventral gray matter of the lumbar spinal cord and a defective glycine cleavage system in three brothers (Bank and Morrow, 1972). Daly *et al.* (1976) consequently measured and studied the regional distribution of GCS in homogenates of the rat CNS in more detail. The distribution of GCS in the various regions agreed with the previous studies indicating lower apparent activity in the medulla–pons and spinal cord (Table 13).

The 25-fold difference in activity suggested the presence of an inhibitor or controlling mechanism in those regions of the CNS in which the activity was low. To examine this possibility, homogenates of the CNS regions were incubated with liver homogenates (Daly *et al.*, 1976). The combined GCS activity of the liver and any region of the CNS was significantly less than the sum of the activities measured separately in each homogenate. This nonadditivity appeared greater in regions in which the GCS activity was low (spinal cord and medulla–pons) than in regions in which the GCS activity was high (telencephalon and cerebellum). In fact, an inverse linear relationship was found between the logarithm of the GCS activity of each area and the percent inhibition of the liver activity (measure of nonadditivity; Figure 8). The "inhibitor" was heat-labile, located in the particulate fractions of the CNS, and nondialyzable. Increased concentrations of NAD in the assay system reversed the effect of the inhibitor (Daly *et al.*, 1976).

It remains to be seen whether this endogenous inhibitor of the GCS within the CNS has any significance in the metabolic and/or transmitter roles of glycine *in vivo* or whether it is merely a serendipitous finding due to tissue homogenization and the *in vitro* assay. The potency of the inhibition, the fact that the GCS activity appears inversely related (exponentially) to the concentration of the inhibitor within the five regions, and the apparent importance of the GCS in the liver (Yoshida and Kikuchi, 1970) suggest that the apparent activity *in vitro* may not reflect either the amounts of the enzyme system *in vivo* or the possible significance of the GCS in the metabolism of glycine within the CNS.

Preliminary experiments in which the contribution of various pathways to glycine degradation was estimated *in vivo* indicate that a significant portion of the glycine in the CNS of the rat is metabolized via the GCS. After intracisternal injection of [2-^{14}C]glycine, the cerebellum and medulla–pons were analyzed for the specific radioactivities of serine and glycine by the method of Shank and Aprison (1970b). In addition, the distribution of radioactivity was determined in the C-2 and C-3 carbons of serine after paper chromatographic isolation and periodate cleavage of this amino acid. (Table 14). The specific radioactivity of serine was highest in the medulla–pons and the estimated total rate of conversion of [2-^{14}C]glycine to [^{14}C]serine was approximately 2.5-fold faster in the medulla–pons than in the cerebellum (Table 14). However, the percentage of label in the C-3 carbon of serine isolated from the cerebellum was twice that from the medulla–pons.

A model was devised to estimate the minimum contribution of the GCS in the conversion of [2-^{14}C]glycine to [^{14}C]serine. If the GCS is coupled to SHMT in this conversion, then the C-3 carbon as well as the C-2 carbon of serine will receive label. If one assumes equilibration of exogenous [2-^{14}C]glycine with the endogenous pools of the glycine acting as

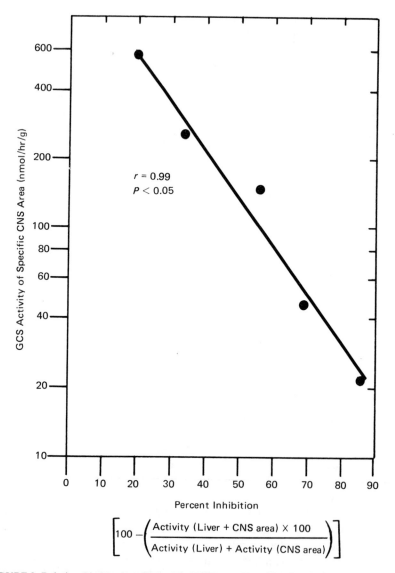

$$\left[100 - \left(\frac{\text{Activity (Liver + CNS area)} \times 100}{\text{Activity (Liver)} + \text{Activity (CNS area)}} \right) \right]$$

FIGURE 8. Relationship between the level of GCS activity in five specific regions of the CNS and the ability of each source of GCS to inhibit liver GCS activity. Homogenates from each CNS region were incubated with homogenates of liver and the nonadditivity of the two activities was calculated from these combined activities and from the activities in aliquots of the homogenates when incubated separately. Note that the ordinate is logarithmic and the levels of GCS in each region are the mean values given in Table 13. The liver homogenate had an activity of 12.7 μmol/hr/g. The percent reductions in the expected (additive) values for the liver and telencephalon, midbrain, cerebellum, medulla–pons, and spinal cord were 20, 56, 34, 69, and 86, respectively. Reprinted with permission from Daly *et al.* (1976).

TABLE 14.   Distribution of Radioactivity in the Cerebellum and Medulla–Pons of the Rat after Intracisternal Injection of [2-^{14}C] Glycine[a]

	Cerebellum	Medulla–Pons
Glycine (dpm/nmol)	913 ± 117	905 ± 66
Serine (dpm/nmol)	504 ± 78	729 ± 87
Flux (Gly → Ser)$_{total}$[b]	2.45	6.12
C-3 serine/C-2 serine	0.23 ± 0.05	0.12 ± 0.03
GCS (%)[c]	46 ± 10	24 ± 6
Flux (Gly → Ser)$_{GCS}$[b]	1.13	1.47
Flux (Gly → Ser)$_{SHMT}$[b]	1.32	4.65

[a] Data are given as mean ± SEM; $N = 5$. Rats were killed 35 min after intracisternal injection of 1.53 μCi [2-^{14}C]glycine (22.5 μCi/μmol; 68 nmol injected).
[b] Flux values (μmol/hr/g) were estimated from the approximation formula of Shank and Aprison (1970a):

$$F = \frac{C_{ser} \Delta S_{ser}}{\Delta t} \bigg/ (\overline{S}_{gly} - \overline{S}_{ser})$$

[c] Estimate of the GCS = 2 (percent radioactivity in C-3 carbon of serine). See text for description of model.

substrate for both SHMT and the GCS, and if one assumes the specific radioactivity of the ^{14}C-THF formed to be the same as these glycine pools, then the label would be equal in both the C-2 and C-3 carbons of serine when the enzymatic activities are coupled. Since this latter assumption would require the endogenous pool of C-THF to be infinitesimally small, the model would lead to an underestimation of a coupled SHMT and GCS. To estimate the contribution of the coupled enzyme, the model would multiply the percentage of radioactivity in the C-3 position by 2—the GCS would be the source of the label in the C-3 carbon and the coupled SHMT would be the source of an equal amount of label in the C-2 carbon. On the other hand, if the GCS did not participate in the conversion of [2-^{14}C]glycine to serine and only SHMT participated in the conversion, then there would be no label found in the C-3 carbon of serine. In either case, the C-1 carbon of serine is not labeled after injection of [2-^{14}C]glycine.

Using such a model the coupled GCS and SHMT were estimated to contribute approximately 46 and 24% of the label in the conversion of [2-^{14}C]glycine to [^{14}C]serine in the cerebellum and medulla–pons (Table 14). The estimated flux rates for the coupled enzymes and SHMT alone were calculated from these percentages and the total estimated flux of [2-^{14}C]glycine to serine. These estimated flux rates for the coupled GCS and SHMT were approximately equal in the cerebellum and medulla–pons (Table 14) in sharp distinction to the ratio of the GCS activities found in these two areas *in vitro* (Table 13). It would appear that the GCS plays a significant role in the conversion of glycine to serine *in vivo* and that the *in vitro* activities do not reflect this significance.

It remains to be seen whether the "inhibitor" of the GCS found during *in vitro* assay (Daly *et al.*, 1976) is an artifact of *in vitro* assay or whether this inhibition of the GCS has any significance in the metabolic and/or transmitter roles of glycine *in vivo*. Recent reports have described multiple forms of folates (Brody *et al.*, 1976) and the soluble location of both transmethylation and folate-interconverting enzymes within the CNS of the rat (Burton and Sallach, 1975; Rassin and Gaull, 1975). SHMT and the GCS probably represent the major mechanism for the generation of the one-carbon pool (Burton and Sallach, 1975) and SHMT appears to be the biosynthetic enzyme for glycine within the CNS (Shank and Aprison, 1970a; Daly and Aprison, 1974). The formation of one-carbon units and glycine within the mitochondria, their utilization within the cytosol, and the necessity for strict control of the levels of glycine in the transmitter pool emphasize the need for regulation in both the metabolism and transport of these compounds within the mitochondrion. A substance inhibiting the activity of the GCS but not that of SHMT would influence the degree of coupling in this enzymatic system. A tightly coupled GCS and SHMT could rapidly degrade glycine without changing the levels of the one-carbon pool, whereas a loosely coupled SHMT could mediate the synthesis of both glycine and one-carbon units from the original carbon skeleton of glucose via serine.

7. OTHER EXPERIMENTAL STUDIES

7.1. Maturation Studies

Different kinds of data (neurochemical, neurophysiological, neuro-pharmacological, and behavioral) are available which provide evidence for the early onset of inhibition in the CNS. Agrawal and Himwich (1970) have reported the glycine levels in whole brain of six different vertebrates varying in age (0, 1, 7, 14, 21, 30 days and adult). They found that in the mouse, rabbit, guinea pig, dog, and cat, the level of cerebral glycine decreased from birth to adult, varying only in the rate at which the decline occurred. There was not much of a change in cerebral glycine in the rat. Davies and Johnston (1974) measured glycine and 16 other amino acids in four brain areas and spinal cord of 10-day-old rats, and found that (1) the content of glycine was higher in the spinal cord and medulla–pons than in the cerebellum and cerebral cortex with the midbrain values being interme-diate, (2) glycine was the only amino acid which showed such a distribution in 10-day-old rats, and (3) the spinal levels of glycine, cystathionine, isoleucine, and leucine from 1- and 10-day-old rats did not differ significantly from adult values, whereas the levels of GABA, taurine, glutamate, and several other amino acids were higher in the young rats than in the adults.

A decline in SHMT activity was reported in extracts from mouse brain during the first 2 weeks of postnatal life (Bridgers, 1968) as well as in five different areas of the rat CNS from 1-, 10- and 91-day-old animals (Davies and Johnston, 1974). SHMT activity decreased in the spinal cord, pons–medulla, and cortex from 1- to 91-day-old animals whereas in the midbrain, the decrease was only from 1 to 10 days. In the cerebellum, the SHMT activity was highest at 10 days and lowest at 91 days. Davies and Johnston (1974) also measured glycine transaminase activity in the same five areas and found that there was a slight increase at 10 days of age over that found at 1 day of age.

Davies et al. (1975) reported a specific K^+-stimulated, Ca^{2+}-dependent release of labeled glycine and GABA from slices of cerebral cortex and spinal cord from animals that were 1 and 10 days old as well as from adult rats. Thus, the data reported by Davies and Johnston (1974) and Davies et al. (1975) support the conclusion of Aprison, Werman, and their co-workers as well as of Curtis and his co-workers that glycine is functioning as an inhibitory transmitter in the spinal cord of the rat even in early postnatal life.

The neuropharmacological and behavioral data have also indicated an early onset of inhibition in the spinal cord of the chick (Stokes and Bignall, 1974; Oppenheim and Reitzel, 1975). By observing the effect of locally applied strychnine on neuronal burst discharges recorded from the spinal cord and sciatic nerve at various ages, Stokes and Bignall (1974) found that this drug enhanced the burst activity from 13 days on in chick embryos; no effect was reported at earlier ages. Oppenheim and Reitzel (1975) studied the development of behavioral sensitivity to strychnine in the chick embryo between day 7 of incubation and day 1 of posthatching. These authors noted that the behavioral signs of strychnine appeared 4–5 days before the drug-induced bioelectrical activity (polyneuronal bursts) recorded from the lumbar spinal cord. Although the data from these two studies do not agree exactly as to "starting time," the data after day 13 are in agreement. Since the polyneuronal burst activity correlates fairly well with movements or behavior, the two measures should reflect similar underlying processes. However, even with the problem of starting time not exactly settled by these studies, it is interesting that Zukin et al. (1975) found that both the high-affinity uptake system of glycine and the [^{3}H]strychnine binding develop between days 14 and 21 in the chick embryo.

Cho *et al.* (1973) have grown spinal cord explants from chick embryos in culture up to 16 days and used this preparation to study the uptake of [^{3}H]glycine and [^{14}C]glutamate. They showed that the rate of accumulation of glycine (and glutamate) increased in the cultures between the ages of 3 and 10 days, thus matching their morphological development. In addition, the uptake system for glycine had a K_m of 41 μM, indicating a high-affinity uptake process, and like other similar systems, required Na$^+$ in the medium. It also was temperature-sensitive and showed saturation kinetics.

7.2. Behavioral Effects of Drug and Metabolite Interactions

7.2.1. Substance P, Morphine, and β, β-Iminodipropionitrile

Stern *et al.* (1974) have reported that the injection of synthetic substance P increases the levels of glycine in both the brain and spinal cord of mice. Otsuka (1977) has recently discussed the role of substance P in the spinal cord and reviewed its role as a sensory transmitter. Since the neurophysiological action of substance P has been reported to be slower than that of glutamate, it is of interest that a biochemical system may also be involved in some of the actions of substance P, as suggested by the reported elevation of glycine levels (Stern *et al.*, 1974). Stern and his co-workers have also reported that (1) substance P possesses sedative activity as well as the ability to antagonize morphine analgesia (Stern and Hadžović, 1973), (2) acute and chronic morphine poisoning caused a decrease in the content of spinal glycine (Stern *et al.*, 1973), and (3) morphine analgesia could be abolished by either substance P or by glycine. Stern and Hadžović (1970) also reported that large doses of glycine (intraperitoneally) reversed the hind limb rigidity produced during aortic occlusion in rats and that substance P could be used in place of glycine.

Stern *et al.* (1974) found that the administration of β, β-iminodipropionitrile (IDPN) to mice caused continuous decrease in spinal levels of glycine over a 20-day period and the excessive motor activity produced in these animals could be antagonized by either substance P or glycine if given within 2 weeks after the last injections of IDPN. However, after 20 days following the last administration of IDPN only glycine was fully effective in reducing the excessive motor activity.

7.2.2. Physiology and Behavior

There are a number of different published papers involving glycine and its possible role in physiological processes in the CNS that have not as yet been studied in depth. These studies are also called to the attention of the reader.

Takano and Neumann (1972) have shown that intravenously injected glycine is capable of inhibiting the stretch reflex tension. They studied this process with the triceps surae muscle of the precollicular decerebrate cat. After the reflex was totally inhibited following an injection of 125 mg/kg of glycine into the jugular vein, it took 90 min to recover. A second dose was less effective than the first.

Pollay (1976) has recently studied the movement of glycine across the blood–brain barrier in the rabbit. He concluded that glycine does not cross the blood–brain barrier by a carrier-mediated process. It would appear from other studies that very little if any glycine crosses this barrier (Oldendorf, 1971). Therefore, the reports of physiological and behavioral effects produced after an injection of glycine must be carefully considered in terms of possible mechanisms.

Piepho and Friedman (1971) reported that there is a 24-hr rhythm in the content of glycine in the pons–medulla and spinal cord of the rat. The levels of glycine were generally higher during the dark phase (12 hr). However, the content of glycine in the medulla was relatively stable during the complete 24-hr cycle. The circadian rhythm was most prominent in the pons, whereas in the cervical, thoracic, and lumbar segments of the spinal cord, glycine levels were lowest during the light phase. The authors suggest that the lower levels of glycine during the lighted portion of the cycle may be secondary to the minimal feeding and motor activity of rats during this period.

7.2.3. Alcohol

While studying the effect of alcohol on the sleeping time as measured by the loss of righting reflex in mice, Blum *et al.* (1972) noted that glycine and its major precursor, serine, significantly enhanced the behavioral effect. The combination of ethanol and glycine resulted in a duration of sleep time that was almost twice the sum of the sleeping time when glycine or ethanol was administered (intraperitoneally) separately. A less marked but still significant synergistic effect was noted with serine. Blum *et al.* (1972) suggest that glycine may be inhibiting glutamine synthetase, thereby increasing glutamate and consequently GABA. The latter inhibitory transmitter has been implicated in the depressant actions of ethanol in the CNS.

7.3. Tissue Culture

In the early 1970s, Hösli and co-workers investigated the role of several putative transmitters employing a different system—spinal neurons from newborn rats grown in tissue culture (Hösli *et al.*, 1971*b*, 1972*a,b*, 1973*a,b*; Hösli and Hösli, 1972). During this period these investigators reported that (1) glycine caused a hyperpolarization with a time course similar to that observed in the cat (Hösli *et al.*, 1971*b*); and (2) localization of [³H]glycine accumulation by neurons and glia in cultures of rat medulla oblongata (Hösli and Hösli, 1972) and rat spinal cord (Hösli *et al.*, 1972*a*) could be demonstrated by autoradiography. In cultures of human and rat spinal cord, Hösli *et al.* (1976) found the membrane potentials of glial cells to be more negative (hyperpolarized) than those recorded from neurons by intracellular techniques. However, the presence of glycine, GABA, glutamic acid, or aspartic acid in the bathing fluid (0.1 mM) produced no consistent effect on the membrane potential of glial cells.

8. A FUNCTIONAL MODEL OF GLYCINERGIC NEUROTRANSMISSION

8.1. Compartmentation in Glycinergic Nerve Endings

In 1975, Aprison and co-workers suggested a working model for the glycinergic nerve ending (see Figure 9) which contained four compartments: mitochondrial, metabolic (cytoplasmic), functional (intracellular transmitter), and free (in cleft). The latter two compartments would comprise the total transmitter pool. Data from Aprison's laboratory showed that glycine can be derived from glucose via serine in the CNS (Shank and Aprison, 1970*a*), and the conversion of serine to glycine occurs in the mitochondria by the action of serine hydroxymethyltransferase, an enzyme that requires tetrahydrofolate as a cofactor (Daly and Aprison, 1974). The degradation of glycine also occurs within the mitochondria and is catalyzed by SHMT and/or the glycine cleavage system (Daly *et al.*, 1976). The newly synthesized glycine is released from the mitochondria into the cytoplasm, a portion of which is then taken into the functional compartment (Aprison *et al.*, 1975). After the propagation of an action potential into the presynaptic terminal, glycine is released into the cleft (free pool). It then diffuses across the junction and interacts with specific receptors on the adjacent postsynaptic membrane which results in an increased influx of Cl^-, or an increased outflow of K^+, or both. This increase in conductance across the postsynaptic membrane usually causes a hyperpolarization of the membrane and renders the postsynaptic cell less excitable. Although inactivation of the free pool of glycine is now thought to occur mainly by reuptake into the presynaptic terminal, some glycine may diffuse from the cleft and be taken up by adjacent neuronal and glial cells.

Neurobiologists agree that there must be some mechanism dependent on presynaptic depolarization that will enable the transmitter to be mobilized and then released into the synaptic cleft. Thus, the concept requires

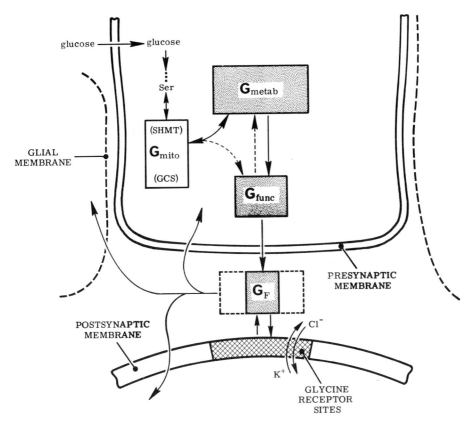

FIGURE 9. A hypothetical simplified model of a glycinergic synapse. The various compartments of glycine referred to are mitochondrial (G_{mito}), metabolic (G_{metab}), functional (G_{func}), and free (G_F). SHMT refers to serine hydroxymethyltransferase, and GCS to the glycine cleavage system. Reprinted with permission from Aprison *et al.* (1975).

the identification of a functional compartment that is the source of the free pool in the synaptic cleft. Some speculations on this concept are now considered.

8.2. Speculations on the Location of the Functional Pool of Glycine

8.2.1. Metabolic–Vesicular Equilibration

The possibility that the functional pool of glycine is associated with synaptic vesicles deserves continued attention for a number of reasons, including (1) available evidence strongly suggests that acetylcholine, nor-epinephrine, and serotonin are stored in such structures; (2) the ratios of released protein components, norepinephrine, and ATP are the same as the ratios in isolated synaptic vesicles; and (3) published data showing no clear association of amino acids with synaptic vesicles may be subject to error on the basis of either unavoidable technical limitations of the procedures employed, or the possibility of equilibration between metabolic (cyto-plasmic) and vesicular pools of glycine.

The following data favor the hypothesis that the functional pool of glycine is associated with synaptic vesicles. First, there is excellent evi-dence indicating that synaptic vesicles are present in glycinergic nerve endings (see figures in Hökfelt and Ljungdahl, 1971; Matus and Dennison, 1971; Ljungdahl and Hökfelt, 1973), and that the vesicles are not spherical but elliptical or flat, a configuration suggested to be common to the presyn-aptic nerve ending of inhibitory synapses (Uchizono, 1965). Second, Holtz-man *et al.* (1971) showed that horseradish peroxidase is taken up into the synaptic vesicles (presumably by pinocytosis) in synapses on lobster stretch muscle and that this process is enhanced by neurally evoked transmitter release. Since these crustacean neuromuscular junctions are thought to utilize GABA or glutamate as transmitters, these observations suggest that these amino acids may be released from vesicles.

Aprison *et al.* (1975) suggested the following explanation for the paucity of positive data showing an association of glutamate, GABA, or glycine with synaptic vesicles in vertebrate preparations: there is an equi-librium between cytoplasmic and vesicular glycine that may be disrupted during the homogenization and isolation procedures. As biosynthesis of glycine occurs in the mitochondria, this amino acid is released into the cytoplasm of the nerve ending and then it may penetrate the membrane of the vesicle until equilibration with the cytoplasmic pool is reached. The vesicular glycine could be released by the process of exocytosis into the synaptic cleft, and the synaptic vesicles would then be re-formed (retrieval process) by invagination and pinching off of the presynaptic membrane (Gray and Willis, 1970). Similar processes for glutamate, GABA, and aspartate may explain why it is so difficult to find amino acids associated with synaptic vesicles. Homogenization of the tissue, centrifugation, and washing of the vesicles would allow the amino acids to diffuse readily out of the vesicles into the media (Mangan and Whittaker, 1966). One additional explanation not discussed by Aprison *et al.* (1975) would be that after cytoplasmic–vesicular equilibration, and if little or no disruption occurs during homogenization and centrifugation, the amount of amino acid found associated with vesicles would be low owing to the latter's inability to concentrate amino acid transmitters. One consequence of the model shown in Figure 9, and the latter idea, is that if glycine was synthesized from labeled serine in the mitochondria, the specific radioactivity of glycine in the cytoplasm and vesicles should be the same as that released.

8.2.2. Cytoplasmic Pool

De Belleroche and Bradford (1977) recently published a study in which they attempted to localize the intrasynaptosomal origin of released transmitters by employing techniques to label amino acid transmitters radioactively in various intrasynaptosomal compartments. They studied the release of GABA, glutamate, and aspartate in synaptosomal preparations from the cerebral cortex of the rat. These data may have a bearing on other amino acid transmitters including glycine in different regions of the CNS (medulla oblongata, lumbar spinal cord, etc.) and therefore deserve some discussion.

De Belleroche and Bradford (1977) measured the specific radioactivities of glutamate, aspartate, and GABA after release induced by KCl (56mM) or veratrine (75 μM). Stimulation with 56 mM K$^+$ produced significant increases in the release of glutamate and GABA compared with that released under control conditions. From measurements of the specific radioactivities of the amino acids, the authors made calculations to obtain estimates of the "synaptosomal source" from which the three amino acids were released. Their data and calculations show a similarity of the specific radioactivities of the soluble cytoplasmic amino acids within the synaptosome to those released by stimulation. The specific radioactivities of vesicular GABA and aspartate were significantly different from both the cytoplasmic pool and that released, whereas the specific radioactivities of glutamate were nonsignificantly different in the vesicular and cytoplasmic pools after K$^+$ stimulation.

The decrease in the cytoplasmic pool size after K$^+$ stimulation could account for at least 80% of the quantity released into the media for all three amino acids. De Belleroche and Bradford (1973, 1977) concluded that the origin of the released amino acids was cytoplasmic rather than vesicular. Furthermore, based on estimates of the turnover rate in synaptic vesicles these authors concluded that the synaptic vesicles did not function as intermediate carriers for the release of cytoplasmic amino acids. This latter conclusion would argue against the metabolic–vesicular equilibration model discussed earlier.

Although the problem of the anatomical and biochemical localization of the functional pool for amino acid transmitters is not resolved, more interest in this problem is evident. It is hoped that as more neurochemists and neurobiologists turn their attention to this difficult problem, it will be clarified and perhaps solved. This recent study of De Belleroche and Bradford (1977) appears to be a step toward this goal.

9. NEUROLOGICAL SIGNIFICANCE

9.1. Hyperglycinemia Syndromes

There are a fairly large number of hereditary disorders involving errors in the metabolism or excretion of glycine. Of specific interest are reports studying the metabolism of glycine in the "nonketotic hyperglycinemia" syndrome. The other large class of disorders involving elevated blood levels of glycine consists of the "ketotic hyperglycinemia" syndrome(s). The clinical basis for the distinction between the two syndromes is the ketonuria and ketoacidosis found in the latter. However, recent studies (Wadlington *et al.*, 1975) have made these findings less clear-cut than originally supposed. The distinction is of great practical value since there is promise that the natural history of the disorders involving ketotic hyperglycinemia can be altered by dietary therapy (Nyhan, 1967), whereas no effective therapy has been found to alter natural history in the nonketotic syndromes (Krieger *et al.*, 1977)—these unfortunate individuals for the most part suffer as yet irreversible psychiatric and neurological retardation which results in early death.

The hyperglycinemia in the ketotic syndromes has been thought to be secondary to primary defects in the metabolism of propionic acid (Hsia *et al.*, 1969), methylmalonic acid (Rosenberg *et al.*, 1968), isovaleric acid (Ando *et al.*, 1971), and isoleucine (Hillman and Keating, 1974). Various products which accumulate because of the primary metabolic defect have been shown to alter glycine metabolism (Hillman *et al.*, 1973; Hillman and Otto, 1974; Ho and Hillman, 1974). The defect in the nonketotic syndromes is thought to involve directly the metabolism of glycine. Studies both *in vivo* (Ando *et al.*, 1968; Bank and Morrow, 1972) and *in vitro* employing liver samples (Tada *et al.*, 1969, 1974; Yoshida *et al.*, 1969; De Groot *et al.*, 1970; Wada *et al.*, 1972; Reploh *et al.*, 1973; Trijbels *et al.*, 1974; Corbeel *et al.*, 1975; Perry *et al.*, 1975a; Farriaux *et al.*, 1976) have suggested that the lesion in nonketotic hyperglycinemia is a defective glycine cleavage system. A recent report failed to detect activity of the GCS in autopsy specimens from the CNS of patients with nonketotic hyperglycinemia (Perry *et al.*, 1975a), but was able to detect the GCS at reduced levels in specimens from patients with unclassified hyperglycinemia (neither ketotic or nonketotic). The metabolism of glyoxylate has been reported to be normal in nonketotic hyperglycinemia (Gerritsen *et al.*, 1969). The GCS has also been shown defective in ketotic hyperglycinemia (Ando *et al.*, 1972; Nishimura *et al.*, 1974; Tada *et al.*, 1974; Corbeel *et al.*, 1975; Motokawa *et al.*, 1977) as well as in cases of unclassified hyperglycinemia (Perry *et al.*, 1975a). Revsin and Morrow (1976) have recently suggested that a decrease in the cellular transport of glycine may be defective in addition to, or instead of, an enzymatic mechanism in the nonketotic syndrome. The nonketotic syndrome was originally thought to be present only with the defect in oxidation of glycine and without altered propionic or methylmalonic acid metabolism (Baumgartner and Wick, 1972; Baumgartner *et al.*, 1975). However, more recent reports have provided evidence for other metabolic defects associated with the nonketotic syndrome (Wada *et al.*, 1972; Krieger and Hart, 1974; Corbeel *et al.*, 1975; De Groot *et al.*, 1975; Geison *et al.*, 1975; Brandt *et al.*, 1976; Farriaux *et al.*, 1976; Kolvraa *et al.*, 1976; Revsin *et al.*, 1977).

What has evolved from case reports are at least two syndromes which overlap both clinically and biochemically. Part of the confusion is undoubtedly due to the similarity in clinical presentation and the ambiguity in the diagnostic criteria for each syndrome. It was originally noted by Levy *et al.* (1972) that the ratio of glycine in the plasma to glycine in the CSF was different in the two syndromes of hyperglycinemia. Recent reports have suggested that this concentration ratio of glycine in plasma to glycine in CSF is the most definitive test for distinguishing the two syndromes (Perry *et al.*, 1975*a,b*; Scriver *et al.*, 1975). The normal lumbar CSF/plasma ratio for glycine has been found to be approximately 0.02—among the lowest of any of the amino acids (Dickinson and Hamilton, 1966; Perry *et al.*, 1975*a,b*; McGale *et al.*, 1977). Values for this ratio in nonketotic hyperglycinemia are usually greater than 0.10 and not uncommonly greater than 0.20 (Perry *et al.*, 1975*b,c*; Scriver *et al.*, 1975; Holmgrem and Blomquist, 1977; Krieger *et al.*, 1977). Values for the ratio in other hyperglycinemias and in a normal subject after an oral glycine load are not different from the ratio in control subjects (Krieger *et al.*, 1977).

Two reports are of special interest in understanding the metabolic regulation and function of glycine within the CNS. Perry *et al.* (1975*b*) have studied the neurochemical lesions in nonketotic hyperglycinemia in the greatest detail to date. The content of glycine in autopsy specimens of patients with nonketotic hyperglycinemia was found to be significantly elevated from controls in all areas of the CNS studied (cerebral cortex, cerebellar cortex, basal ganglia, and spinal cord) but not in these areas in specimens from patients with nonclassified hyperglycinemia. A normal level of glycine in the brain of a patient who died with ketotic hyperglycinemia had been previously reported by Ando and Nyhan (1974). Perry *et al.* (1975*b*) found reduced activity of the GCS in the brains of the patients with nonclassified hyperglycinemia, but could not detect any enzymatic activity in the brains of the patients with nonketotic hyperglycinemia. The GCS activity was reduced in the livers of both groups of patients. There appears to be some merit in the proposal of the term "glycine encephalopathy" by

Perry's group for nonketotic hyperglycinemia although this syndrome appears to be quite heterogeneous (see earlier).

Bank and Morrow (1972) studied three brothers with hyperglycinemia. This report is unique with regard to both the late appearance of symptoms and the apparent localization of the neuropathological lesion. These brothers were asymptomatic to the ages of 2, 10, and 18 years, respectively. At the time of the study, they were apparently normal mentally with neurological deficits limited to the lower extremities. These deficits were consistent with both upper and lower motoneuron lesions and were clinically localized to the ventrolateral gray matter of the spinal cord, the area normally having the highest levels of glycine in the neuraxis. All three patients had marked hyperglycinemia and the two brothers studied had distinctly abnormal conversion of intravenously administered $[1\text{-}^{14}C]$glycine to $^{14}CO_2$. It is very interesting in view of the neurotransmitter role of glycine that an apparent systemic defect in glycine metabolism was manifested in an isolated spinal cord lesion. The CSF/plasma ratio of glycine in the two brothers studied (0.02–0.03) would indicate that the disorder was not nonketotic hyperglycinemia.

The biochemical lesions are not clear in the hyperglycinemic syndromes. It has been suggested that long-standing elevation of plasma glycine by itself may be a benign process without neurological or psychiatric sequelae (Pavone *et al.*, 1975) although it has been reported that an acute glycine load in newborn rats produced respiratory depression and convulsions (De Groot *et al.*, 1977). There appears to be an elevation of glycine levels within the CNS only in nonketotic hyperglycinemia and desensitization of the glycine receptor by chronically elevated levels of glycine in the extracellular fluid of the CNS has been postulated as the pathophysiologic basis of the neurological deficits (Ransom and Nelson, 1976). Although difficult to reconcile with the concept of desensitization, the promising preliminary report of clinical improvement in a patient treated with oral strychnine would also implicate the postsynaptic glycine receptor in the pathogenesis of nonketotic hyperglycinemia (Gitzelmann *et al.*, 1977).

In nonketotic hyperglycinemia there is no measurable activity of the GCS in the CNS and reduced activity peripherally (liver), whereas in other hyperglycinemias, activity of the GCS can be measured at reduced levels both within the CNS and peripherally. Although the total activity of SHMT activity has been measured in liver homogenates from patients with hyperglycinemia (Yoshida *et al.*, 1969), no report has appeared in which the investigators have studied the individual activities of the cytoplasmic and mitochondrial isoenzymes in the hyperglycinemia syndromes. Since SHMT within the CNS appears to be localized mainly if not exclusively in the mitochondrial fraction (Daly and Aprison, 1974) (see also Section 6.3) and a significant portion of the GCS within the CNS is coupled to SHMT (Table 14), this "coupled" SHMT may be a limiting factor in the metabolism of glycine. Since the CNS levels of glycine are elevated in nonketotic hyperglycinemia (Perry *et al.*, 1975*b*) and glycine is synthesized mainly via serine (Shank and Aprison, 1970*a,b*), there may be a selective inhibition of this enzyme in the conversion of glycine to serine within the CNS. Another possibility is that there may be an endogenous inhibitor(s) of the GCS in the hyperglycinemia syndromes similar to that found in rat CNS *in vitro* (Daly *et al.*, 1976). However, Perry *et al.* (1975*b*) sought but did not find such an inhibitor. What is clear is that more enzymatic studies are needed to clarify the metabolic defect in the syndromes and that these studies should include the measurement of both isoenzymatic forms of SHMT as well as the GCS.

9.2. Studies of Spasticity

Interruption of descending motor tracts can produce a spastic paralysis in the muscles innervated by spinal segments below the level of the lesion. This classic upper motor neuron paralysis occurs in experimental animals whose spinal cords have been transected but only after a variable period of spinal shock characterized by flaccid paralysis and areflexia. Spasticity is considered a release phenomenon consisting of a number of clinical signs: hypertonicity, hyperreflexia, clonus, clasp-knife rigidity, decreased superficial reflexes, and the Babinski response. A number of recent reports have provided neurochemical evidence for the disruption of several neurotransmitter systems mediating segmental inhibition after experimentally produced spasticity.

Hall *et al.* (1976) measured the content of several amino acids in the ventral gray matter in the lumbar enlargement of the canine spinal cord at various times after thoracic transection. There was a drop in the levels of glycine and aspartate evident at 1 week posttransection. The levels continued to decline until 8 weeks, at which time the values were approximately 40 and 50% of controls, respectively. The levels of GABA and glutamate remained constant until 8 weeks posttransection, at which time the levels were approximately 67 and 75% of controls, respectively. The experimental animals developed signs of spasticity between 3 and 6 weeks posttransection. Therefore, it would appear that the levels of glycine and aspartate in the ventral gray were more closely associated with development of the clinical signs of spasticity than the levels of GABA or glutamate.

It is interesting to speculate that spinal transection disrupted the interneuronal pool within the ventral gray matter which utilizes glycine and probably aspartate as transmitters (Davidoff *et al.*, 1967*b*) and that the disruption may be responsible for some of the clinical components of spasticity. There have been several reports (see Hall *et al.,* 1976) describing decreased postsynaptic and recurrent inhibition in spinal spasticity. There is very good evidence that glycine is at least one of the neurotransmitters mediating these inhibitions in the spinal cord (see earlier). Further support for the same role of glycinergic transmission in producing spasticity is provided by the clinical improvement of spasticity with oral administration of glycine in humans (Stern and Bokonjić, 1974) or with intramuscular administration of glycine in dogs (Smith *et al.,* 1977). In this latter study, the systemic administration of glycine was able to increase its level in the lumbosacral spinal segments studied.

We do not wish to imply that alterations in recurrent or postsynaptic inhibition and in the levels of glycine are the total answer to the question of the neurochemical basis of spasticity. There are numerous other hypotheses which have been proposed to explain the pathophysiologic mechanisms involved (see Hall *et al.,* 1976; Smith *et al.,* 1976). A disruption of presynaptic inhibition with altered levels of GABA in the spinal dorsal gray is among the most prominent of these (Smith *et al.,* 1976). However, these studies do provide evidence for a role of the spinal amino acid transmitters, including glycine, in spinal spasticity. Further neurochemical investigations are needed especially in view of the promising clinical trials with systemic glycine administration (Stern and Bokonjić, 1974; Smith *et al.,* 1977).

10. CONCLUDING REMARKS

Since Aprison and Werman (1965) predicted that glycine was a major postsynaptic inhibitory transmitter in the cat spinal cord, many studies have confirmed and extended their observations. Thus, we now know from neurochemical, neurophysiological, and neuropharmacological data that glycine functions as an inhibitory transmitter not only in the spinal cord, but probably also at specific synapses in the medulla oblongata, pons, tectum, and retina. Along with the metabolic roles for glycine (shown in Figure 1), we can add its important functional role (Figure 10).

It is our hope that the basic research reviewed herein will not only foster more research elucidating the role of glycine in neurotransmission, but will also foster a closer association between basic and clinical investigations. Further, we hope that this closer association will result in benefits applicable directly to patient management. The preliminary reports describing such clinical benefits in tetanus, hyperglycinemia, and spasticity are very encouraging that this association may be fruitful.

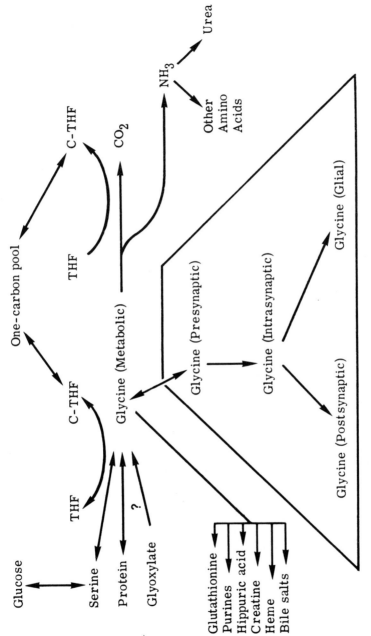

FIGURE 10. Fate of glycine in the metabolic and functional pools and interaction between the two pools.

ACKNOWLEDGMENT

The studies from our laboratories reviewed herein are currently supported in part by a grant from the National Institute of Mental Health (MHO3225).

11. REFERENCES

Agrawal, H. C., and Himwich, W. A., 1970, Amino acids, proteins and monoamines of developing brain, in: *Developmental Neurobiology* (W. A. Himwich, ed.), pp. 287–310, Thomas, Springfield, Ill.

Aitken, J. T., and Bridger, J. E., 1961, Neuron size and neuron population density in the lumbosacral region of the cat's spinal cord, *J. Anat.* **95**:38–53.

Ames, A., III, and Pollen, D. A., 1969, Neurotransmission in central nervous tissue: A study of isolated rabbit retina, *J. Neurophysiol.* **32**:424–442.

Andersen, P., Eccles, J. C., and Schmidt, R. F., 1962, Presynaptic inhibition in the cuneate nucleus, *Nature* **194**:741–743.

Andersen, P., Eccles, J. C., Loyning, Y., and Voorhoeve, P. E., 1963, Strychnine-resistant central inhibition, *Nature* **200**:843–845.

Andersen, P., Eccles, J. C., Oshima, K., and Schmidt, R. F., 1964, Mechanism of synaptic transmission in the cuneate nucleus, *J. Neurophysiol.* **27**:1096–1116.

Ando, T., and Nyhan, W. L., 1974, Propionic acidemia and the ketotic hyperglycinemia syndrome, in: *Heritable Disorders of Amino Acid Metabolism* (W. L. Nyhan, ed.), pp. 37–60, Wiley, New York.

Ando, T., Nyhan, W. L., Gerritsen, T., Gong, L., Heiner, D. C., and Bray, P. F., 1968, Metabolism of glycine in the nonketotic form of hyperglycinemia, *Pediatr. Res.* **2**:254–263.

Ando, T., Klinberg, W. G., Ward, A. N., Rasmusseen, K., and Nyhan, W. L., 1971, Isovaleric acidemia presenting with altered metabolism of glycine, *Pediatr. Res.* **5**:478–486.

Ando, T., Nyhan, W. L., Connor, J. D., Rasmusseen, K., Donnell, G., Barnes, N., Cottom, D., and Hull, D., 1972, The oxidation of glycine and propionic acid in propionic acidemia with ketotic hyperglycinemia, *Pediatr. Res.* **6**:576–583.

Aprison, M. H., 1970a, Evidence of the release of [^{14}C]glycine from hemisectioned toad spinal cord with dorsal root stimulation, *Pharmacologist* **12**:222.

Aprison, M. H., 1970b, Studies on the release of glycine in the isolated spinal cord of the toad, *Trans. Am. Soc. Neurochem.* **1**:25.

Aprison, M. H., 1971, Biochemical aspects of inhibitory mechanisms in the CNS, in: Proceedings of the VIII International Union of Physiological Sciences.

Aprison, M. H., 1978, Glycine as a neurotransmitter, in: *Psychopharmacology: A Generation of Progress* (M. A. Lipton, A. Di Mascio, and K. F. Killam, eds.), pp. 333–346, Raven Press, New York.

Aprison, M. H., and McBride, W. J., 1973, Evidence for the net accumulation of glycine into a synaptosomal fraction isolated from the telencephalon and spinal cord of the rat, *Life Sci.* **12**:449–458.

Aprison, M. H., and Werman, R., 1965, The distribution of glycine in cat spinal cord and roots, *Life Sci.* **4**:2075–2083.

Aprison, M. H., and Werman, R., 1968, A combined neurochemical and neurophysiological approach to the identification of central nervous system neurotransmitters, in: *Neurosciences Research* (S. Ehrenpreis and O. C. Solnitzky, eds.), Vol. 1, pp. 143–174, Academic Press, New York.

Aprison, M. H., Shank, R. P., Davidoff, R. A., and Werman, R., 1968, The distribution of glycine, a neurotransmitter suspect in the central nervous system of several vertebrate species, *Life Sci.* **7**:583–590.

Aprison, M. H., Shank, R. P., and Davidoff, R. A., 1969, A comparison of the concentration of glycine, a transmitter suspect, in different areas of the brain and spinal cord in seven different vertebrates, *Comp. Biochem. Physiol.* **28**:1345–1355.

Aprison, M. H., Davidoff, R. A., and Werman, R., 1970, Glycine: Its metabolic and possible transmitter roles in nervous tissue, in: *Handbook of Neurochemistry* (A. Lajtha, ed.), Vol. 3, pp. 381–397, Plenum Press, New York.

Aprison, M. H., McBride, W. J., and Freeman, A. R., 1973, The distribution of several amino acids in specific ganglia and nerve bundles of the lobster, *J. Neurochem.* **21**:87–95.

Aprison, M. H., Daly, E. C., Shank, R. P., and McBride, W. J., 1975, Neurochemical evidence for glycine as a transmitter and a model for its intrasynaptosomal compartmentation, in: *Metabolic Compartmentation and Neurotransmission* (S. Berl, D. D. Clarke, and D. Schneider, eds.), pp. 37–63, Plenum Press, New York.

Balcar, V. J., and Johnston, G. A. R., 1973, High affinity uptake of transmitters. Studies of the uptake of L-aspartate, GABA, L-glutamate, and glycine in cat spinal cord, *J. Neurochem.* **20**:529–539.

Bank, W. J., and Morrow, G., 1972, A familial spinal cord disorder with hyperglycinemia, *Arch. Neurol.* **27**:136–144.

Banna, N. R., and Jabbur, S. J., 1969, Pharmacological studies on inhibition in the cuneate nucleus of the cat, *Int. J. Neuropharmacol.* **8**:299–307.

Banos, G., Daniel, P. M., Moorhouse, S. R., and Pratt, O. E., 1975, The requirements of the brain for some amino acids, *J. Physiol. (Lond.)* **246**:539–548.

Barker, J. L., Nicoll, R. A., and Padjen, A., 1975, Studies on convulsants in the isolated frog spinal cord. I. Antagonism of amino acid response, *J. Physiol. (Lond.)* **245**:521–536.

Baumgartner, E. R., and Wick, H., 1972, Normal propionate metabolism in nonketotic hyperglycinemia, *N. Engl. J. Med.* **286**:784–785.

Baumgartner, E. R., Bachman, C., Brechbuhler, T., and Wick, H., 1975, Acute neonatal nonketotic hyperglycinemia: Normal propionate and methylmalonate metabolism, *Pediatr. Res.* **9**:559–564.

Beart, P. M., and Bilal, K. B., 1976, Compartmentation and release of glycine *in vitro*, *Neurosci. Abstr.* **2**:594.

Belcher, G., Davis, J., and Ryall, R. W., 1976, Glycine-mediated inhibitory transmission of group 1A-excited inhibitory interneurons by Renshaw cells, *J. Physiol. (Lond.)* **256**:651–662.

Belcheva, S., and Vitanova, L., 1974, Effects of some antagonists of the inhibitory transmitters on biological activity of retinal cells, *Aggressologie* **15**:461–469.

Benecke, R., Takano, K., Schmidt, J., and Henatsch, H.-D., 1977, Tetanus toxin-induced actions on spinal Renshaw cells and Ia-inhibitory interneurones during development of local tetanus in the cat, *Exp. Brain Res.* **27**:271–286.

Bennett, J. P., Jr., Logan, W. J., and Snyder, S. H., 1972, Amino acid neurotransmitter candidates: Sodium-dependent high-affinity uptake by unique synaptosomal fractions, *Science* **178**:997–999.

Benuck, M., Stern, F., and Lajtha, A., 1971, Transamination of amino acids in homogenates of rat brain, *J. Neurochem.* **8**:1555–1567.

Benuck, M., Stern, F., and Lajtha, A., 1972, Regional and subcellular distribution of amino-transferases in rat brain, *J. Neurochem.* **19**:949–957.

Berger, S. J., Carter, J. G., and Lowry, O. H., 1977a, The distribution of glycine, GABA, glutamate and aspartate in rabbit spinal cord, cerebellum and hippocampus, *J. Neurochem.* **28**:149–158.

Berger, S. J., McDaniel, M. L., Carter, J. G., and Lowry, O. H., 1977b, Distribution of four potential transmitter amino acids in monkey retina, *J. Neurochem.* **28**:159–163.

Biscoe, T. J., and Curtis, D. R., 1967, Strychnine and cortical inhibition, *Nature* **214**:914–915.

Biscoe, T. J., Duggan, A. W., and Lodge, D., 1972, Antagonism between bicuculline, strychnine, and picrotoxin and depressant amino acids in the rat nervous system, *Comp. Gen. Pharmacol.* **3**:423–433.

Bisti, S., Iosif, G., Marchesi, G. F., and Strata, P., 1971, Pharmacological properties of inhibition in the cerebellar cortex, *Exp. Brain Res.* **14**:24–37.

Blasberg, R., and Lajtha, A., 1965, Substrate specificity of steady state amino acid transport in mouse brain slices, *Arch. Biochem. Biophys.* **112**:361–377.

Blasberg, R., and Lajtha, A., 1966, Heterogeneity of the mediated transport systems of amino acid uptake in brain, *Brain Res.* **1**:86–104.

Blum, K., Wallace, J. E., and Geller, I., 1972, Synergy of ethanol and putative neurotransmitters: Glycine and serine, *Science* **176**:292–294.

Boehme, D. H., Fordice, M. W., Marks, N., and Vogel, W., 1973, Distribution of glycine in human spinal cord and selected regions of brain, *Brain Res.* **50**:353–359.

Boehme, D. H., Marks, N., and Fordice, M. W., 1976, Glycine levels in the degenerated human spinal cord, *J. Neurol. Sci.* **27**:347–352.

Boyd, E. S., Meritt, D. A., and Gardner, C., 1966, The effect of convulsant drugs on transmission through the cuneate nucleus, *J. Pharmacol. Exp. Ther.* **154**:398–409.

Bradford, H. F., 1969, Respiration *in vitro* of synaptosomes from mammalian cerebral cortex, *J. Neurochem.* **16**:675–684.

Bradford, H. F., 1970, Metabolic response of synaptosomes to electrical stimulation: Release of amino acids, *Brain Res.* **19**:239–247.

Bradford, H. F., and Thomas, A. J., 1969, Metabolism of glucose and glutamate by synaptosomes from mammalian cerebral cortex, *J. Neurochem.* **16**:1495–1504.

Bradford, H. F., Bennett, G. W., and Thomas, A. J., 1973, Depolarizing stimuli and the release of physiologically active amino acids from suspensions of mammalian synaptosomes, *J. Neurochem.* **21**:495–505.

Bradley, K., Easton, D. M., and Eccles, J. C., 1953, An investigation of primary or direct inhibition, *J. Physiol.* **122**:474–488.

Brandt, N. J., Rasmussen, K., Brandt, S., Kolvraa, S., and Schonheyder, F., 1976, D-Glyceric-acidaemia and nonketotic hyperglycinaemia, *Acta Paediatr. Scand.* **65**:17–22.

Bridgers, W. F., 1965, The biosynthesis of serine in mouse brain extracts, *J. Biol. Chem.* **240**:4591–4597.

Bridgers, W. F., 1967, Mouse brain phosphoserine phosphohydrolase and phosphotransferase, *J. Biol. Chem.* **242**:2080–2085.

Bridgers, W. F., 1968, Serine transhydroxymethylase in developing mouse brain, *J. Neurochem.* **15**:1325–1328.

Broderick, D. S., Candland, K. L., North, J. A., and Mangum, J. H., 1972, The isolation of serine transhydroxymethylase from bovine brain, *Arch. Biochem. Biophys.* **148**:196–198.

Brody, T., Shin, Y. S., and Stokstad, E. L. R., 1976, Rat brain folate identification, *J. Neurochem.* **27**:409–413.

Brooks, V. B., Curtis, D. R., and Eccles, J. C., 1957, The action of tetanus toxin on the inhibition of motoneurones, *J. Physiol.* **135**:655–672.

Bruin, W. J., Frantz, B. M., and Sallach, H. J., 1973, The occurrence of a glycine cleavage system in mammalian brain, *J. Neurochem.* **20**:1649–1658.

Burkhardt, D. A., 1972, Effects of picrotoxin and strychnine upon electrical activity of the proximal retina, *Brain Res.* **43**:246–249.

Burton, E. G., and Sallach, H. J., 1975, Methylenetetrahydrofolate reductase in the rat central nervous system: Intracellular and regional distribution, *Arch. Biochem. Biophys.* **166**:483–494.

Cho, Y. D., Martin, R. O., and Tunnicliff, G., 1973, Uptake of [^{3}H]glycine and [^{14}C]glutamate by cultures of chick spinal cord, *J. Physiol.* **235**:437–446.

Christensen, H. N., Cooper, P. E., Johnson, R. D., and Lynch, E. L., 1947, Glycine and alanine concentrations of body fluids, experimental modification, *J. Biol. Chem.* **168**:191–196.

Cohen, A. I., McDaniel, M. L., and Orr, H. T., 1973, Absolute levels of some free amino acids in normal and biologically fractioned retinas, *Invest. Ophthalmol.* **12**:686–693.

Coombs, J. S., Eccles, J. C., and Fatt, P., 1955, The inhibitory suppression of reflex discharges from motoneurones, *J. Physiol. (Lond.)* **130**:396–413.

Corbeel, L., Tada, K., Colombo, J. P., Eeckels, R., Eggermont, E., Jaekan, J., Den Tandt, W., Harvengt, L., Delhaye, J., and Deloecker, W., 1975, Methylmalonic acidaemia and nonketotic hyperglycinaemia: Clinical and biochemical aspects, *Arch. Dis. Child.* **50**:103–109.

Corbett, J. L., and Harris, P. J., 1973, Studies on the sympathetic nervous system in tetanus, *Nauyn-Schmiedebergs Arch. Pharmacol.* **276**:447–460.

Crawford, J. M., and Curtis, D. R., 1964, The excitation and depression of mammalian cortical neurones by amino acids, *Br. J. Pharmacol. Chemother.* **23**:313–329.

Crawford, J. M., Curtis, D. R., Voorhoeve, P. E., and Wilson, V. J., 1963, Strychnine and cortical inhibition, *Nature* **200**:845–846.

Curtis, D. R., 1959, Pharmacological investigations upon the inhibition of spinal motoneurones, *J. Physiol. (Lond.)* **145**:175–192.

Curtis, D. R., 1962, The depression of spinal inhibition by electrophoretically administered strychnine, *Int. J. Neuropharmacol.* **1**:239–250.

Curtis, D. R., 1963, The pharmacology of central and peripheral inhibition, *Pharmacol. Rev.* **15**:333–364.

Curtis, D. R., and DeGroat, W. C., 1968, Tetanus toxin and spinal inhibition, *Brain Res.* **10**:208–212.

Curtis, D. R., and Johnston, G. A., 1970, Strychnine, glycine and vertebrate postsynaptic inhibition, *Nature* **225**:1258.

Curtis, D. R., and Johnston, G. A. R., 1974, Amino acid transmitters in the mammalian central nervous system, *Ergebn. Physiol.* **69**:98–188.

Curtis, D. R., and Watkins, J. C., 1960, The excitation and depression of spinal neurons by structurally related amino acids, *J. Neurochem.* **6**:117–141.

Curtis, D. R., and Watkins, J. C., 1963, Acidic amino acids with strong excitatory actions on mammalian neurones, *J. Physiol. (Lond.)* **166**:1–14.

Curtis, D. R., and Watkins, J. C., 1965, The pharmacology of amino acids related to gamma-aminobutyric acid, *Pharmacol. Rev.* **17**:347–392.

Curtis, D. R., Phillis, J. W., and Watkins, J. C., 1959, The depression of spinal neurones by γ-amino-*n*-butyric acid and β-alanine, *J. Physiol. (Lond.)* **146**:185–203.

Curtis, D. R., Phillis, J. W., and Watkins, J. C., 1960, The chemical excitation of spinal neurones by certain acidic amino acids, *J. Physiol. (Lond.)* **150**:656–682.

Curtis, D. R., Hösli, L., Johnston, G. A. R., and Johnston, I. H., 1968*a*, The hyperpolarization of spinal interneurones by glycine and related amino acids, *Exp. Brain Res.* **5**:235–258.

Curtis, D. R., Hösli, L., and Johnston, G. A. R., 1968*b*, A pharmacological study of the depression of spinal neurones by glycine and related amino acids, *Exp. Brain Res.* **6**:1–18.

Curtis, D. R., Duggan, A. W., and Johnston, G. A. R., 1971, The specificity of strychine as a glycine antagonist in the mammalian spinal cord, *Exp. Brain Res.* **12**:547–565.

Curtis, D. R., Felix, D., Game, C. J. A., and McCulloch, R. M., 1973, Tetanus toxin and the synaptic release of GABA, *Brain Res.* **51**:358–362.

Curtis, D. R., Game, C. J. A., and Lodge, D., 1976*a*, The *in vivo* inactivation of GABA and other inhibitory amino acids in the cat nervous system, *Exp. Brain Res.* **25**:413–428.

Curtis, D. R., Game, C. J. A., and Lodge, D., 1976*b*, Benzodiazepines and central glycine receptors, *Br. J. Pharmacol.* **56**:307–311.

Curtis, D. R., Game, C. J. A., Lodge, D., and McCulloch, R. M., 1976*c*, A pharmacological study of Renshaw cell inhibition, *J. Physiol. (Lond.)* **258**:227–242.

Curtis, D. R., Lodge, D., Johnston, G. A. R., and Brand, S. J., 1976*d*, Central actions of benzodiazepines, *Brain Res.* **118**:344–347.

Cutler, R. W. P., 1975, Glycine release from rat spinal cord, American Society of Neurochemistry, Abstract, 6th Meeting, p. 191.

Cutler, R. W. P., Hammerstad, J. P., Cornick, L. R., and Murray, J. E., 1971, Efflux of amino acid neurotransmitters from rat spinal cord slices. I. Factors influencing the spontaneous efflux of [^{14}C]glycine and ^{3}H-GABA, *Brain Res.* **35**:337–355.

Cutler, R. W. P., Murray, J. E., and Hammerstad, J. P., 1972, Role of mediated transport in the electrically induced release of [^{14}C]glycine from slices of rat spinal cord, *J. Neurochem.* **19**:539–542.

Daly, E. C., and Aprison, M. H., 1974, Distribution of serine hydroxymethyltransferase and glycine transaminase in several areas of the central nervous system of the rat, *J. Neurochem.* **22**:877–885.

Daly, E. C., Nadi, N. S., and Aprison, M. H., 1976, Regional distribution and properties of the glycine cleavage system within the central nervous system of the rat: Evidence for an endogenous inhibitor during *in vitro* assay, *J. Neurochem.* **26**:179–185.

Davidoff, R. A., and Adair, R., 1976, GABA and glycine transport in frog CNS: High affinity uptake and potassium-evoked release *in vitro*, *Brain Res.* **118**:403–415.

Davidoff, R. A., Shank, R. P., Graham, L. T., Jr., Aprison, M. H., and Werman, R., 1967*a*, Association of glycine with spinal interneurons, *Nature* **214**:680–681.

Davidoff, R. A., Graham, L. T., Jr., Shank, R. P., Werman, R., and Aprison, M. H., 1967*b*, Changes in amino acid concentrations associated with loss of spinal interneurons, *J. Neurochem.* **14**:1025–1031.

Davidoff, R. A., Aprison, M. H., and Werman, R., 1969, The effects of strychnine on the inhibition of interneurons by glycine and γ-aminobutyric acid, *Int. J. Neuropharmacol.* **8**:191–194.

Davidson, N., and Southwick, C. A. P., 1971, Amino acids and presynaptic inhibition in the rat cuneate nucleus, *J. Physiol. (Lond.)* **219**:689–708.

Davidson, N., and Suckling, E. E., 1967, Studies on corticofugal inhibition in the rat dorsal column nuclei, *Fed. Proc.* **26**:491.

Davies, L. P., and Johnston, G. A. R., 1973, Serine hydroxymethyltransferase in the central nervous system regional and subcellular distribution studies, *Brain Res.* **54**:149–156.

Davies, L. P., and Johnston, G. A. R., 1974, Postnatal changes in the levels of glycine and the activities of serine hydroxymethyltransferase and glycine:2-oxoglutarate aminotransferase in the rat central nervous system, *J. Neurochem.* **22**:107–112.

Davies, L. P., Johnston, G. A. R., and Stephanson, A. L., 1975, Postnatal changes in the potassium-stimulated, calcium-dependent release of radioactive GABA and glycine from slices of rat central nervous tissue, *J. Neurochem.* **25**:387–392.

Davis, R., and Huffmann, R. D., 1969, Pharmacology of the brachium conjunctivum-red nucleus synaptic system in the baboon, *Fed. Proc.* **28**:775.

Davson, H., 1967, *Physiology of the Cerebrospinal Fluid,* Little, Brown, Boston, Mass.

De Belleroche, J. S., and Bradford, H. F., 1972, Metabolism of beds of mammalian cortical synaptosomes: Response to depolarizing influences, *J. Neurochem.* **19**:585–602.

De Belleroche, J. S., and Bradford, H. F., 1973, Amino acids in synaptic vesicles from mammalian cerebral cortex: A reappraisal, *J. Neurochem.* **21**:441–451.

De Belleroche, J. S., and Bradford, H. F., 1977, On the site of origin of transmitter amino acids released by depolarization of nerve terminals *in vitro, J. Neurochem.* **29**:335–343.

Deffner, G. G. J., 1961, The dialyzable free organic constituents of squid blood; a comparison with nerve axoplasm, *Biochim. Biophys. Acta* **47**:378–388.

DeGroat, W. C., 1970, The effects of glycine, GABA and strychnine on sacral parasympathetic preganglionic neurones, *Brain Res.* **18**:542–544.

De Groot, C. J., Troelstra, J. A., and Hommes, F. A., 1970, Nonketotic hyperglycinemia: An *in vitro* study of the glycine-serine conversion in liver of three patients and the effect of dietary methionine, *Pediatr. Res.* **4**:238–243.

De Groot, C. J., Vandenberg, H., and Hommes, F. A., 1975, Studies on valine sensitivity in nonketotic hyperglycinemia, *Helv. Paediatr. Acta* **30**:247–254.

De Groot, C. J., Hommes, F. A., and Touwen, B. C. L., 1977, The altered toxicity of glycine in nonketotic hyperglycinemia, *Hum. Hered.* **27**:178.

DeMarchi, W. J., and Johnston, G. A. R., 1969, The oxidation of glycine by D-amino acid oxidase in extracts of mammalian central nervous tissue, *J. Neurochem.* **16**:335–361.

Dennison, M. E., Jordan, C. C., and Webster, R. A., 1976, Distribution and localization of tritiated amino acids by autoradiography in the cat spinal cord *in vivo, J. Physiol. (Lond.)* **258**:55P–56P.

De Robertis, E., Pellegrino De Iraldi, A., Rodriquez De Lores Arnaiz, G., and Salganicoff, L., 1962, Cholinergic and noncholinergic nerve endings in rat brain. I. Isolation and subcellular distribution of acetylcholine and acetylcholinesterase, *J. Neurochem.* **9**:23–35.

Diamond, J., Roper, S., and Yasargil, G. M., 1973, The membrane effects, and sensitivity to strychnine, of neural inhibition of the mauthner cell, and its inhibition by glycine and GABA, *J. Physiol.* **232**:87–111.

Dickinson, J. C., and Hamilton, P. B., 1966, The free amino acids of human spinal fluid determined by ion exchange chromatography, *J. Neurochem.* **13**:1179–1187.

Dimfel, W., and Habermann, E., 1973, Histoautoradiographic localization of ^{125}I-labelled tetanus toxin in rat spinal cord, *Nauyn-Schmiedebergs Arch. Pharmacol.* **280**:177–182.

Dray, A., and Straughan, D. W., 1976, Benzodiazepines: GABA and glycine receptors on single neurons in the rat medulla, *J. Pharm. Pharmacol.* **28**:314–315.

Dudzinski, D. S., and Cutler, R. W. P., 1974, Spinal subarachnoid perfusion in the rat: Glycine transport from spinal fluid, *J. Neurochem.* **22**:355–361.

Duggan, A. W., and McLennan, H., 1971, Bicuculline and inhibition in the thalamus, *Brain Res.* **25**:188–191.

Duggan, A. W., Lodge, D., and Biscoe, T. J., 1973, The inhibition of hypoglossal motoneurones by impulses in the glossopharyngeal nerve of the rat, *Exp. Brain Res.* **17**:261–270.

Eccles, J. C. (ed.), 1964, *The Physiology of Synapses,* Springer-Verlag, Berlin and New York.

Eccles, J. C., Fatt, P., and Koketsu, K., 1954, Cholinergic and inhibitory synapses in a pathway from motor-axon collaterals to motoneurons, *J. Physiol. (Lond.)* **126**:524–562.

Edwardson, J. A., Bennett, G. W., and Bradford, H. F., 1972, Release of amino acids in neurosecretory substances after stimulation of nerve-endings (synaptosomes isolated from the hypothalamus), *Nature* **240**:554–556.

Ehinger, B., and Lindberg-Bauer, B., 1976, Light-evoked release of glycine from cat and rabbit retina, *Brain Res.* **113**:535–549.

Fagg, G. E., Jordon, C. C., and Webster, R. A., 1976, The release of endogenous amino acids from the cat spinal cord, *Br. J. Pharmacol.* **58**:440P–441P.

Farriaux, J. P., Morel, P., and Hommes, F. A., 1976, Nonketotic hyperglycinemia with increased propionic acid excretion and hyperammonemia, *N. Engl. J. Med.* **294**:558.

Fedineć, A. A., 1967, Absorption and distribution of tetanus toxin in experimental animals, in: *Principles of Tetanus* (L. Echmann, ed.), pp. 169–176, Huber, Bern.

Fedineć, A. A., and Shank, R. P., 1971, Effect of tetanus toxin on the content of glycine, gamma-aminobutyric acid, glutamate, glutamine and aspartate in rat spinal cord, *J. Neurochem.* **18**:2229–2234.

Feld, R. D., and Sallach, H. J., 1974, The regulation of D-glycerate dehydrogenase from porcine spinal cord, *Brain Res.* **73**:558–562.

Felix, D., and McLennan, H., 1971, The effect of bicuculline on the inhibition of mitral cells of the olfactory bulb, *Brain Res.* **25**:661–664.

Filipovic, N., Stern, P., and Fuks, Z., 1976, Effects of serine on morphine-dependent mice, *Pharmacology* **14**:247–255.

Franklin, G. M., Dudzinski, D. S., and Cutler, R. W. P., 1975, Amino acid transport into the cerebrospinal fluid of the rat, *J. Neurochem.* **24**:367–372.

Freeman, A. R., 1973, Electrophysiological analysis of the actions of strychnine, bicuculline and picrotoxin on the axonal membrane, *J. Neurobiol.* **4**:567–582.

Frontali, N., 1964, Brain glutamic acid decarboxylase and synthesis of γ-aminobutyric acid in vertebrate and invertebrate species, in: *Comparative Neurochemistry* (D. Richter, ed.), pp. 185–192, Macmillan, New York.

Gahwiler, B. H., 1976, Spontaneous bioelectric activity of cultured Purkinje cells during exposure to glutamate, glycine, and strychnine, *J. Neurobiol.* **7**:97–107.

Gaitonde, M. K., Fayein, N. A., and Johnson, A. L., 1975, Decreased metabolism *in vivo* of glucose into amino acids of the brain of thiamine-deficient rats after treatment with pyrithiamine, *J. Neurochem.* **24**:1215–1223.

Galindo, A., Krnjević, K., and Schwartz, S., 1967, Micro-iontophoretic studies on neurones in the cuneate nucleus, *J. Physiol. (Lond.)* **192**:359–377.

Gaull, G. E., von Berg, W., Räihä, N. C. R., and Sturman, J. A., 1973, Development of methyltransferase activities of human fetal tissues, *Pediatr. Res.* **7**:527–533.

Geison, R. L., O'Neill Rowley, B., and Gerritsen, T., 1975, Urinary organic acid analysis in nonketotic hyperglycinemia: Nonspecific occurrence of free benzoic acid due to a β-streptococcus infection, *Clin. Chim. Acta* **60**:137–142.

Gelfan, S., and Tarlov, I. M., 1963, Altered neuron population in L₇ segment of dogs with experimental hind-limb rigidity, *Am. J. Physiol.* **205**:606–616.

Geller, H. M., and Woodward, D. J., 1974, Responses of cultured cerebellar neurons to iontophoretically applied amino acids, *Brain Res.* **74**:67–80.

Gerritsen, T., Nyhan, W. L., Rehberg, M. L., and Ando, T., 1969, Metabolism of glyoxylate in nonketotic hyperglycinemia, *Pediatr. Res.* **3**:269–274.

Gilles, R., and Schoffeniels, E., 1964, Action de la veratrine, de la cocaine et de la stimulation électrique sur la synthèse et sur le pool des acides amines de la chaine nerveuse ventrale du homard, *Biochim. Biophys. Acta* **82**:525–537.

Gitzelmann, R., Cuenod, M., Otten, A., Steinmann, B., and Dumermuth, G., 1977, Nonketotic hyperglycinemia treated with strychnine, *Pediatr. Res.* **11**:1016.

Graham, L. T., Jr., and Aprison, M. H., 1966, Fluorometric determination of aspartate, glutamate and γ-aminobutyrate in nerve tissue by using enzymic methods, *Anal. Biochem.* **15**:487–497.

Graham, L. T., Jr., Shank, R. P., Werman, R., and Aprison, M. H., 1967, Distribution of some synaptic transmitter candidates in cat spinal cord: Glutamic acid, aspartic acid, γ-aminobutyric acid, glycine and glutamine, *J. Neurochem.* **14**:465–472.

Gray, E. G., and Whittaker, V. P., 1962, The isolation of nerve endings from brain: An electron microscopic study of cell fragments derived by homogenization and centrifugation, *J. Anat.* **96**:79–88.

Gray, E. G., and Willis, R. A., 1970, On synaptic vesicles, complex vesicles and dense projections, *Brain Res.* **24**:149–168.

Gregson, N. A., and Williams, P. L., 1969, A comparative study of brain and liver mitochondria from newborn and adult rats, *J. Neurochem.* **16**:617–626.

Gushchin, S., Kozhechkin, S. N., and Sverdlov, Y. S., 1969, Presynaptic nature of depression by tetanus toxin of postsynaptic inhibition, *Dokl. Akad. Nauk. (U.S.S.R.)* **187**:604–606 (English transl.).

Haas, H. L., and Hösli, L., 1973*a*, The depression of brain stem neurones by taurine and its interaction with strychnine and bicuculline, *Brain Res.* **52**:399–402.

Haas, H. L., and Hösli, L., 1973*b*, Strychnine and inhibition of bulbar reticular neurones, *Experientia* **29**:542–544.

Habermann, E., 1973, Interaction of labelled tetanus toxin and toxoid with substituents of rat brain and spinal cord *in vitro*, *Nauyn-Schmiedebergs Arch. Pharmacol.* **276**:341–359.

Habermann, E., and Wellhöner, H. H., 1974, Advances in tetanus research, *Klin. Wochenschr.* **52**:255–265.

Habermann, E., Dimfel, W., and Raker, K. O., 1973, Interaction of labelled tetanus toxin with substructures of rat spinal cord *in vivo*, *Nauyn-Schmiedebergs Arch. Pharmacol.* **276**:361–373.

Hadžović, S., and Brankov, K., 1974, Inhibitory transmitters in tetanus therapy, *Nauyn-Schmiedebergs Arch. Pharmacol.* **248**:R27.

Hall, P. V., Smith, J. E., Campbell, R. L., Felten, D. L., and Aprison, M. H., 1976, Neurochemical correlates of spasticity, *Life Sci.* **18**:1467–1472.

Hammerstad, J. P., Murray, J. E., and Cutler, R. W. P., 1971, Efflux of amino acid neurotransmitters from rat spinal cord slices. II. Factors influencing the electrically induced efflux of [^{14}C]glycine and ^{3}H-GABA, *Brain Res.* **35**:357–367.

Hedrick, J. L., and Sallach, H. J., 1964, The nonoxidative decarboxylation of hydroxypyruvate in mammalian systems, *Arch. Biochem. Biophys.* **105**:261–269.

Hill, R. G., Simmonds, M. A., and Straughan, D. W., 1973, Amino acid antagonists and the depression of cuneate neurones by γ-aminobutyric acid (GABA) and glycine, *Br. J. Pharmaol.* **47**:642–643P.

Hill, R. G., Simmonds, M. A., and Straughan, D. W., 1976, Antagonism of γ-aminobutyric acid and glycine by convulsants in the cuneate nucleus of cat, *Br. J. Pharmacol.* **56**:9–19.

Hillman, R. E., and Keating, J. P., 1974, Beta-ketothiolase deficiency as a cause of the "ketotic hyperglycinemia syndrome," *Pediatrics* **53**:221–225.

Hillman, R. E., and Otto, E. F., 1974, Inhibition of glycine-serine interconversion in cultured human fibroblasts by products of isoleucine catabolism, *Pediatr. Res.* **8**:941–945.

Hillman, R. E., Sowers, L. H., and Cohen, J. L., 1973, Inhibition of glycine oxidation in cultured fibroblasts by isoleucine, *Pediatr. Res.* **7**:945–947.

Ho, C. K., and Hillman, R. E., 1974, Studies on ketotic hyperglycinemia-inhibitors of serine hydroxymethyltransferase, *Pediatr. Res.* **8**:433.

Hökfelt, T., and Ljungdahl, A., 1971, Light and electron microscopic autoradiography on spinal cord slices after incubation with labelled glycine, *Brain Res.* **32**:189–194.

Holmgren, G., and Blomquist, H. K., 1977, Nonketotic hyperglycinemia in two sibs with mild psychoneurological symptoms, *Neuropaediatric* **8**:67–72.

Holtzman, E., Freeman, A. R., and Kashner, L. A., 1971, Stimulation-dependent alterations in peroxidase uptake at lobster neuromuscular junctions, *Science* **173**:733–736.

Hopkin, J. M., and Neal, M. J., 1970, The release of ^{14}C-Glycine from electrically stimulated rat spinal cord slices, *Proc. Br. Pharmacol. Soc.* **4**:136–137P.

Hopkin, J. M., and Neal, M. J., 1971, Effect of electrical stimulation and high potassium concentrations on the efflux of (^{14}C)glycine from slices of spinal cord, *Br. J. Pharmacol.* **42**:215–223.

Hösli, L., and Haas, H. L., 1972, The hyperpolarization of neurones of the medulla oblongata by glycine. *Experientia* **28**:1057–1058.

Hösli, L., and Hösli, E., 1972, Autoradiographic localization of the uptake of glycine in cultures of rat medulla oblongata, *Brain Res.* **45**:612–616.

Hösli, L., Tebēcis, A. K., and Schonwetter, H. P., 1971*a*, A comparison of the effects of monoamines on neurones of the bulbar reticular formation, *Brain Res.* **25**:357–370.

Hösli, L., Andrès, P. F., and Hösli, E., 1971*b*, Effects of glycine on spinal neurones grown in tissue culture, *Brain Res.* **34**:399–402.

Hösli, E., Ljungdahl, Å., Hökfelt, T., and Hösli, L., 1972*a*, Spinal cord tissue cultures—A model for autoradiographic studies on uptake of putative neurotransmitters such as glycine and GABA, *Experientia* **28**:1342–1344.

Hösli, L., Andrès, P. F., and Hösli, E., 1972*b*, Effects of potassium on the membrane potential of spinal neurones in tissue culture, *Pflugers Arch. Ges. Physiol.* **333**:362–365.

Hösli, L., Hösli, E., and Andrès, P. F., 1973*a*, Nervous tissue culture—A model to study action and uptake of putative neurotransmitters such as amino acids, *Brain Res.* **62**:597–602.

Hösli, L., Hösli, E., and Andrès, P. F., 1973*b*, Uptake and action of glycine in cultures of central nervous tissue from rat, in: *Central Nervous System—Studies on Metabolic Regulation and Function* (E. Genazzani and H. Herken, eds.), pp. 77–83, Springer-Verlag, Berlin and New York.

Hösli, L., Andrès, P. F., and Hösli, E., 1976, Action of amino acid transmitters on glial cells in tissue culture, *Neurosci. Lett.* **2**:223–227.

Hsia, Y. E., Scully, K. J., and Rosenberg, L. E., 1969, Defective propionate carboxylation in ketotic hyperglycinemia, *Lancet* **i**:757–758.

Humoller, F. L., Mahler, D. J., and Parker, M. M., 1966, Distribution of amino acids between plasma and spinal fluid, *Int. J. Neuropsychiatry* **2**:293–297.

Iliffe, T. M., McAdoo, D. J., Beyer, C. B., and Haber, B., 1977, Amino acid concentration in the aplysia nervous system: Neurons with high glycine concentrations, *J. Neurochem.* **28**:1037–1042.

Iversen, L. L., and Bloom, F. E., 1972, Studies of the uptake of ^{3}H-GABA and [^{3}H]glycine in slices and homogenates of rat brain and spinal cord by electron microscopic autoradiography, *Brain Res.* **41**:131–143.

Johnston, G. A. R., 1968, The intraspinal distribution of some depressant amino acids, *J. Neurochem.* **15**:1013–1017.

Johnston, G. A. R., and Iversen, L. L., 1971, Glycine uptake in the central nervous system slices and homogenates: Evidence for different uptake mechanisms in spinal cord and cerebral cortex, *J. Neurochem.* **18**:1951–1961.

Johnston, G. A. R., and Vitali, M. V., 1969*a*, Glycine producing transaminase activity in extracts of spinal cord, *Brain Res.* **15**:471–472.

Johnston, G. A. R., and Vitali, M. V., 1969*b*, Glycine-2-oxoglutarate transaminase in rat cerebral cortex, *Brain Res.* **15**:201–208.

Johnston, G. A. R., DeGroat, W. C., and Curtis, D. R., 1969, Tetanus toxin and amino acid levels in cat spinal cord, *J. Neurochem.* **16**:797–800.

Johnston, G. A. R., Vitali, M. V., and Alexander, H. M., 1970, Regional and subcellular distribution studies on glycine:2-oxoglutarate transaminase activity in cat spinal cord, *Brain Res.* **20**:361–367.

Jones, D. G., and Bradford, H. F., 1971, Observations on the morphology of mammalian synaptosomes following their incubation and electrical stimulation, *Brain Res.* **28**:491–499.

Jordan, C. C., and Webster, R. A., 1971, Release of acetylcholine and ^{14}C-glycine from the cat spinal cord *in vivo*, *Br. J. Pharmacol.* **43**:441P.

Kaeser, H., and Saner, A., 1970, The effect of tetanus toxin on neuromuscular transmission, *Eur. Neurol.* **3**:193–205.

Kawamura, H., and Provini, L., 1970, Depression of cerebellar Purkinje cells by microiontophoretic application of GABA and related amino acids, *Brain Res.* **24**:293–304.

Kelly, J. S., and Krnjević, K., 1969, The action of glycine on cortical neurones, *Exp. Brain Res.* **9**:155–163.

Kelly, J. S., and Renaud, L. P., 1971, Postsynaptic inhibition in the cuneate blocked by GABA antagonists, *Nature New Biol.* **232**:25–26.

Kelly, J. S., and Renaud, L. P., 1973a, On the pharmacology of the γ-aminobutyric acid receptors on cuneo-thalamic relay cells of the cat, *Br. J. Pharmacol.* **48**:369–386.

Kelly, J. S., and Renaud, L. P., 1973b, On the pharmacology of the glycine receptors on the cuneo-thalamic relay cells in the cat, *Br. J. Pharmacol.* **48**:387–395.

Kelly, J. S., and Renaud, L. P., 1973c, On the pharmacology of ascending, descending and recurrent postsynaptic inhibition of cuneothalamic relay cells in the cat, *Br. J. Pharmacol.* **48**:396–408.

Kennedy, A. J., Neal, M. J., and Lolley, R. N., 1977, The distribution of amino acids within the rat retina, *J. Neurochem.* **29**:157–159.

Kikuchi, G., 1973, The glycine cleavage system: Composition reaction mechanism and physiological significance, *Mol. Cell. Biol.* **1**:169–187.

King, L. E., and Fedineć, A. A., 1974, Pathogenesis of local tetanus in rats: Neural ascent of tetanus toxin, *Nauyn-Schmiedebergs Arch. Pharmacol.* **281**:391–401.

Koechlin, B. A., 1955, On the chemical composition of the axoplasm of squid giant nerve fibers with particular reference to its ion pattern, *J. Biophys. Biochem. Cytol.* **1**:511–529.

Koenig, H., 1958, An autoradiographic study of nucleic acid and protein turnover in the mammalian neuraxis, *J. Biophys. Biochem. Cytol.* **4**:785–792.

Kolvraa, S., Rasmussen, K., and Brandt, N. J., 1976, D-Glyceric acidemia: Biochemical studies of a new syndrome, *Pediatr. Res.* **10**:825–830.

Kondrashova, M. N., and Rodionova, M. A., 1971, Realization of the glyoxylate cycle in animal cell mitochondria, *Dokl. Akad. Nauk SSSR,* **196**:1225–1227.

Korol, S., and Owens, G. W., 1974, Glycine, strychnine and retinal inhibition, *Experientia* **30**:1161–1162.

Krieger, I., and Hart, Z. H., 1974, Valine-sensitive nonketotic hyperglycinemia, *J. Pediatr.* **85**:43–48.

Krieger, I., Winbaum, E. S., and Eisenbrey, A. B., 1977, Cerebrospinal fluid glycine in nonketotic hyperglycinemia. Effect of treatment with sodium benzoate and a ventricular shunt, *Metabolism* **26**:517–524.

Krnjević, K., and Phillis, J. W., 1963, Iontophoretic studies of neurones in the mammalian cerebral cortex, *J. Physiol. (Lond.)* **165**:274–304.

Krnjević, K., and Schwartz, S., 1966, Cortical inhibition and GABA, *Fed. Proc.* **25**:627.

Krnjević, K., Randic, M., and Straughan, D. W., 1966, Pharmacology of cortical inhibition, *J. Physiol. (Lond.)* **184**:78–105.

Krnjević, K., Puil, E., and Werman, R., 1977, GABA and glycine actions on spinal motoneurons, *Can. J. Physiol. Pharmacol.* **55**:658–669.

Kryzhanovsky, G. N., 1973, The mechanism of action of tetanus toxin: Effect on synaptic processes and some particular features of toxin binding by nervous tissue, *Nauyn-Schmiedebergs Arch. Pharmacol.* **276**:247–270.

Kryzhanovsky, G. N., 1975, Present data on the pathogenesis of tetanus, *Prog. Drug Res.* **19**:301–313.

Kryzhanovsky, G. N., and Sheykhon, F. D., 1973, Descending supraspinal effect in tetanus intoxication of the spinal cord, *Exp. Neurol.* **38**:110–122.

Kuno, M., and Muneoka, A., 1962, Further studies on site of action of systematic omega-amino acids in the spinal cord, *Jap. J. Physiol.* **12**:397–410.

Laborit, H., Baron, C., London, A., and Olympie, J., 1971, Central nervous activity and comparative general pharmacology of glyoxylate, glycolate and glycoaldehyde, *Agressologie* **12**:187–211.

Lajtha, A., and Toth, J., 1961, The brain barrier system. II. Uptake and transport of amino acids by the brain, *J. Neurochem.* **8**:216–225.

Lajtha, A., and Toth, J., 1963, The brain barrier system. V. Stereospecificity of amino acid uptake, exchange and efflux, *J. Neurochem.* **10**:909–920.

Lamothe, C., Thuret, F., and Laborit, H., 1971, The action of glyoxylic acid, glycolic acid and glycoaldehyde, *in vivo* and *in vitro,* on some phases of energy metabolism in cerebral cortex, liver and myocardial slices of the rat, *Agressologie* **12**:233–240.

Lane, J. D., Smith, J. E., Hall, P. V., Campbell, R. L., and Aprison, M. H., 1977, Levels of taurine in eight areas of the canine lumbar spinal cord, Abstract, 6th International Meeting of the International Society of Neurochemistry.

Larson, M. D., 1969, An analysis of the action of strychnine on the recurrent IPSP and amino acid induced inhibitions in the cat spinal cord, *Brain Res.* **15**:185–200.

Levy, H. L., Nishimura, R. N., Erickson, A. M., and Janowska, S. E., 1972, Hyperglycinemia: *In vivo* comparison of nonketotic and ketotic (propionic acidemia) forms. I. CSF glycine and blood/CSF glycine, *Pediatr. Res.* **6**:400.

Lewis, P. R., 1952, The free amino acids of invertebrate nerve, *Biochem. J.* **52**:330–338.

Liang, C. C., 1962, Studies on experimental thiamine deficiency. Trends of keto acid formation and detection of glyoxylic acid, *Biochem. J.* **82**:429–434.

Ljungdahl, Å., and Hökfelt, T., 1973, Autoradiographic uptake patterns of [³H]GABA and [³H]glycine in central nervous tissues with special reference to the cat spinal cord, *Brain Res.* **62**:587–590.

Logan, W. J., and Snyder, S. H., 1971, Glycine, glutamic and aspartic acids: Unique high affinity uptake systems in central nervous tissue of the rat, *Nature* **234**:297–299.

Logan, W. J., and Snyder, S. H., 1972, High affinity uptake systems for glycine, glutamic and aspartic acids in synaptosomes of rat central nervous tissues, *Brain Res.* **42**:413–431.

Mangan, J. L., and Whittaker, V. P., 1966, The distribution of free amino acids in subcellular fractions of guinea pig brain, *Biochem. J.* **98**:128–137.

Matus, A. I., and Dennison, M. E., 1971, Autoradiographic localization of tritiated glycine at "flat vesicle" synapses in spinal cord, *Brain Res.* **32**:195–197.

Matus, A. I., and Dennison, M. E., 1972, An autoradiographic study of uptake of exogenous glycine by vertebrate spinal cord slices *in vitro, J. Neurocytol.* **1**:27–34.

McBride, W. J., Daly, E., and Aprison, M. H., 1973, Interconversion of glycine and serine in a synaptosome fraction isolated from the spinal cord, medulla oblongata, telencephalon, and cerebellum of the rat, *J. Neurobiol.* **4**:557–566.

McBride, W. J., Shank, R. P., Freeman, A. R., and Aprison, M. H., 1974, Levels of free amino acids in excitatory, inhibitory and sensory axons of the walking limbs of the lobster, *Life Sci.* **14**:1109–1120.

McClain, L. D., Carl, G. F., and Bridgers, W. F., 1975, Distribution of folic acid coenzymes and folate-dependent enzymes in mouse brain, *J. Neurochem.* **24**:719–722.

McGale, E. H. F., Pye, I. F., Stonier, C., Hutchinson, E. C., and Aber, G. M., 1977, Studies on the interrelationship between cerebrospinal fluid and plasma amino acid concentrations in normal individuals, *J. Neurochem.* **29**:291–297.

McLaughlin, B. J., Barber, R., Saito, K., Roberts, E., and Yu, J. Y., 1975, Immunocytochemical localization of glutamate decarboxylase in rat spinal cord, *J. Comp. Neurol.* **164**:305–321.

Mellanby, J., and Whittaker, V. P., 1968, The fixation of tetanus toxin by synaptic membranes, *J. Neurochem.* **15**:205–208.

Mellanby, J., van Heyningen, W. E., and Whittaker, V. P., 1965, Fixation of tetanus toxin by subcellular fractions of brain, *J. Neurochem.* **12**:77–79.

Mitchell, J. F., and Phillis, J. W., 1962, Cholinergic transmission in the frog spinal cord, *Br. J. Pharmacol. Chemother.* **19**:534–542.

Miyata, Y., and Otsuka, M., 1975, Quantitative histochemistry of γ-aminobutyric acid in cat spinal cord with special reference to presynaptic inhibition, *J. Neurochem.* **25**:239–244.

Morimoto, T., Takata, M., and Kawamura, Y., 1968, Effect of lingual nerve stimulation on hypoglossal motoneurons, *Exp. Neurol.* **22**:174–190.

Motokawa, Y., and Kikuchi, G., 1971, Glycine metabolism in rat liver mitochondria: V. Intramitochondrial localization of the reversible glycine cleavage system and serine hydroxymethyltransferase, *Arch. Biochem. Biophys.* **146**:461–466.

Motokawa, Y., Kikuchi, G., Narisawa, K., and Arakawa, T., 1977, Reduced level of glycine cleavage system in the liver of hyperglycinemia patients, *Clin. Chim. Acta* **79**:173–181.

Mulder, A. H., and Snyder, S. H., 1974, Potassium-induced release of amino acids from cerebral cortex and spinal cord slices of the rat, *Brain Res.* **76**:297–308.

Murakami, M., Ohtsu, K., and Ohtsuka, T., 1972, Effects of chemicals on receptors and horizontal cells in the retina, *J. Physiol. (Lond.)* **227**:899–913.

Murayama, S., and Smith, C. M., 1965, Rigidity of hind limbs of cats produced by occulsion of spinal cord blood supply, *Neurology* **15**:565–579.

Murray, J. E., and Cutler, R. W. P., 1970, Clearance of glycine from cat cerebrospinal fluid: Faster clearance from spinal subarachnoid than from ventricular compartment, *J. Neurochem.* **17**:703–704.

Nakano, Y., Fujioka, M., and Wada, H., 1968, Studies on serine hydroxymethylase isoenzymes from rat liver, *Biochim. Biophys. Acta* **159**:19–26.

Neal, M. J., 1969, Uptake of [¹⁴C]glycine by rat spinal cord, *Br. J. Pharmacol.* **36**:205P–206P.

Neal, M. J., 1971, The uptake of [¹⁴C]glycine by slices of mammalian spinal cord, *J. Physiol. (Lond.)* **215**:103–117.

Neal, M. J., and Pickles, H., 1969, Uptake of [¹⁴C]glycine by spinal cord, *Nature* **223**:679.

Neal, M. J., Peacock, D. J., and White, R. D., 1973, Kinetic analysis of amino acid uptake by the rat retina *in vitro*, *Br. J. Pharmacol.* **47**:656–657.

Nelson-Krause, D. C., and Howard, B. D., 1976, Release of glycine and GABA from synaptosomes prepared from rat central nervous tissue, *Fed. Proc.* **35**:543.

Nicoll, R. A., and Barker, J. L., 1971, The pharmacology of recurrent inhibition in the supraoptic neurosecretory system, *Brain Res.* **35**:501–511.

Nishimura, Y., Tada, K., and Arakawa, T., 1974, Coexistence of defective activity in glycine-cleavage reaction and propionyl-CoA carboxylase in the liver of a hyperglycinemic child, *Tohoku J. Exp. Med.* **113**:267–271.

Nyhan, W. L., 1967, Treatment of hyperglycinemia, *Am. J. Dis. Child.* **113**:129–133.

Obata, K., 1965, Pharmacological study on postsynaptic inhibition of Deiters' neurons, Abstract, 23rd International Congress of Physiological Sciences, p. 406.

Obata, K., Takeda, K., and Shinozaki, H., 1970, Further study on pharmacological properties of the cerebellar-induced inhibition of Deiters' neurones, *Exp. Brain Res.* **11**:327–342.

Oldendorf, W. H., 1971, Brain uptake of radiolabeled amino acids, amines, and hexoses after arterial injection. *Am. J. Physiol.* **221**:1629–1639.

Oppenheim, R. W., and Reitzel, J., 1975, Ontogeny of behavioral sensitivity to strychnine in the chick embryo: Evidence for the early onset of CNS inhibition, *Brain Behav. Evol.* **11**:130–159.

Ordoñez, L. A., and Wurtman, R. J., 1973, Enzymes catalyzing the *de novo* synthesis of methyl groups in the brain and other tissues of the rat, *J. Neurochem.* **21**:1447–1455.

Osborne, R. H., and Bradford, H. F., 1973, Tetanus toxin inhibits amino acid release from nerve ending *in vitro*, *Nature New Biol.* **244**:157–158.

Osborne, R. H., Bradford, H. F., and Jones, D. G., 1973, Patterns of amino acid release from nerve-endings isolated from spinal cord and medulla, *J. Neurochem.* **21**:407–419.

Otsuka, M., 1977, Substance P and sensory transmitter, in: *Advances in Neurochemistry* (B. W. Agranoff and M. H. Aprison, eds.), Vol. 2, pp. 193–211, Plenum Press, New York.

Pavone, L., Mollica, F., and Levy, H. L., 1975, Asymptomatic type II hyperprolinaemia associated with hyperglicinaemia in three sibs, *Arch. Dis. Child.* **50**:637–641.

Perry, T. L., Berry, K., Hansen, S., Diamond, S., and Mok, C., 1971*a*, Regional distribution of amino acids in human brain obtained at autopsy, *J. Neurochem.* **18**:513–519.

Perry, T. L., Hansen, S., Berry, K., Mok, C., and Lesk, D., 1971*b*, Free amino acids and related compounds in biopsies of human brain, *J. Neurochem.* **18**:521–528.

Perry, T. L., Hansen, S., and Kennedy, J., 1975*a*, CSF amino acids and plasma–CSF amino acid ratio in adults, *J. Neurochem.* **24**:587–589.

Perry, T. L., Urquhart, N., Maclean, J., Evans, M. E., Hansen, S., Davidson, A. G. F., Applegarth, D. A., Macleod, P. J., and Lock, J. E., 1975*b*, Nonketotic hyperglycinemia glycine accumulation due to absence of glycine cleavage in brain, *N. Engl. J. Med.* **292**:1269–1272.

Perry, T. L., Urquhart, N., Maclean, J., and Hansen, J., 1975*c*, Reply to the letter of Sciver, C. R., Sprague, W., and Harwood, S. P., *N. Engl. J. Med.* **293**:778.

Piepho, R. W., and Friedman, A. H., 1971, Twenty-four hour rhythms in the glycine content of rat hindbrain and spinal cord, *Life Sci.* **10**:1355–1362.

Pollay, M., 1976, Movement of glycine across the blood–brain barrier of the rabbit, *J. Neurobiol.* **7**:123–128.

Precht, W., Baker, R., and Okada, Y., 1973, Evidence for GABA as the synaptic transmitter of the inhibitory vestibulo-ocular pathway, *Exp. Brain Res.* **18**:415–428.

Price, D. L., Griffin, J., Young, A., Peck, K., and Stocks, A., 1975, Tetanus toxin: Direct evidence for retrograde intraaxonal transport, *Science* **188**:945–947.

Price, D. L., Stocks, A., Griffin, J. W., Young, A., and Peck, K., 1976, Glycine-specific synapses in rat spinal cord: Identification by electron microscope autoradiography, *J. Cell Biol.* **68**:389–395.

Price, D. L., Griffin, J. W., and Peck, K., 1977, Tetanus toxin: Evidence for binding at presynaptic nerve endings, *Brain Res.* **121**:379–384.

Purpura, D. P., Girado, M., Smith, T. G., Callan, D. A., and Grundfest, H., 1959, Structure–activity determinants of pharmacological effects of amino acids and related compounds on central synapses, *J. Neurochem.* **3**:238–266.

Ransom, B. R., and Nelson, P. G., 1976, Possible pathophysiology of neurologic abnormalities associated with nonketotic hyperglycinemia, *N. Engl. J. Med.* **294**:1295–1296.

Rassin, D. K., and Gaull, G. E., 1975, Subcellular distribution of enzymes of transmethylation and transsulphuration in rat brain, *J. Neurochem.* **24**:969–978.

Reploh, H., Grobe, H., Dickmann, L., Palm, D., v. Bassewitz, D. B., and Jenett, W., 1973, The clinical findings in a patient with nonketotic hyperglycinemia, *Z. Kinderkeilkd.* **114**:191–204.

Reubi, J. C., and Cúenod, M., 1976, Release of exogenous glycine in the pigeon optic tectum during stimulation of a midbrain nucleus, *Brain Res.* **112**:347–361.

Revsin, B., and Morrow, G., 1976, Glycine transport in normal and nonketotic hyperglycinemic human diploid fibroblasts, *Exp. Cell Res.* **100**:95–103.

Revsin, B., Lebowitz, J., and Morrow, G., 1977, Effect of valine on propionate metabolism in control and hyperglycinemia fibroblasts and in rat liver, *Pediatr. Res.* **11**:749–753.

Rexed, B., 1954, A cytoarchitectonic atlas of the spinal cord in the cat, *J. Comp. Neurol.* **100**:297–379.

Richardson, T. W., Aprison, M. H., and Werman, R., 1965, An automatic direct-current operating temperature-control device, *J. Appl. Physiol.* **20**:1355–1356.

Roberts, P. J., 1974, The release of amino acids with proposed neurotransmitter function from the cuneate and gracile nuclei of the rat *in vivo, Brain Res.* **67**:419–428.

Roberts, P. J., and Mitchell, J. F., 1972, The release of amino acids from the hemisected spinal cord during stimulation, *J. Neurochem.* **19**:2473–2481.

Romano, M., and Cerra, M., 1967, Further studies on the toxicity of glyoxylate in the rat, *Gazz. Biochem.* **16**:354–358.

Roper, S., and Diamond, J., 1970, Strychnine antagonism and glycine: A reply, *Nature* **225**:1259.

Roper, S., Diamond, J., and Yasargil, G., 1969, Does strychnine block inhibition postsynaptically?, *Nature* **223**:1168–1169.

Rosenberg, L. E., Lilljequist, A., and Hsia, Y. E., 1968, Methylmalonic acidiria: An inborn error leading to metabolic acidosis, long-chain ketouria and intermittent hyperglycinemia, *N. Engl. J. Med.* **278**:1319–1322.

Ryall, R. W., Piercey, M. F., and Polosa, C., 1972, Strychnine-resistant mutual inhibition of Renshaw cells, *Brain Res.* **41**:119–129.

Sato, T., Kochi, H., Sato, N., and Kikuchi, G., 1969, Glycine metabolism by rat liver mitochondria, *J. Biochem.* **65**:77–83.

Scriver, C. R., Spraque, W., and Horwood, S. P., 1975, Plasma-CSF glycine in normal and nonketotic hyperglycinemic subjects (letter), *N. Engl. J. Med.* **293**:778.

Schwab, M. E., and Thoenen, H., 1976, Electron microscopic evidence for a transsynaptic migration of tetanus toxin in spinal cord motoneurons: An autoradiographic and morphometric study, *Brain Res.* **105**:213–227.

Schwab, M. E., and Thoenen, H., 1977, Selective transsynaptic migration of tetanus toxin after retrograde axonal transport in peripheral sympathetic nerves: A comparison with nerve growth factor, *Brain Res.* **122**:459–474.

Schwander, J., and Lamarche, M., 1972, Inhibition of oxygen consumption in rat brain homogenate by sodium glyoxylate, *C.R. Seances Soc. Biol.* **166**:186–189.

Semba, T., and Kano, M., 1969, Glycine in the spinal cord of cats with local tetanus rigidity, *Science* **164**:571–572.

Shank, R. P., and Aprison, M. H., 1970*a*, The metabolism of glycine and serine in eight different areas of the rat central nervous system. *J. Neurochem.* **17**:1461–1475.

Shank, R. P., and Aprison, M. H., 1970*b*, Method for multiple analyses of concentration and specific radioactivity of individual amino acids in nervous tissue extracts, *Anal. Biochem.* **35**:136–145.

Shank, R. P., Aprison, M. H., and Baxter, C. F., 1973, Precursors of glycine in the central nervous system: Comparison of specific activities in glycine and other amino acids after administration of [U-^{14}C]glucose, [3,4^{14}C]glucose, [1-^{14}C]glucose, [U-^{14}C]serine or [1,5^{14}C]citrate to the rat, *Brain Res.* **52**:301–308.

Shaw, R. K., and Heine, J. D., 1965, Ninhydrin positive substances present in different areas of normal rat brain, *J. Neurochem.* **12**:151–155.

Sky-Peck, H. H., Rosenbloom, C., and Winzler, R. J., 1966, Incorporation of glucose into the protein-bound amino acids of one-day-old mouse brain *in vitro, J. Neurochem.* **13**:223–228.

Smith, J. E., Hall, P. V., Campbell, R. L., Jones, A. R., and Aprison, M. H., 1976, Levels of γ-aminobutyric acid in the dorsal grey lumbar spinal cord during the development of experimental spinal spacticity, *Life Sci.* **19**:1525–1530.

Smith, J. E., Hall, P. V., Galvin, M. R., Jones, A. R., and Campbell, R. L., 1977, The effects of glycine replacement on canine spinal spasticity, *Trans. Am. Soc. Neurochem.* **8**:210.

Snodgrass, S. R., Cutler, R. W. P., Kang, E. S., and Lorenzo, A. V., 1969, Transport of neutral amino acids from feline cerebrospinal fluid, *Am. J. Physiol.* **217**:974–980.

Snyder, S. H., 1975, The glycine synaptic receptor in the mammalian central nervous system, *Br. J. Pharmacol.* **53**:473–484.

Snyder, S. H., and Enna, S. J., 1975, The role of central glycine receptors in the pharmacologic actions of benzodiazepines, *Adv. Biochem. Psychopharmacol.* **14**:81–91.

Snyder, S. H., Logan, W. J., Bennett, J. P., and Arregui, A., 1973*a*, Amino acids as central nervous transmitters: Biochemical studies, in: *Neurosciences Research, Vol. 5: Chemical Approaches to Brain Function* (S. Ehrenpreis and I. J. Kopin, eds.), pp. 131–157, Academic Press, New York.

Snyder, S. H., Young, A. B., Bennett, J. P., and Mulder, A. H., 1973*b*, Synaptic biochemistry of amino acids, *Fed. Proc.* **32**:2039–2047.

Starr, H. S., 1973, Effect of dark adaptation on GABA system in retina, *Brain Res.* **59**:331–337.

Stern, P., and Bokonjić, R., 1974, Glycine therapy in 7 cases of spasticity, a pilot study, *Pharmacology* **12**:117–119.

Stern, P., and Hadžović, J., 1970, Effect of glycine on experimental hindlimb rigidity in rats, *Life Sci.* **9**:955–959.

Stern, P., and Hadžović, J., 1973, Pharmacological analysis of central actions of substance P, *Arch. Int. Pharmacodyn.* **202**:259–262.

Stern, P., Ćatović, S., and Filipovic, N., 1973, The metabolism of glycine in mice treated acutely and chronically with morphine, *Pharmacology* **10**:97–103.

Stern, P., Ćatović, S., and Stern, M., 1974, Mechanism of action of substance P, *Naunyn-Schmiedebergs Arch. Pharmacol.* **281**:233–239.

Stokes, B. T., and Bignall, K. E., 1974, The emergence of inhibition in the chick embryo spinal cord, *Brain Res.* **77**:231–242.

Straschill, M., 1968, Action of drugs on single neurons in the cat's retina, *Vision Res.* **8**:35–47.

Straughan, D. W., 1974, Convulsant drugs: Amino acid antagonism and central inhibition, *Neuropharmacology* **13**:495–508.

Tada, K., Narisawa, K., Yoshida, T., Konno, T., Yokayama, Y., Nakagawa, H., Tanno, K., Mochizuki, K., Arakawa, T., Yoshida, T., and Kikuchi, G., 1969, Hyperglycinemia: A defect in glycine cleavage reaction, *Tohoku J. Exp. Med.* **98**:289.

Tada, K., Corbeel, L. M., Eeckels, R., and Eggermont, E., 1974, A block in glycine cleavage reaction as a common mechanism in ketotic and nonketotic hyperglycinemia, *Pediatr. Res.* **8**:721–723.

Takano, K., and Neumann, K., 1972, Effect of glycine upon stretch reflex tension, *Brain Res.* **36**:474–475.

Tebēcis, A. K., and DiMaria, A., 1972, Strychnine-sensitive inhibition in the medullary reticular formation: Evidence for glycine as an inhibitory transmitter, *Brain Res.* **40**:373–383.

Tebēcis, A. K., and Ishikawa, T., 1973, Glycine and GABA as inhibitory transmitters in the medullary reticular formation studies involving intra- and extracellular recording, *Pflugers Arch.* **338**:273–278.

Tebécis, A. K., and Phillis, J. W., 1969, The use of convulsants in studying possible functions of amino acids in the toad spinal cord, *Comp. Biochem. Physiol.* **28**:1303.

Tebēcis, A. K., Hösli, L., and Haas, H., 1971, Bicuculline and the depression of medullary reticular neurones by GABA and glycine, *Experientia* **27**:548.

Ten Bruggencate, G., and Engberg, I., 1968, Analysis of glycine actions on spinal interneurones by intracellular recording, *Brain Res.* **11**:446–450.

Ten Bruggencate, G., and Engberg, I., 1971, Iontophoretic studies in Deiters' nucleus of the inhibitory actions of GABA and related amino acids and the interactions of strychnine and picrotoxin, *Brain Res.* **25**:431–448.

Ten Bruggencate, G., and Sonnhof, U., 1972, Effects of glycine and GABA, and blocking actions of strychnine and picrotoxin in the hypoglossus nucleus, *Arch. Ges. Physiol.* **334**:240–252.

Trijbels, J. M. F., Monnens, L. A. H., van der Zee, S. P. M., Vrenken, J. A. Th., Sengers, R. C. A., and Schretlen, E. D. A. M., 1974, A patient with nonketotic hyperglycinemia: Biochemical findings and therapeutic approaches, *Pediatr. Res.* **8**:598–605.

Tsukada, Y., Nagata, Y., Hirano, S., and Matsutani, T., 1963, Active transport of amino acid into cerebral cortex slices, *J. Neurochem.* **10**:241–256.

Tureen, L. L., 1936, Effect of experimental temporary vascular occlusion on the spinal cord. I. Correlation between structural and functional changes, *A.M.A. Arch. Neurol. Psychiatry* **35**:789–807.

Uchizono, K., 1965, Characteristics of excitatory and inhibitory synapses in the central nervous system of the cat, *Nature* **207**:642–643.

Uhr, M. L., 1973, Glycine decarboxylation in the central nervous system. *J. Neurochem.* **20**:1005–1009.

Uhr, M. L., and Sneddon, M. K., 1971, Glycine and serine inhibition of *d*-glycerate dehydrogenase and 3-phosphoglycerate dehydrogenase of rat brain, *FEBS Lett.* **17**:137–140.

Uhr, M. L., and Sneddon, M. K., 1972, The regional distribution of *d*-glycerate dehydrogenase and 3-phosphoglycerate dehydrogenase in the cat central nervous system: Correlation with glycine levels, *J. Neurochem.* **19**:1495–1500.

van Heyningen, W. E., 1974, Gangliosides as membrane receptors for tetanus toxin, cholera toxin and serotonin, *Nature* **249**:415–417.

Voaden, M. J., Marshall, J., and Murani, N., 1974, The uptake of [³H]-γ-aminobutyric acid and [³H]glycine by the isolated retina of the frog, *Brain Res.* **67**:115–132.

Wada, Y., Tada, K., Takada, G., Omura, K., Yoshida, T., Kuniya, T., Aoyama, T., Hakui, T., and Harada, S., 1972, Hyperglycinemia associated with hyperammonemia: *In vitro* glycine cleavage in liver, *Pediatr. Res.* **6**:622–625.

Wadlington, W. B., Kilroy, A., Ando, T., Sweetman, L., and Nyhan, W. L., 1975, Hyperglycinemia and propionyl CoA carboxylase deficiency and episodic severe illness without consistent ketosis, *J. Pediatr.* **86**:707–712.

Werman, R., 1972, CNS cellular level: Membranes, *Annu. Rev. Physiol.* **34**:337–374.

Werman, R., and Aprison, M. H., 1968, Glycine: The search for a spinal cord inhibitory transmitter, in: *Structure and Functions of Inhibitory Neuronal Mechanisms* (C. von Euler, S. Skoglund, and U. Soderberg, eds.), pp. 473–486, Pergamon Press, Oxford.

Werman, R., Davidoff, R. A., and Aprison, M. H., 1966, Glycine and postsynaptic inhibition in cat spinal cord, *Physiologist* **9**:318.

Werman, R., Davidoff, R. A., and Aprison, M. H., 1967, Inhibition of motoneurones by iontophoresis of glycine, *Nature* **214**:681–683.

Werman, R., Davidoff, R. A., and Aprison, M. H., 1968, Inhibitory action of glycine on spinal neurons in the cat, *J. Neurophysiol.* **31**:81–95.

Wiechert, P., 1963, Über die Permeabilität der Blut-liquao-schranke für einige Aminosäuren, *Acta Biol. Med. Germ.* **10**:305–310.

Wiechert, P., and Schroter, P., 1964, Der Einfluss von γ-Aminobuttersaure, L-Glutaminsaure und Glycin auf die Blut-hirn-schranke und die Enzymaktivitaten des Kaninchengehirnes, *Acta Biol. Med. Germ.* **12**:475–580.

Wilson, V. J., Diecke, F. P. J., and Talbot, W. H., 1960, Action of tetanus toxin on conditioning of spinal motoneurones, *J. Neurophysiol.* **23**:659–666.

Yagi, K., and Sawaki, Y., 1975, Recurrent inhibition and facilitation: Demonstration in the tubero-infundibular system and effects of strychnine and picrotoxin, *Brain Res.* **84**:155–159.

Yoshida, T., and Kikuchi, G., 1970, Major pathways of glycine and serine catabolism in rat liver, *Arch. Biochem. Biophys.* **139**:380–392.

Yoshida, T., and Kikuchi, G., 1973, Major pathways of serine and glycine catabolism in various organs of the rat and cock, *J. Biochem.* **73**:1013–1022.

Yoshida, T., Kikuchi, G., Tada, K., Narisawa, K., and Arakawa, T., 1969, Physiological significance of glycine cleavage system in human liver as revealed by the study of a case of hyperglycinemia, *Biochem. Biophys. Res. Commun.* **35**:577–583.

Young, A. B., and Snyder, S. H., 1973, Strychnine binding associated with glycine receptors of the central nervous system, *Proc. Natl. Acad. Sci. U.S.A.* **70**:2832–2836.

Young, A. B., and Snyder, S. H., 1974a, Strychnine binding in rat spinal cord membranes associated with the synaptic glycine receptor: Cooperativity of glycine interactions, *Mol. Pharmacol.* **10**:790–809.

Young, A. B., and Snyder, S. H., 1974b, The glycine synaptic receptor—Evidence that strychnine binding is associated with the ionic conductance mechanism, *Proc. Natl. Acad. Sci. U.S.A.* **71**:4002–4005.

Young, A. B., Zukin, S. R., and Snyder, S. H., 1974, Interaction of benzodiazepines with central nervous glycine receptors: Possible mechanism of action, *Proc. Natl. Acad. Sci. U.S.A.* **71**:2246–2250.

Zacks, S. J., and Sheff, M. F., 1970, Pathobiological aspects of the action of tetanus toxin in the nervous system and skeletal muscle, *Neurosci. Res.* **3**:210–287.

Zukin, S. R., Young, A. B., and Snyder, S. H., 1975, Development of the synaptic glycine receptor in chick embryo spinal cord, *Brain Res.* **83**:525–530.

INDEX